COMMUNITY HEALTH NURSING

Frameworks for Practice

COMMUNITY HEALTH NURSING

Frameworks for Practice

Edited by

Pam Gastrell MPhil, BA, RN, RM, RHV, DN, RNT, Cert Ed

Director of Studies, Primary Health Care Nursing, University of Southampton

Judy Edwards OBE, BSc (Econ), RN, RHV, PGCE

Co-Course Director, Community Health Studies, University of Wales College of Medicine, Cardiff

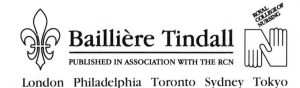

Baillière Tindall

PUBLISHED IN ASSOCIATION WITH THE RCN

London Philadelphia Toronto Sydney Tokyo

Baillière Tindall
W. B. Saunders Company Ltd

24–28 Oval Road
London NW1 7DX

The Curtis Center
Independence Square West
Philadelphia, PA 19106-3399, USA

Harcourt Brace & Company
55 Horner Avenue
Toronto, Ontario M8Z 4X6, Canada

Harcourt Brace & Company, Australia
30–52 Smidmore Street
Marrickville, NSW 2204, Australia

Harcourt Brace & Company, Japan
Ichibancho Central Building, 22–1 Ichibancho
Chiyoda-ku, Tokyo 102, Japan

© 1996 Baillière Tindall
Second printing 1997

A catalogue record of this book is available from the British Library

ISBN 0-7020-1890-2

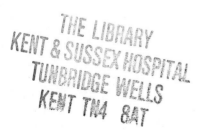
Typeset by WestKey Ltd, Falmouth, Cornwall
Printed and bound by The Bath Press

CONTENTS

CONTRIBUTORS

Graham Allan, BA, MA, PhD
Reader in Sociology, University of Southampton.

Kate Billingham, MA, RN, RSCN, RHV
Director of Public Health Nursing/Senior Lecturer in Applied Research, Sheffield Health/University of Sheffield.

Maggie Boyd, RGN, RM, RHV, MPH
Nurse Advisor, Merton, Sutton and Wandsworth Health Authority, Wilson Hospital, Mitcham, Surrey.

Judith Boxer, RMN, CQSW, RNT
Nurse Lecturer, School of Nursing, Faculty of Medicine, University of Sheffield.

Michael L Burr, Md, FFPHM
Consultant Senior Lecturer, Centre for Applied Public Health Medicine, University of Wales College of Medicine, Cardiff.

David R Cohen, BCom, MPhil
Professor of Health Economics, University of Glamorgan, Mid Glamorgan.

Lesley M Coles, BA, RGN, DN, RM, RHV, RNT, Cert Ed
Lecturer in Health Studies, Primary Health Care Nursing, Sociology and Social Policy, University of Southampton.

Sarah Cowley, BA, PhD, PGDE, RGN, RCNT, RHV, HVT
Senior Lecturer, King's College London.

Graham Crow, BA, MA, PhD,
Lecturer in Sociology, University of Southampton.

Jeffrey Dauvin, RGN, RCNT, RNT, BA (OU)
Teaching Fellow, School of Nursing and Midwifery, University of Southampton.

Tessa Davies, SRN, BSc (Hons)
Teaching Fellow, Department of Sociology and Social Policy, University of Southampton.

Judy Edwards, OBE, BSc (Econ), RN, RHV, PGCE
Co-Course Director, Community Health Studies, University of Wales College of Medicine, Cardiff.

Neil Frude, PhD, MPhil, FBPsS
Senior Lecturer in Psychology, School of Psychology, University of Wales, Cardiff.

Pam Gastrell, MPhil, BA, RN, RMN, RHV, DN, RNT, Cert Ed
Primary Health Care Nursing, University of Southampton.

Steve George, MD, MSc, MFPHM
Senior Lecturer in Public Health Medicine, Institute of Public Health, University of Southampton.

Judy Gillow, RGN, RHV, Cert ed, RNT, Diploma in Community Care
Primary Healthcare Manager, Whitecroft Hospital, Isle of Wight.

Elizabeth Gould, BA (Hons), RGN, RHV
Rhondda Health Unit, MPH, Senior Nurse, Rhondda NHS Trust, Llwynypia Hospital, Rhondda.

David N Greensmith, LLB (Exeter)
Solicitor, Partner, Morgan Bruce, Cardiff.

Michael Hardey, BA (Hons), MA
Lecturer, University of Southampton.

Kate Jolly, MB, ChB, MRCGP, MSc (Public Health)
Lecturer in Public Health Medicine, Institute of Public Health Medicine, Southampton General Hospital, Southampton.

Dee A Jones, BSc (Econ), DPM, GMIPM, PhD
Director of Research Team for the Care of Elderly People, University of Wales College of Medicine, Llandough Hospital, Penarth.

Mark Jones, MSc, BSc (Hons) Nursing, RN, RHV (Hgr.Dip)
Community Health Adviser, Royal College of Nursing of the United Kingdom, London.

Gary F McCulloch, BA (Hons), RMN
Health Promotion Specialist – Mental Health, Sheffield Health, Sheffield.

Brian Millar, RN, DN (Lond), MN (Wales), PGCE
Lecturer in Nursing, School of Nursing Studies, University of Wales College of Medicine, Cardiff.

Elizabeth J Muir, MSc (Econ), Dip Ed, MC Inst. Marketing
Managing Director, The Alternative Marketing Department Ltd, Cardiff.

Stephen Peckham, BSc (Hons), MA (Econ)
Research Fellow, Institute for Health Policy Studies, University of Southampton, Southampton.

Elizabeth Porter, BA, PGCEA, SRN, SCM, HV, FWT Cert
Lecturer in Health Studies, Primary Health Care Nursing, University of Southampton.

Colin Pritchard, FRSA, MA, AAPSW
Professor, Director Mental Health and Professor of Social Work Studies, University of Southampton.

Jim Richardson, BA, RGN, RSCN, PGCE (FE)
Lecturer in Nursing Studies, School of Nursing Studies, University of Wales College of Medicine, Cardiff.

June E Smail, RGN, RM, DN, Cert Ed
Practice Nurse Manager, South Glamorgan F.H.S.A., Cardiff.

Simon A Smail, MA, BM, Bch, FFRCGP, DCH, DORCOG
Sub-Dean and Adviser in General Practice for Wales, University of Wales College of Medicine, Cardiff.

Eileen Thomas, RGN, RHV, MA (Ed)
Senior Lecturer in Public Health Nursing, Institute of Public Health Medicine, Southampton General Hospital.

Tony Thompson, RMN, RNMH, DN (Lond), Cert E, BEd (Hons), RNT, MA
Head of Professional Studies, The Ashworth Centre for Studies in Forensic Mental Health Care, Ashworth Hospital, Liverpool.

FOREWORD

A number of changes in health and social policy in recent years have given increased prominence to the contribution of primary care and community health services. Indeed the publication of EL(94)79, announcing the shift towards a 'primary care-led NHS', marked an intention to reorientate the whole of the National Health Service in favour of a primary-care perspective. The ability to achieve a transformation of this magnitude will rest, in part, upon the capacity and skills of community health nurses and they have found themselves in the spotlight as never before. In order to understand the significance of these shifts it is essential to see them within the broader context of changing health needs, Government policy and professional practice. This book is, therefore, a timely contribution to the debate. The chapters range from discussions of socio-political trends at the international level to analyses of innovative practice in community settings in the UK.

The community health nurse at the end of the twentieth century is at the centre of radical and fast-moving developments both in society at large and in the organization of health care. The demographic, social and economic changes described in this book have had a direct impact upon family life and upon the demand for health services. Primary care professionals, particularly community health nurses, are crucial in satisfying and channelling those demands.

Not only have the boundaries around community health services shifted, but the demarcation lines, roles and responsibilities *within* them have also changed markedly. It is clear that healthy community nursing services, in the future, must draw upon the strengths of all the professional groups involved, to enrich the range and quality of services available to patients and their families. This is a formidable challenge but one which the authors have demonstrated is achievable, where there is clarity of aims and vision.

In anticipating developments in community health nursing in the next century, it is important to understand the context within which these services have evolved in the past. This book is valuable in describing that bigger picture and in analysing the 'frameworks' for practice which will shape the future.

Joan Higgins
Professor of Health Policy
University of Manchester

EDITORS' INTRODUCTION

Political and organizational changes within the National Health Service point to the growing importance of inter-disciplinary preparation for community health nursing practice so that the nursing resources available for primary health care and community care are utilized and managed in the most cost effective and efficient way (DOH 1993; 1994; 1995; NHSME 1993; 1994). Such government documents not only draw attention to the need for greater flexibility within community nursing, but also to the more active and participatory role expected from patients, clients and carers, to the importance of a public health perspective for all nurses and to the challenges associated with the development of evidence-based practice.

By raising the level of educational preparation to meet the future needs and requirements for community health care nursing, the importance of specialist nursing contributions to primary and community health care are also recognized by the United Kingdom Central Council for Nursing, Midwifery and Health Visiting.

This broad-based text is designed to support graduate level studies undertaken by qualified community nurses who have achieved university diploma status and those who have obtained registration following a 'Project 2000'/diploma programme.

The overall aim of this book is to provide a stimulating resource for both students and educators and, in particular, to support the work of the community practice teacher. In that sense it poses questions and issues for reflection, seminars and debate, as well as offering referenced and recommended reading to promote depth and breadth of study.

We have chosen to adopt a 'framework' approach to educational and professional development, in order to demonstrate the linking elements between and within areas such as health and social policy development and social science research. The relationship between public health and primary care development is raised in different ways in different chapters, recognizing the need to work within the framework of local policy developments and that effective teamwork remains the cornerstone for the efficient deployment of scarce resources.

The concept of family is reviewed and placed in the context of the family as a provider of health care, as well as the unit for nursing assessment. The significance of information systems and effective forms of communication for describing the purpose and anticipated benefits or outcomes of individual and family care, are raised with special reference to value for money and service evaluation.

The overlap which is evident in some parts of the book, is intended. It allows for users who are busy or are putting the text alongside other material, to access all relevant information from a single chapter, each of which provides introductory key points and a concluding summary.

Structure and Organization of the Book

The book seeks to address issues of concern common to all those preparing to work in a community or primary care setting. Each section of the book adopts a particular 'framework' for stimulating thinking and critical analysis, exploring some aspect of the health care system, including the social and political context in which health services are developing and changing, together with the implications for professional practice. An introduction to each section provides an overview of the content and each chapter concludes with a summary of the key areas of discussion and recommendations for further reading.

Some important contemporary issues are raised, particularly with reference to understanding and communicating value for money, the significance of drawing together public health and primary care perspectives, and the need for practice development to be underpinned by reliable research. In this context examples of service modifications likely to be beneficial to patients, clients and carers have been included, alongside some critical discussion which questions the reality of quality health care from both the public and practising nurse perspectives.

Beginning with the pressures which drive change, the first section explores policies, demography, the changing role of general practice and the influence of epidemiological research. The second section considers the family from social science and nursing perspectives, highlighting the significance of the family as a source of ill health as well as a resource for enhancing health and quality of life.

The third and fourth sections consider professional issues that influence and facilitate change, such as educational developments, legal and ethical matters and the importance of leadership and team building. Some thought-provoking discussion appears when the 'shifting of boundaries' provides the heading for discussion. However, while it is recognized that a common philosophy guides the professional practice of community nursing (UKCC 1994) and that recurrent themes are present in the guiding principles, the particular value of each area of specialist practice has not been specifically identified. The examples of specific areas of clinical practice reviewed include the role of public health nursing in community development; the role of the practice nurse in the changing environment of primary health care; the origin and development of the nurse practitioner and the paediatric nurse in the community.

The final section focuses on the dilemmas and challenges facing community health nurses in an evolving health service which is being affected by an internal market with the role of general practitioners becoming increasingly influential. The critical issues concerning the value of health promotion, the complexity of community care with special reference to resource allocation, are explored separately. The chapter on *Value for Money* provides thought-provoking issues for everyone taking a critical look at practice and service development. Michael Hardey takes an interesting and rather different perspective, looking at the development of scientific knowledge and questioning whether this knowledge or aspects of social control are influencing and shaping the practice of community nursing.

Other important questions raised for community health nurses to consider, include:

- Do we describe the distinctive features of specialist practice in ways which predict the different and predictable benefits for the recipient (the patient/client), the user (GPs, social services, schools) and the purchaser (Health Service Commissioners, fundholding practices)?

- Do we have clearly stated service goals which are both measurable and achievable and reflect concerns for the most cost effective use of scarce resources?
- Are we able to evaluate service effectiveness using the information systems currently available?
- If not, what needs to be done to ensure that the contribution of community nursing services is recognized locally and nationally, as contributing to the priority health goals for primary and community care?
- What needs to be done by management, what needs to be done by the primary care team and what needs to be done by individual community nurses to develop a reliable data base for service evaluation?

To this end the book concludes with two chapters that explore the advantages and disadvantages of adopting a marketing perspective, together with the dilemmas and challenges of planning and managing health services in a marketing environment. Both chapters focus on aspects of communication which are particularly critical for demonstrating the actual and potential value of a community health nursing service in a negotiating or contracting situation, finishing with suggestions for how nurses could participate in the design and development of a marketing plan for a specialist community nursing service.

REFERENCES

Department of Health (DOH) (1993) *Vision for the Future.* London: HMSO.

DOH (1994) *Working in Partnership: a collaborative approach to care.* London: HMSO.

DOH (1995) *Making it Happen (SNMAC).* London: HMSO.

National Health Service Management Executive (NHSME) (1993) *New World, New Opportunities.* London: HMSO.

NHSME (1994) *Testing the Vision.* BAPS: The DSS Distribution Centre, Lancs.

UKCC (1994) *The Future of Professional Practice Following Registration.* London: UKCC.

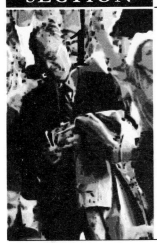

PRESSURES FOR CHANGE

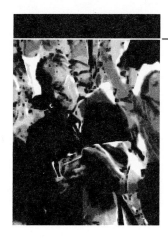

INTRODUCTION

The material contained in this introductory section seeks to set the scene for the reader. The first three chapters consider various contextual issues concerning demographic changes and the policy pressures to move the focus of the National Health Service from secondary care to primary health care and care in the community. The subsequent chapters provide examples to demonstrate the relationship between policy development, epidemiological studies, priority health care issues and practice developments.

The section opens with a review of National Health Service policy developments, the lead up to the current reforms, their introduction and impact. Against this background the second chapter explores the effect of demographic and social factors on health and health care and the inevitability of some form of rationing. The complexities concerning decisions about service priorities are considered and the chapter concludes with a discussion on the likely impact of new medical knowledge and the impact of population changes on primary health care. These themes are taken up in chapter three where the focus and organization of primary health care are reviewed from the general practitioner perspective, including the impact of policy changes and more specifically, general practice fundholding in relation to patient care and community nursing development.

The closing chapters of this section seek to demonstrate the relationship between policies, epidemiology, primary and community health care and in this context, examples are drawn from the prevention and treatment of coronary heart disease, the care of older people and mental health issues in the community.

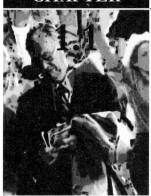

NHS POLICY DEVELOPMENTS

Stephen Peckham

KEY ISSUES

- Background to the 1991 NHS reforms
- The increasing importance of primary care and general practice
- Changing structures in the NHS
- Accountability and control in the NHS
- Implications for health professionals in general practice

INTRODUCTION

The NHS retains its position as a key topic of political debate and media interest with much discussion around whether the recent reforms to the health service are working or not. Do we believe ministers and those within the NHS who point to improved services and more patients treated or should we listen to the sceptical voices which point to the breaking up of the NHS, differing levels of service for patients and under funding? In some senses the jury, is still out on the success or otherwise of the reforms (Robinson and Le Grand, 1994) and the debate about the future of the reforms is just beginning to take shape (Ham, 1994). However, the introduction of the reforms and the changes that have flowed from them are having an important impact on the structure of the health service and how it works. In particular these changes continue to impact on the primary health care sector and, with the government's continued commitment to the expansion of general practice fundholding, the position of community health services.

This chapter will briefly examine the lead up to the reforms and their introduction and impact. In particular the impact of recent changes in the organization of the NHS will be explored which have developed from the two policy paradigms of the internal market and the emphasis on a primary care led NHS. In addition, other key policy issues of the 1990s will be discussed including the influence of *The Health of the Nation* (DOH, 1992a), issues of accountability and the position of the consumer or health care user.

The Context of the NHS Reforms

The 'Crisis in Health'

It is possible to examine the introduction of the NHS reforms from a number of perspectives, some of which are discussed in Robinson and Le Grand's (1994) book on evaluating the reforms. However, to place the discussion of the reforms within the community health service perspective the discussion here will focus on the elements of what has been described as the 'crisis in health'. Many of the features of this 'crisis' are visible in all industrialized countries and have their root in concerns about the rapidly escalating costs of health care (Saltman and Otter, 1992), although the 'crisis' reflects concern about a range of issues of which those given in Box 1.1.1 can be seen as the most significant.

Many of these issues have particular significance for community health services but first we must examine how these factors contributed to the reform of the UK health service in the late 1980s.

The Background to the Reforms

The Conservative government of the 1980s had a particular philosophy which placed the need for a strong economy before social welfare issues. They also had a distrust of public bureaucracy and were keen to see the private sector undertake many of the functions of public services (Butler, 1992). During the 1980s changes in the NHS reflected such views with the development of contracting out of services such as laundry and other domestic services, the introduction of income earning initiatives such as shops in hospitals and an increasing emphasis on introducing cost identification and management (for example the resource management initiative). Also, following the Griffiths Report of 1983, general management was introduced into the NHS to enhance strategic management of the service – representing something of an 'about face' for the government and their views on inefficient bureaucracy. We can see these moves as part of an increasing managerialist perspective which was gradually being introduced into all of the UK public sector during the 1980s.

The political temperature was raised further in the late 1980s with the House of Commons Health and Social Services Committee on funding the NHS in 1987/88 and, perhaps more importantly, the media concern following the Birmingham Children's Hospital scandal in 1987. At the same time the government had set up a working group on the NHS to determine how to make the NHS more efficient, given that there would be no new money. The context of this debate was clearly one of improving the performance of the NHS.

Box 1.1.1 Factors in the crisis in health

- Demographic changes – the UK has an ageing population while at the same time a reduction in the proportion of the population of working age, leading to an increasing demand for health care at a time when health systems will be limited in their ability to respond to this demand.
- Epidemiological transition – a move from a major preoccupation with infectious diseases to one concerned with chronic conditions.
- Changing relationships between patients and health care professionals.
- Concern with social factors – the biomedical or curative approach to health is being questioned with a search for a broader approach which takes into account social factors, recognizes the harmful effects of the environment and shifts the emphasis on to prevention of ill health.
- Continuing concerns about inequalities of health and the recognition that these are deep seated.
- The ever widening gap between demands made on health care services and the resources which the government is prepared to make available.

As the working group was meeting, key changes were taking place in parts of the NHS. Firstly in London the teaching hospitals were beginning to charge for out of district work and in East Anglia a pilot market based scheme influenced by the work of Alan Enthoven had been established. Enthoven had advocated in 1985 that a market in health care could be introduced in the UK by separating purchasers and providers. Clearly such a view fitted well with the rhetoric of the government and, as we have seen, the reliance on markets was philosophically attractive to a government who saw public bureaucracies as inefficient and the private market as more efficient.

Working for Patients

These themes can be seen as permeating *Working for Patients*, the White Paper which was the product of the government's deliberations on the NHS. The preferred solution was to introduce an internal market into the NHS with district health authorities and family health services authorities becoming purchasers and hospitals, community units and general practitioners being the providers. In addition to this separation of responsibilities a new purchaser was introduced, the *general practitioner fundholder* (GPFH).

The internal market was to achieve three key objectives (Box 1.1.2).

There were also a range of other goals and objectives such as increased patient choice, closer cooperation with the private sector, increased involvement in management by doctors and nurses, shorter waiting times, a reduction in the variations in waiting times and prescribing costs and increased financial investment in primary care.

The publication of the *Working for Patients* White Paper sparked off a huge propaganda battle which threatened to destabilize the government's plans for the NHS but which was unable to halt the introduction of the internal market (Butler, 1992). Key criticisms of the proposals were made by the medical and nursing professions, public service unions and the Labour and Liberal Parties. Concerns were expressed about the applicability of market mechanisms to the NHS, the introduction of a two tier service within general practice, the curbing of doctors' clinical freedoms and fears about the privatization of the NHS. It should also be noted that although there were concerns about the cost of the NHS, international comparisons show that total expenditure on health care in the UK is substantially less than that in other industrialized nations, as can be seen from Table 1.1.1.

Yet key indicators of the nation's health show that the UK population is not significantly different to other these countries. Thus it could be argued that the NHS offers good value for money compared to other countries. In essence this is a political argument about how much should be expended on health care. It does not, however, provide an answer to the pressures associated with the 'crisis in health' outlined above and it is probably true to say that any government will always be faced by the need to ration health care services as demand always exceeds what can be achieved with available resources.

Box 1.1.2. Key objectives of the internal market

1. Improved efficiency through market mechanisms, such as competition between providers and better productive processes achieved with increased local responsibility.
2. Improved effectiveness, through purchasing processes designed to ensure identification of need and appropriate determination of service specifications.
3. Increased clinical accountability.

Source: Office of Health Economics, *Compendium of Health Statistics 1992*, Tables 2.3 and 2.6.

Table 1.1.1 International comparisons of health care expenditure (percentage of GDP at market prices, 1990)

Country	Public expenditure on health	Total expenditure on health
Australia	5.2	5.6
Austria	5.6	8.4
Belgium	6.1	7.4
Canada	6.7	9.0
Denmark	5.2	6.2
Finland	6.2	7.4
France	6.6	8.9
Germany	5.9	8.1
Greece	4.0	5.3
Ireland	5.8	7.1
Italy	5.9	7.6
Japan	4.9	6.5
Netherlands	5.9	8.1
New Zealand	5.9	7.2
Norway	6.9	7.2
Portugal	4.1	6.7
Spain	5.2	6.6
Sweden	7.8	8.7
Switzerland	5.1	7.4
United Kingdom	5.2	6.1
United States	5.2	12.4

Another key concern was that the White Paper had little to do with health as it focused primarily on organization. It was partly in response to these criticisms that the *Health of the Nation* White Paper was published in 1992 setting targets for health in areas such as coronary heart disease, cancer, suicide, sexual health and accidents. It is also possible to view the *Health of the Nation* targets as part of the changes within the NHS relating to the division of policy and operational matters between the government and DOH and the NHS itself. This has been a development during the 1980s which underwrote the reforms, but is still a continuing process. In order to understand these broader changes it is essential that we now examine the structure of the reformed NHS.

Interestingly, while there has been this formal separation of purchasing and providing the GP fundholding proposals allowed for a combined purchaser/provider of health care. However, the hope was that the GP fundholder would purchase care more effectively and cheaply taking into consideration the patients' wishes. Proponents of the scheme would argue that given the internal market and separation of the consumer from the purchaser, GP fundholding provides a way forward in meeting consumer preferences (articulated by the GP) and focused attention on reducing costs and thus represents the key hope in achieving the government's aims of consumer choice and market efficiency outlined in *Working for Patients*. As such we have seen the gradual expansion of the GP fundholding scheme over the last four years (Glennerster *et al.*, 1994).

The Reformed NHS

The structure of the reformed NHS, and the continued debate over the roles of the various elements of the NHS, reflect the tension between the desire to keep a centralized NHS and the development of an internal market which is a more decentralized and fragmented structure. The new structure established self-governing hospital and community trusts, health care purchasers in the form of district health authorities (DHAs) and family health services authorities (FHSAs) (the old family practitioner committees, and introduced the concept of general practitioner fundholding where GPs would be able to purchase certain services (such as elective surgery) direct from health care providers for their patients. At the centre there was a formal distinction between the Department of Health, which would focus on policy issues, and the NHS Management Executive, which had developed from the managerial reforms in the 1980s and the establishment of the NHS Board.

Health boards of purchasers and providers were slimmed down and reflected a more business orientation with clear responsibility for managing the organization, particularly so with the trusts where independent status brought responsibility for managing budgets, staffing, activity etc. Regions were still important in terms of overall resource allocation, policy development and organizational development but with the new structure there were concerns that providers should be held accountable through a separate provider structure and this led to the establishment of the seven Executive outposts which roughly mirrored the regional structure. These outposts were responsible for provider development and monitoring thus splitting the role of the regions, which then focused primarily on purchasing.

The structure established in 1991 is shown in Figure 1.1.1. As will be discussed later in this chapter the importance, and roles, of each of these constituent parts has been changing since the introduction of the reforms.

Figure 1.1.1. The structure of the NHS post 1991

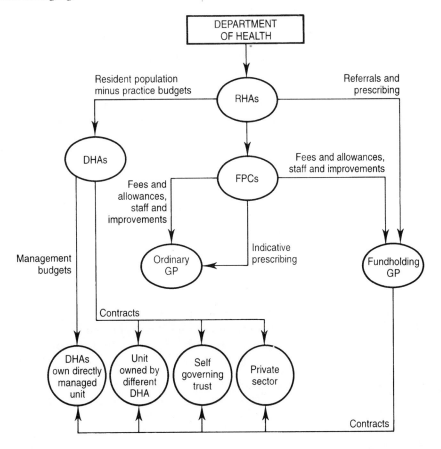

While considerable emphasis had been placed on the concept of the separation of purchasing and providing, the introduction of the reforms was far more cautious with the concept of 'steady state' being a dominant feature of the first year of the reforms. Thus the new system was not encouraged to operate as a fullblown market but rather there was an emphasis on continuity. In fact what we have seen since the development of the internal market is an increasing emphasis on provider and purchaser cooperation rather than the pursuit of a free market. The key to the improvement of the NHS was to be the improved efficiency of providers and the focus on needs based purchasing. However, to date there has been little evidence of competition between providers except in marginal activities, and purchasing skills are still being developed. In fact the development of purchasing has been a major consideration of the NHS Executive.

Key structural changes have also been influenced by the development of a primary health care led NHS and an emphasis on general practitioner developing a purchasing role, either through fundholding or other collaborative mechanisms. The impact of these changes in general practice have been significant, forcing the merger of DHAs and FHSAs or at least closer working relationships and providing impetus to enlarge DHA purchasers. Given the crucial position of the development of primary care which is now at the heart of changes in the NHS it is perhaps useful to examine how this has come about.

Primary Care Moves Centre Stage

Promoting Primary Care Clearly the gradual re-emergence of the role of primary care has been one of the key trends over the last 10 years. The establishment of the NHS in 1948 placed an increasing focus on the role and importance of hospitals but during the 1970s and early 1980s, culminating in the Government Green Paper *Promoting Better Health*, and re-emphasized in *Working for Patients*, the role for primary care was clearly mapped out. Key concerns about primary care emanated from the desire to control access to expensive acute based health care by emphasizing the gatekeeper role of GPs and concerns over the lack of ability to control the demand led expenditure of general practice. GP fundholding, the 1991 Contract and the more recent development of Total Fundholding can all be seen as having developed from these concerns (Glennerster *et al.*, 1994). However, it is also clear that the effectiveness of the UK's health care model with primary care gatekeepers has been one of the factors responsible for keeping overall costs down and has been the envy of other countries.

There has, over the last few years, been an interest in shifting services into the primary care sector away from the large acute hospitals. It is perhaps pertinent to note that the definition of primary care most commonly used relates to general practice. Within this context we can see that a primary care led NHS refers to the development of general practice as a focus for the purchasing and delivery of health care (NHSE, 1994). Within such a scenario the emphasis of the *Cumberlege Report* (DHSS 1986) on locality based delivery of care can be seen as a blip in the movement towards a focus on general practice.

There are many reasons why it is considered useful to shift investment from secondary to primary health care. These fall into two broad categories:

1. Those relating to the inappropriate use of hospital facilities.
2. Those relating to a desire to enhance the scope and standards of primary health care.

Encompassing both of these there is also a desire to provide more cost-effective care.

In terms of enhancing primary care Taylor (1991) has suggested that the main issues are:

- Opportunities to improve patients' access to care in the contexts of:
  (a) initial GP contact;
  (b) other services in the community obtained via the GP;
  (c) hospital care following GP contact;
  (d) GP and other community service care received after discharge from hospital.
- Opportunities to improve cooperation and the effective 'sharing of care' between doctors and other service providers, including consultants, nurses working in the community and hospital/community liaison posts, health visitors, midwives, community psychiatric nurses and social services staff.
- Opportunities to raise clinical and patient support standards in the context of conditions and services like diabetes, epilepsy, childhood asthma, depression and antenatal care.
- Opportunities to promote an enhanced sense of confidence, self-esteem, control and/or ownership amongst individuals involved in primary care, whether they be patients or service providers.

The Cost Issue

A key consideration within this debate has been the relative costs of primary and secondary care. While secondary care consumes twice the amount of resources that primary care does, it treats only a tenth of the episodes of ill health that are treated within primary care. Clearly we can see an incentive for shifting health care into the primary care sector (Taylor, 1991). This should also be seen in the context of the continuing movement in hospital care.

> . . . towards the delivery of progressively more high-cost, high-technology interventions involving shorter patient stays on concentrated secondary care sites. (Taylor, 1991:7)

At the same time there has been increasing focus on the cost of prescribing drugs, differing referral rates by GPs, the role of GPs and community health workers (especially relating to health promotion, for example) and the quality of care to older people, 'socially disadvantaged people' and terminally ill people. Some of these issues have been addressed through the use of generic drugs, restricted lists, the 1990 GP Contract and through the fundholding scheme. However, despite these approaches prescribing costs are still rising faster than other costs.

The GP contract, GP fundholding and the purchaser/provider split have brought many of these issues to the fore and provide a focus for moving the debate forward in relation to health gain, accessibility of services, provision of flexible services, purchasing care for localities, developing more cost-effective health care services and moving the responsibility for the provision of care between providers. The actual potential of such developments remains hotly disputed with little evaluation having been undertaken (Robinson and Le Grand, 1994). This situation is, however, changing with the pilots for total purchasing being fully evaluated over the first two years. There have, however, been calls from policy analysts for future health care policy decisions to be based more on evidence (Ham *et al.*, 1995).

It must be recognized though, that any shift across the boundary raises serious implications for those working in the NHS. Even the small shifts that have taken place have already raised issues about the appropriate membership of primary health care teams, what skill mix is appropriate in general practice and the need to examine traditional patterns of care such as the GP's gatekeeper role. Add to these the current debates about nurse training and role and the changing arrangements for contracting community nurses within fundholding practices, it is possible to begin to see that a number of changes are exacerbating each other and leaving many people working in primary care feeling very vulnerable. On the other hand, of course, many people see this situation as an opportunity to develop new patterns of care perhaps along the lines of the Lyme Regis Community Care Unit in Dorset. Here the general practice has developed into a small community services unit which both provides a range of health and social care and purchases secondary care (Robinson, 1993).

General Practice
Fundholding

Any discussion about the future direction of primary health care services is now firmly entrenched in the development of general practice fundholding which has seen a remarkable move up the political and policy agenda since its inception in the late 1980s and minor role in *Working for Patients*. Fundholding has become to be seen as one of key forces for change within the reformed NHS. Advocates of fundholding talk about its closeness to the patient, providing a patient focused approach to purchasing, freedom for GPs to provide better services for their patients and freedom to influence patterns of health care provision by community and acute units (Glennerster *et al.*, 1994).

The research on fundholding does not provide unequivocal evidence of its success. However, the government remains committed to the scheme and has gradually extended it since its inception in 1991 in both scope – with 50 pilot total fundholding projects – and to encompass more GPs with the reduction in list size and the concept of community fundholding. What is clear is the fact that this scheme, which was included in *Working for Patients* at the last minute to provide a more radical edge to the reforms, has created a substantial amount of controversy (Whitehead, 1994) but has also fundamentally changed patterns of service delivery in some areas of health care (Glennerster *et al.*, 1994).

Key questions about the efficiency and effectiveness of fundholding remain to be answered, in particular the issue of transaction costs – the cost of setting up and monitoring contracts and patient care. These would seem to be high because of the individualized nature of general practice. Whether total purchasing and different forms of contracting can overcome these remains to be seen. What is not in question is the fact that fundholding is changing the nature of relationships within the primary care sector with the development of contracting for community nursing services – and in places increased direct employment of nursing staff – and the increased level of community services now being based within general practice the role of Community Health Services is under threat (Browning, 1995). In addition a focus at practice level will require a re-evaluation of roles within the practice team.

Changing Structures

One key consequence of the reforms and the increasing power and growth of GP purchasing has then been the wholesale restructuring of the NHS at the provider, purchaser, regional and central levels. The creation of purchasing authorities has led to a merger mania which reduced the number of DHAs from 183 in 1993 to around a hundred in 1994. These mergers have also resulted in new configurations of joint DHA/FHSA purchasers formalized from 1 April 1996, radically changing the administrative structure of the NHS. Purchasers have become larger because of the pressure on keeping management costs down but also because more purchasing functions are being devolved to general practitioners.

In 1994 major changes were also announced in the role and structure of regional health authorities. Set up in 1974 to provide strategic management within the NHS their role came to be questioned following the introduction of the reforms. In particular the idea of managed approaches to health care delivery were at odds with the logic of the internal market and the freedom of purchasers and providers.

What we are in fact seeing is a dual process of increasing centralization of the controlling mechanisms of the NHS while at the same time developing a fragmented structure through purchasers and self-controlling providers. This tension is at the heart of many of the public sector changes in the UK during the last 15 years and finds its roots in the desire to separate the policy development and formulation processes from operational activities. The lesson from the NHS and other areas of government (such as the prison service) make it clear that such a separation is not easy to achieve. While ministers may wish to leave day-to-day operational decisions to managers public perceptions and political necessity mean that there will always be an interest in such matters. In fact ministers have not been shy in taking credit for improvements or good news within the service, but have tended to use the NHS Executive as a shield against bad news.

Accountability and Control

These fundamental changes taking place within the NHS affect the way it is controlled and held accountable. These include the adoption of market mechanisms, the role of commissioning managers in whom control is vested and the increased emphasis on primary care and the role of general practitioners and other primary care staff. These latter changes require differing forms of accountability structure for nurses, as acknowledged by the recent NHSME *New Deal* document, and GPs which is addressed in the accountability framework (NHSE, 1995).

Although the NHS has traditionally been viewed as being held accountable centrally through the Secretary of State for Health, in reality accountability has always been something of a patchwork quilt with management and organizational structures using different accountability mechanisms to clinical and nursing staff who have their own professional bodies. In addition, there is also the Health Service Ombudsman whose remit covers dealing with instances of maladministration, and Community Health Councils (CHCs) who have provided some sense of local accountability. It must be recognized, however, that the centralized political accountability has provided the key focus of attention as can be seen by crises in service provision in the early 1990s to which the then Secretary of State felt she needed to respond. These included the problems with the London Ambulance Service, supervision of people in the community with mental health problems, and cases of fraud and probity of board members and NHS staff.

Currently the key debates within the NHS focus on whether the market mechanism can provide an appropriate route for accountability and how traditional routes of accountability through management and professional structures can be maintained in a fragmented NHS. This is of particular concern to community staff who may see their jobs transferred to general practice. A more fundamental question which also has to be asked is who are fundholding general practitioners accountable to? Clearly they must meet financial and administrative criteria and targets set by regions and the NHSE, but who monitors the level of care, types of care provided and decisions made within the practice? While in the consultation document the NHSE has suggested a stronger role for local people it is not clear how this is to be achieved and based on existing practice little progress in this form of accountability has been made within general practice (Peckham, 1994).

There are also significant questions which remained to be answered with regard to clinical accountability. While the reforms have made clinicians more accountable to their employing organizations it is clear that accountability to patients has not been strengthened. The *Patient's Charters* (1992, 1995) do provide some definitive level of standards but these do not relate to quality of care and do not confer any substantial rights. For example, the Charter right to information is limited by a clinician's freedom to decide what information to give.

Attention has also been drawn to the increasing secretiveness of the NHS (Longley, 1993). Secretive trust boards, fewer DHA/FHSA meetings, smaller boards, the demise of regions resulting in the loss of regional boards and there is some discussion that CHCs may in future be funded directly by the NHSE. This would mean that the watchdogs are being funded by the agency they should be holding to account! Add to this the lack of accountability structures for GPs and it is possible to see some credence to these arguments.

Clearly the market is not seen as a suitable replacement for these forms of account-ability and the growing interest in openness, corporate governance and accountability to the public are just some of the suggested approaches to improve NHS accountability. The problem is the development of effective mechanisms for such accountability. Recent moves by the NHSE to establish appointment panels for board members and the discussion documents on corporate governance and GP account-ability are clear signs of a new level of caution. How effective these approaches will be remains to be seen. Also the level of political interest in the NHS is unlikely to diminish and therefore there will remain strong vestiges of central accountability.

Perhaps the most unknown factor is how public accountability through consumer and community involvement will develop. Current pressure to achieve responsive-ness to consumers and the emphasis on developing charter type standards are clearly creating a different environment within the NHS. There is much discussion about appropriate mechanisms for achieving involvement in health care, particularly those aspects of purchasing which create fierce debate such as the rationing or prioritizing of health care.

Future Scenarios

The only clear message from the recent changes to the NHS is that they have not stopped yet and despite ministerial protestations to the fact that a time of tranquillity and stability is needed, the changes are likely to continue as market mechanisms become more prominent. Essentially there is a dichotomy between the desire for a centrally coordinated service and a fragmented market based one. Currently the two exist side by side but how far this is tenable in the future is not clear. The debate currently centres around the need for a managed market but to what extent it is possible to define the degree of management will remain a contested issue.

The continuing emphasis on general practice fundholding is leading to a greater degree of diversification with GPs becoming more likely to make resource allocation decisions for individual patients. In addition the focus on general practice is likely to mean the reconfiguration of both hospital and community based services. Already we can see changing relationships within the primary health care team and tensions developing between area based approaches, envisaged by Cumberlege, and the focus on the practice list. General practice based health care will challenge existing professional structures and the role of the newly developed health authority purchasers. With increased employment of nursing staff within general practice existing management and career structures will change. Also the boundaries between staff in general practice could become more confused and we are beginning to see this with the current nurse practitioner projects (Gordon and Hadley, 1996; Meads, 1996).

The big question must be the extent to which general practice is willing to take on the new role in the NHS currently being envisaged. It is clear that any development of general practice will bring tighter controls. One of the principles with fundholding and 1990 GP contract is the increased introduction of cash limited budgets, it does not seem impossible that, if total fundholding is universally introduced, general practice will become cash limited service rather than based on a fee for service. Also, any increase in responsibility or workload in general practice requires a rethink of roles and responsibilities, not only of the GPs but also other practice staff, nursing and administrative, particularly if divisions between general medical services (GMS) fundholding budgets and other contracts are abolished.

At the heart of much of the current debate is the issue of accountability. Regions have been drawn into the web of the central NHS Executive and will act more as the executive arm of central government in future. With purchasing being focused more and more on general practice there is a clear problem of how GPs can be held accountable for purchasing decisions and what the role of the health authority will be (NHSE, 1995).

CONCLUSIONS

Writing a chapter on health policy outlining what is happening is still like trying to take a snapshot at a moving target. The pace of change within the NHS is greater than anything since the formation of the NHS in 1948. We can only watch as these changes unfold as the implications of current organizational reorganization and the development of general practice based purchasing are not yet clear. What is clear, though, is that these changes have an energy of their own and as they embed into the NHS it will become increasingly difficult for their effects to be reversed, thus posing a problem for the Labour Party should they become the next government. Currently the Labour Party is rethinking its opposition to fundholding and the NHS reforms. They, like the British Medical Association, may have to work within the framework of the reforms unless they wish to push through another major reorganization. What seems likely is that the concept of purchasing and providing is here to stay, as will be some form of general practice purchasing, but what the exact form would be under a future Labour government still requires some crystal ball gazing. The next few years will, though, present significant challenges to health care professionals and managers. In particular there must begin to be a debate about roles and responsibilities. Nurse practitioners are the start of this process, as are discussions about generic nursing and the need to address the boundaries of medical and social care. But, it is also a challenge to the medical profession with a need for GPs, in particular, to examine their role within primary health care.

SUMMARY

- The 'crisis in health' and government views about market mechanisms for organizing the health service in this country were the key drivers in shaping the NHS reforms.

■ While not a key part of the reforms, the changes in primary care, particularly the development of fundholding, have had significant effects on the continuing development of delivery and purchasing structures of the NHS.

■ The impact of the reforms and the process of change introduced by the government in 1991 has led to fundamental changes in accountability and organizational structures which have led to changes at district and regional health authority levels.

■ The concept of purchasing and providing would seem to be well embedded in the NHS and the basic concept of such a split is likely to remain, irrespective of which political party is in government.

DISCUSSION QUESTIONS

◆ To what extent can the internal market provide the improved effectiveness in terms of cost savings and consumer responsiveness outlined in *Working for Patients*?

◆ Will the continued development of general practice fundholding undermine the principle of equal access to health care within the NHS?

◆ What is the future role for community health service units in the NHS? How have they been affected by general practice fundholding? Will they continue to exist?

◆ To what extent will an emphasis on the development of purchasing and providing at practice level lead to changes in the roles of community nursing staff and general practitioners?

◆ How far would it be possible for a new government to change fundamentally the internal market system as it has developed?

FURTHER READING

Glennerster H, Matsaganis M, Owens P and Hancock S (1994) *Implementing GP Fundholding. Wild Card or Winning Hand?* Buckingham: Open University Press.
While suffering from a number of methodological weaknesses, as an evaluation of fundholding this study does provide a very good guide to the development of general practice fundholding. It is worth balancing this with some more critical reading such as the chapter by Whitehead in Robinson and Le Grand.

Gordon P and Hadley J (eds) (1996) *Extending Primary Care*. Oxford: Radcliffe Medical Press.
This book provides an attempt to analyse some of the current developments in primary care, including looking at what is meant by primary care.

Harrison S and Pollitt C (1994) *Controlling Health Professionals. The Future of Work and Organization in the NHS*. Buckingham: Open University Press.
One of the key aspects of the reforms has been the increased managerial control over health professionals. This book sets the context for these changes and discusses the impact on health care professions.

Klein R (1996) *The Politics of the NHS*, 3rd edn. London: Longman.
Klein is an excellent guide to the politics and policies which shape the way the NHS works. He provides a good history and political analysis of the UK health care system and contains some illuminating material about recent changes in the structure and organization of the NHS.

Meads G (ed) (1996) *Future Options for General Practice.* Oxford: Radcliffe Medical Press.
This is an excellent collection of articles which provide an overview of many current UK developments. Raises lots of issues about the future direction that primary care might take.

O'Keefe E, Ottewill R and Wall A (1992) *Community Health: Issues in Management.* Sunderland: Business Education Publishers.
Although a little out of date given the rapid development of fundholding this book provides an excellent introduction to many issues relating to community health services.

Robinson R and Le Grand J (Eds). (1994) *Evaluating the NHS Reforms.* London: King's Fund Institute.
In the absence of any formal evaluations of the 1990 NHS reforms this book is perhaps the next best thing. It draws together the findings of a number of King's Fund projects on aspects of the reforms together with commentaries on the background to the reforms and one on equity by Margaret Whitehead.

REFERENCES

Browning R (1995) The future of community health trusts. *Primary Care Management* **5:** 7-10.

Butler J (1992) *Patients, Policies and Politics: Before and After Working for Patients.* Buckingham: Open University Press.

DHSS (1986) *Neighbourhood Nursing: A Focus For Care.* London: HMSO.

DOH (1987) *Promoting Better Health: The Government's Programme for Improving Primary Health Care.* Cm 249. London: HMSO.

DOH (1989) *Working For Patients.* CM555. London: HMSO.

DOH (1992a) *The Health of the Nation.* London: HMSO.

DOH (1992b) *The Patient's Charter.* London: HMSO.

DOH (1995) *The Patient's Charter and You.* London: HMSO.

Enthoven AC (1985) National Health Service: some reforms that might be politically feasible. *Economist* **295** (7399): 19-22.

Exworthy M (1993) *Community Nursing: A background paper exploring current issues.* Briefing Paper No9, Wessex Research Consortium, Institute for Health Policy Studies, University of Southampton.

Glennerster H, Matsaganis M, Owens P and Hancock S (1994) *Implementing GP Fundholding. Wild Card or Winning Hand?* Buckingham: Open University Press.

Gordon P and Hadley J (eds) (1996) *Extending Primary Care.* Oxford: Radcliffe Medical Press.

Griffiths R (1983) *Report of the NHS Management Inquiry.* London: DHSS.

Ham C (1994) Where now for the reforms? *British Medical Journal* **309:** 351-352.

Ham C, Hunter DJ and Robinson R (1995) Evidence based policy-making. *British Medical Journal* **310:** 71-72.

Harrison S and Pollitt C (1994) *Controlling Health Professionals. The Future of Work and Organization in the NHS.* Buckingham: Open University Press.

Klein R (1996) *The Politics of the NHS*, 3rd edn London: Longman.

Labour Party (1994) *Health 2000 The health and wealth of the nation in the 21st century.*

Longley D (1993) *Public Law and Health Service Accountability.* Buckingham: Open University Press.

NHSE (1995) *An Accountability Framework for GP Fundholding.* Leeds: NHSE.

Meads G (ed) (1996) *Future Options for General Practice.* Oxford: Radcliffe Medical Press.

O'Keefe E, Ottewill R and Wall A (1992) *Community Health: Issues in Management.* Sunderland: Business Education Publishers.

Ottewill R and Wall A (1990) *The Growth and Development of the Community Health Services.* Sunderland: Business Education Publishers.

Peckham S (1994) Local voices and primary care. *Critical Public Health* **5**(2): 36-40.

Robinson B (1993) Power to the localities; An integrated approach to health and social care delivery. *Primary Care Management* **3**(11): 2-3.

Robinson R and Le Grand J (Eds) (1994) *Evaluating the NHS Reforms.* London: King's Fund Institute.

Saltman B and Otter C (1992) *Planned Markets and Public Competition.* Buckingham: Open University Press.

Taylor D (1991) *Developing Primary Care: Opportunities for the 1990s.* London: King's Fund Institute.

Whitehead M (1994) Is is Fair?: Evaluating the equity implications of the NHS reforms. In R Robinson and J Le Grand (Eds) *Evaluating the NHS Reforms.* London: King's Fund Institute.

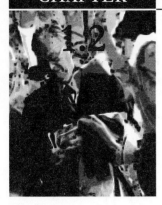

DEMOGRAPHIC CHANGES

Kate Jolly and Steve George

KEY ISSUES

- The effect of ageing on health and disease
- The changing pattern of disease
- The significance of ethnicity for health
- The implications for women of community care
- An introduction to the concept of rationing
- The development of service priorities
- The impact of population characteristics and new knowledge on the role of primary care

INTRODUCTION

This chapter considers the effects of demographic and social factors on health and health care. It discusses the inevitability of some form of rationing and considers methods of determining service priorities. These factors, together with new medical knowledge and NHS policy developments all affect the role and provision of primary care.

The Effect of Ageing on Health and Disease

Life expectancy has increased markedly during this century. A newborn male had a life expectancy of 73.2 years in 1991 compared to 45.5 years in 1901; a newborn female in 1991 had a life expectancy of 78.8 years compared to 49 years in 1901. A major contribution to the increase in life expectancy has been the fall in deaths during infancy. Figure 1.2.1 shows that the fall in perinatal and infant mortality rates in England has continued even in recent years.

A consequence of our increased longevity, associated with a falling birth rate, is the rising proportion of elderly persons in the population. Eighteen per cent of the population are now over pensionable age, and the proportion of people aged over 85 years has increased by 49% between 1981 and 1991. This rise in the very elderly population is illustrated by the increase in the number of telegrams sent out by Buckingham Palace to mark people's one hundredth birthday – from 302 in 1955 to 4703 in 1993. As a result of the longer life expectancy of women 66% of people aged 75 years and over are female. Adult women make greater use of medical services than men of the same age.

Figure 1.2.1. Perinatal and infant mortality rates in England 1960–1992. PMR = perinatal mortality rate (number of stillbirths and deaths under one week per 1000 live and stillbirths). IMR = infant mortality rate (number of deaths under one year per 1000 live births).

Source: OPCS. In 1992 198 stillbirths were excluded following the introduction of new legislation on 1 October 1992

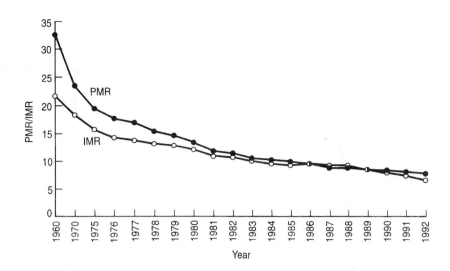

Older people experience more illness. The 1991 census asked people whether they suffered from long-term illness. Figure 1.2.2 illustrates how the percentage of people living in Great Britain with a limiting long-term illness rises to almost 70% of those aged 85 years and over.

The rising prevalence of long-term illness with age is mirrored by hospital discharge rates (except in children – who use more hospital services than young adults). Hospital discharge rates per year in 1985 rose from 7.5% at 30 years to 20% at 75 years and 40% in those aged 85 years and above. With increasing numbers of elderly this has major implications for resource use.

As people age the pattern of disease from which they suffer changes. Major causes of death such as circulatory disease and cancer become more common, as do diseases of the musculoskeletal system, which are a considerable cause of ill health. Accidents are common in the elderly, with one-third of all people aged 65 years and over experiencing one or more falls each year.

Over a third (36% in 1985) of people over 65 years now live alone, compared with 22% in 1962. This is largely at the expense of people living with relatives. The resulting social isolation inevitably increases the need for social and health care.

Figure 1.2.2.
Proportion of the population with a limiting long-term illness, 1991. pen = pensionable age (60 for women and 65 for men).

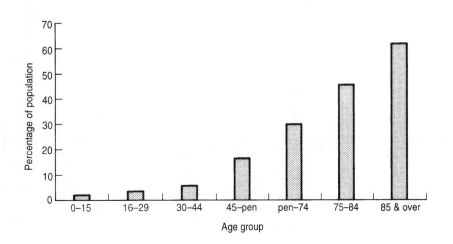

Source: OPCS

The Changing Pattern of Disease

The Decline of Infectious Disease

The major change in the pattern of disease since the last century has been the decline of infectious diseases and the increased prevalence of chronic non-infectious disease. Infectious diseases do still present some challenges, as illustrated by the HIV virus and the associated opportunistic infections which arise in immunocompromised individuals, but their impact on the population has been much reduced since the mid nineteenth century.

Improved standards of living appear to have been the main cause of the decline of mortality from infectious disease, since deaths from many diseases, such as tuberculosis, had fallen considerably prior to the introduction of effective treatments. Medical interventions have played a role, particularly for diseases such as diphtheria and poliomyelitis, but overall the contribution of medicine to increased life expectancy has been very small (McKeown, 1979).

The Quantity of Life – Causes of Mortality

The aims of the health service have often been described as 'adding years to life and life to years'. The main causes of death in the late twentieth century are those that are most prevalent in older people. The major cause of death is ischaemic heart disease, followed by cerebrovascular disease (stroke) and cancers. These are all problems particularly associated with ageing. Ischaemic heart disease is the main cause of death for both males and females aged 55 years and over.

The maximum lifespan of a human being appears to be fairly fixed, at somewhere between 115 and 120 years. No one has ever survived longer than this, and there is unlikely to be enormous scope for increasing longevity as such. *Average* life expectancy, however, also takes into account all those who die prematurely, and premature deaths in childhood and mid-life offer ample scope for prevention. A useful indicator of premature mortality which takes account of all deaths to people aged 15 to 64 years is 'years of working life lost'. Years of working life lost for England and Wales and for 1992 are shown in the following Box 1.2.1. The percentages are of the total years of working life lost in males or females due to the disease in question.

The Quality of Life – Causes of Disability

Improving the quality of life in older people involves alleviating those problems which often cause disability rather than death. Increasingly, disability caused by congenital and infectious disease is being replaced by that caused by chronic disease of neurological, musculoskeletal or cardiorespiratory origin. Arthritis, hearing and visual loss and mental illness all become more common with age. This is a major challenge for providers of care.

Box 1.2.1. Years of working life lost for England and Wales for 1992

Males aged 15–64	%
• Circulatory disease	24
• Cancers	22
• Accidental deaths	16
Females aged 15–64	
• Cancers	41
• Circulatory disease	15
• Accidental deaths	8

Social Inequalities

Many of the chronic diseases common in our society are considered to be diseases of affluence and are less prevalent in developing countries. However, with very few exceptions (such as some cancers), almost all causes of death are more common in people who are in social classes IV and V. Despite falls in death from ischaemic heart disease the gap between social classes I and V has not narrowed and may even be widening.

Ethnicity and Health

Studies of migrants living in a new country show that the diseases which affect first generation immigrants mirror those of their country of origin, taking into account the fact that this a selectively healthy group. The pattern of disease of subsequent generations tends to move towards that experienced by the host country's population. The United Kingdom is an increasingly multicultural society, with people of many different racial origins. Whilst the majority of illness suffered by residents of 'non-white' racial origins is similar to that of the white population there are some important differences.

Until the 1991 census there was little information about the numbers of people who perceived themselves to be in a particular ethnic group. In 1991 slightly over 3 million people (5.5% of the UK population) described themselves as belonging to an ethnic group other than white. The largest single group was Indian, making up 1.5% of the total population; three black groups (African, Caribbean and others) made up 1.6% and Pakistanis 0.9%. The age structure of the ethnic minority populations is much younger than that of the white population, with only 1% of the people who belong to an ethnic minority group aged 65 years and over.

While some cancers are less common in ethnic minority groups, some other diseases are more common. Mortality from coronary heart disease is raised in people from the Indian sub-continent, a fact which is not adequately explained by patterns of conventional risk factors. Non-insulin dependent diabetes is more common in people of both Asian and Caribbean origins and may partially explain the high mortality from coronary heart disease. Mortality from stroke is markedly raised in people of Caribbean origin and less so in people of African or Asian origins. Tuberculosis has 25 times the incidence rate in people from the Indian sub-continent compared to the white population. Hepatitis B is endemic in the Far East and some parts of the Caribbean resulting in a chronic carrier state in some people with these origins. Both tuberculosis and hepatitis B can be prevented by offering immunization to newborn children from high risk ethnic minority groups. Certain blood disorders, sickle cell disease and thalassaemia are more common in a number of racial groups. Schizophrenia appears to have a higher incidence among people of Caribbean origin living in England.

Patterns of service usage also differ between the white population and some ethnic minority groups. For instance, women of Asian origin have a particularly low uptake of cervical and breast screening programmes, with the result that some women may present with advanced cancer which could have been cured if detected earlier.

The challenge for providers of health care is to ensure equality of access for people from all racial backgrounds and to provide services in a culturally sensitive manner. In geographical areas with a high proportion of people of a particular ethnic origin special services may be required.

The Implications for Women of 'Community Care'

Women are going to be affected by the move towards community care both as the main receivers and providers of care.

Women as Receivers of Community Care

A higher proportion of the elderly are women and more elderly women live alone than men. Data from the 1986 General Household Survey showed that 61% of women aged 85 years and over lived alone compared with 37% of men, and that 33% of women aged 65–69 years lived alone compared to 13% of men of the same age. Much long-term care that was previously provided by the health service has now been redefined as social care and the recipients are means tested. This is likely to reduce the range of care options available to elderly women.

Women as Providers of Community Care

Community care involves both care in the community and care by the community, largely women. Women are the main carers of elderly relatives. An increasing proportion of women are in paid employment, 61% in 1981 compared to 30% in 1921. This means that fewer women are available to provide care, or they do so in addition to working and looking after their own families, which is likely to increase stress and ill health. The rise in women of working age in employment also results in the providers of voluntary care being increasingly elderly themselves. The rising proportion of women deferring childbirth into their thirties and forties will result in these women having both young children and dependent parents.

The 'Care in the Community' policy encourages people to be cared for in their own homes. It has removed the right to financial assistance to live in residential care. This is likely to increase the burden on informal carers.

An Introduction to the Concept of Rationing

To someone brought up in the tradition of the 1948 National Health Service Act, the concept of 'rationing' seems at first alien. A health service free at the point of contact is central to the philosophy of most who choose to work in the British National Health Service (NHS). 'Rationing' arouses images of better quality services going to those who can afford to pay, while those who cannot have to put up with second best or, worse still, no health service at all. However, this need not be the case and, as we shall see, some form of rationing of health services is not only essential but inevitable.

In order to understand why, it is necessary to become familiar with a term used by economists, that of 'opportunity cost'. This means simply that if money is spent on one thing, it cannot be spent on something else (Mooney *et al.*, 1980). Obviously, there is never an infinite amount of money to spend, however much we choose to allocate to health, so we always have to choose what to spend our money on.

What Do We Mean By Rationing?

Klein (1992) describes four different dimensions to rationing:

1. Decisions about the allocation of resources to broad sectors or client groups. These decisions can be at a high level, say, allocating budgets between the Department of Health and the Ministry of Defence, or at a lower level, where the choice could be between distributing health care between elderly people and children, or between a new maternity unit and a new children's orthopaedic service.

2. Decisions about the allocation of resources to specific forms of treatment (particularly those which require investment in new facilities). Here, the choice may lie between, say, surgery and lithotripsy (ultrasound shock wave therapy) for kidney stones, or between two different antibiotics for the treatment of urinary tract infection. The common feature in both cases is that the choice is between alternative treatments for the same condition. This is a central difference between choices within this dimension and choices within the previous dimension.

3. Decisions about how to prioritize access to treatment between different patients. The choice here is necessitated by the fact that a treatment is available, but that there is not enough to go round to satisfy demand. The choice is therefore between different individuals for the same treatment. A typical case might be renal dialysis for patients in chronic renal failure.

4. Decisions about how much to invest in individual patients once access has been achieved. This could be for different reasons. For instance, the decision might be whether or not to 'switch off' someone in a long-lasting coma and whose life is maintained by a life support machine, and in doing so, mobilize extra resources which might be used to treat someone else. However, another example might be to reduce the number and type of investigations given routinely to patients being admitted to hospital, in order to save resources which might be used to treat a larger number of patients overall.

An area which often causes confusion is the difference between 'rationing', and 'refusal to treat on clinical grounds'. The latter depends on the balance in the individual patient between treating and not treating. If we are considering an operative procedure, it makes obvious sense not to carry out the procedure if the risk of death during or immediately following operation outweighs the increased possibility of survival in the long term, or if there is no health benefit to the patient and only a financial cost to be borne.

How Should We Make Rationing Decisions?

Logically, resources should be distributed in order to purchase those services that will ensure the maximum health gain to the population. To do this we would need to know the true need for each type of intervention, the cost in terms of resources used, and the benefit in terms of health gained for every health intervention, including some which are slightly removed from health care such as the provision of affordable housing and a minimum wage to those that need it. Armed with such information we would be able to work out the best mix of interventions needed to maximize health gain. However, although much work is being done on this front, history shows that the way in which resources have been distributed in the past has not generally been determined by this logical process.

How Have We Made Rationing Decisions In The Past?

When the NHS was formed in 1948 it was anticipated that as time passed the stock of available ill health would be used up and the amount of money that would have to be spent on the NHS would gradually decrease. This has proved to be untrue. In most industrialized countries the proportion of gross national product (GNP - that is, the total income of a country) spent on health care doubled in the three decades between 1960 and 1990. In the USA some 16% of GNP is spent on health care (compared to 6% in the UK) and this is predicted to reach 20% by the turn of the century (Stevens and Raftery, 1994). However, rising health care costs cannot wholly be explained by the rise in the number of elderly people and the consequent rise in demand for health and social services.

The original aim of the NHS was not only to provide a health service free at the point of contact, but to provide 'the best' possible medical care for everyone. 'The best' is interpreted almost invariably to mean 'the latest' or 'the most technologically advanced' by the majority of health care professionals, and it is their natural desire to see that all their patients get what they consider to be the current state of the art treatment. This has led to a rapid acceleration of the scope of medical treatment. Many of the therapies now on offer were not even imagined in 1948. Moreover, as successive new treatments become routine, we move on to finding cures or controlling measures for maladies thought formerly to be incurable or uncontrollable, or to treating problems that were deemed previously too minor to be worthy of consideration. Consequently, we will never reach a state where the whole population has 'perfect health', and the cost of health care rises inexorably.

It is difficult for the providers of a particular health intervention, be it a new operation, drug or piece of technology, to assess objectively the benefits brought about by its use. In order to overcome the difficulties encountered in researching into a new intervention, a health care professional will often develop an almost religious belief in its worth. The result is that over 80% of the health interventions used in the NHS have never been tested in terms of their effectiveness (Smith, 1991). Further, in order to get such an intervention into practice, people will utilize a number of political techniques, such as 'shroud waving' (the prophecy of the terrible consequences of the intervention not being introduced) or merely shouting louder than everybody else ('planning by decibels').

Practical Attempts At Rationing

The area of 'resource allocation' has been one of intense interest for health service researchers, and health economists in particular, for some years. The ideal, according to one widely quoted school, is to develop a single index (that is, a single scale of measurement) by which to measure health, and to convert all known research into measurements on that scale. A simple way of doing this is to measure the years survived by people following a health intervention, and to compare it with the number of years survived by those not receiving the intervention. Of course, this does not take into account the quality of life of people following an intervention.

In order to try to account for quality of life, an index has been developed which incorporates quality of life, as measured on the Rosser Disability/Distress Scale (Rosser and Kind, 1972). This index is known as the quality adjusted life year, or 'QALY'. An ideal life year has a value of one, and this amount becomes less as the year becomes 'less healthy'. According to these assumptions, it makes sense, therefore, to aim to gain as many QALYs as possible for a given resource input. However, many criticisms have been levelled at QALYs. They make perfect sense where the group of patients to be treated is the same, and we are merely assessing alternative treatments for the same condition, but difficulties start when we are comparing treatments which would benefit different groups. As an example, older people have a natural disadvantage when it comes to resource allocation, in that they will be expected to live for a shorter period of time whatever the intervention, even if their post-intervention mortality and morbidity is no worse than that of their younger competitors. An intervention will always produce fewer QALYs if it is applied to older people. On the other hand, it has been argued that older people have had 'a fair innings', and that treatment should naturally be given to younger people who have not had the benefit of so many years of life previously (Lockwood, 1988). The quality dimension also counts, however. Take the case of people with, say, renal failure. It might be considered that one year of life with renal failure is not worth the same as one year of life in perfect health (although the person with renal failure might be quick to point out that it is better than no life at all). Again, the affected individual is at a disadvantage. The alternative, however, is to allocate all treatment on the basis of random choice – 'the toss of a coin'.

We come now to the concept of 'needs assessment'. 'Need' for a health intervention (that is, the ability to benefit from the intervention) can be assessed using the three methods shown in Box 1.2.2.

Each method has its pros and cons. Comparison with other places may be the only information we have at the moment for a variety of services. However, if the basic truth is that the service does nobody any good, wherever provided, comparison will eventually fail. Consensus seems to offer a way in which all parties can be satisfied, but we will always be faced by problems of competing moral and philosophical standpoints, and by a certain degree of self-interest. The ability to argue a case, based upon their degree of education and knowledge gives certain groups an unfair advantage. Conversely the general public may be less well able than health professionals to distinguish between their need for an intervention (as defined above) and their demand for it, which is based on the desire to be healthy, but without expert knowledge of the effectiveness of the intervention. A good example here is lung cancer, where the major effective intervention would be stopping people smoking, perhaps by banning tobacco advertising, but where much is still spent on attempts at curative interventions which are ineffective in over 80% of patients (Stevens and Raftery, 1994). Epidemiology is the ideal, but we are several years from this ideal situation.

What Shall We Do In The Interim?

Epidemiological methods by which we can set priorities are in their infancy, but a start has been made. In the meantime, changes to services offered need to be made incrementally, with new information on effectiveness being incorporated as it becomes available. Consensus is important in this process, but it is important that the distinction is made between need and demand for services, and attempts made to educate people about services which are demanded but which have been proven to be ineffective. Only in this way can we arrive at a fairer distribution of resources.

Factors that Impact on the Role of Primary Care

Demand for primary care is affected by three main areas: population characteristics, new medical knowledge and political and policy changes.

Box 1.2.2. Methods for assessing need

- Comparison – that is, by seeing what is provided elsewhere
- Consensus – that is, by asking different groups of people (purchasers, providers, and most importantly patients) what they want, and coming to an agreement
- Epidemiology – by assessing scientifically the burden of disease and the cost-effectiveness of interventions to control it – this is the ideal situation described above.

Policy Changes

Many recent policies have affected both the provision of and demand for primary care. These include 'Care in the Community', fundholding by general practitioners, the NHS focus on primary care, the shift in emphasis towards prevention, the 'Patient's Charter' and the changing structure of the primary health care team, which was affected by allowances to encourage group practices and the employment of receptionists and practice nurses. These changes are discussed in Chapters 1 and 3.

Population Characteristics

Population characteristics have largely acted to increase the workload of primary health care teams. The ageing population suffers from more illness and diseases of a chronic nature. Unemployment increases chronic illness and people in the lower socioeconomic classes have a higher mortality from most causes. Other social changes, such as more women in employment, increased distance between families and more lone-parent households, have reduced people's ability to cope without professional help. The increased levels of car ownership in society may act to reduce access to primary care in both general practice surgeries and accident and emergency departments, if these services become reliant on people being able to present themselves.

New Medical Knowledge

New medical knowledge has led to more diagnostic tests, treatments and screening being done in primary care. The boundaries between primary and secondary care are shifting. General practice no longer acts as a filter, whereby the majority of people requiring treatment are referred to hospital. This change has been aided by the increased range of drug treatments available and the ability of general practitioners to have open access to hospital investigations, such as X-rays, pathology tests and endoscopies. Research which has shown the ability of primary care to manage many chronic diseases, such as hypertension, asthma and diabetes, has led to an increasing participation of practice nurses in the management of these diseases. This has been associated with a recent interest in the development of guidelines for the management of specific problems. The increased prominence of health promotion and screening has increased the role of practice nurses within the primary health care team. It is important that professionals recognize the different ethical responsibilities between treating an illness presented by a patient and looking for pre-symptomatic disease or risk factors for disease. Professionals involved in screening will need to be adequately trained so they can explain the implications of the test.

Earlier discharges from hospital, the increasing use of day surgery and the care of increasingly frail people in the community will not only increase the direct contact of the primary health care team, but will also increase the need for liaison between health and social services. Members of the primary health care team will act as the key worker for particular individuals.

CONCLUSION

Many influences are acting to increase the amount of care provided in the community. This will inevitably place demands on both lay and professional providers of care. This will require new work practices, good communication between professionals and a willingness to consider altering the boundaries between the various professional groups.

SUMMARY

■ The ageing population will lead to an increased prevalence of chronic disease and increased pressure on resources.

■ Access to health services is an issue of importance for all sectors of society, particularly people from ethnic minority groups.

■ Women will be affected by the move towards community care as both the main providers of care and as the main recipients.

■ Resources will always be limited so it is inevitable that methods for prioritizing health care will have to be developed.

■ Primary care is affected by the demography of the population, new medical advances and policies. General practice fundholding will have a particularly large impact on the provision and organization of community services.

DISCUSSION QUESTIONS

◆ Consider the constraints for community nurses wishing to contribute to research into the outcomes of care provided in the community. How might these be overcome?

◆ What are the training requirements of community nurses to meet the challenges of new medical knowledge and policies?

◆ Think of someone you know well, a friend or relative, but not yourself, who requires regular medical treatment or care of some sort. How would you like the decision to be made regarding the resources needed for their treatment or care?

FURTHER READING

Hughes J and Gordon P (1992) *Hospitals and Primary Care, Breaking the Boundaries.* London: King's Fund. This is a working paper for the King's Fund Commission on the Future of Acute Services in London. It explores the interface between hospitals and primary care and describes innovative ways of providing more services in the community.

Robinson R (1993) Economic evaluation and health care. *British Medical Journal.* **307:** 670-673, 726-728, 793-795, 859-862, 924-926.

This series of articles provides a clear introduction to basic health economics and explains costs and the various forms of cost-benefit analyses.

Smith A and Jacobson B (1988) *The Nation's Health: A Strategy for the 1990s.* London: King's Fund. This report provides an overview of the epidemiological trends of the major diseases affecting the UK population and considers how mortality rates can be reduced and improvements achieved in health related behaviours.

REFERENCES

Department of Health (1991) *The Patient's Charter.* London: HMSO.

Klein R (1992) Warning signals from Oregon: the different dimensions of rationing need untangling. *British Medical Journal* **304:** 1457-1458.

Lockwood M (1988) Quality of life and resource allocation. In S Mendus and JM Bell (Eds) *Philosophy and Medical Welfare.* Cambridge: Cambridge University Press.

McKeown T (1979) *The Role of Medicine.* Oxford: Blackwell.

Mooney GH, Russell EM and Weir RD (1980) *Choices for Health Care*: Chapter One, pp 1-9. London: Macmillan Press.

The National Health Service and Community Care Act (1990). London: HMSO.

Office of Population Censuses and Surveys, Social Services Division (1986) *General Household Survey.* London: HMSO.

Rosser R.M and Kind P (1972) The measurement of hospital output. *International Journal of Epidemiology* **1:** 361-368.

Smith R (1991) Where is the wisdom . . . ? *British Medical Journal* **303:** 798-N799.

Stevens A and Raftery J (Eds), (1994) *Health Care Needs Assessment: the epidemiologically based needs assessment reviews.* Oxford: Radcliffe Medical Press.

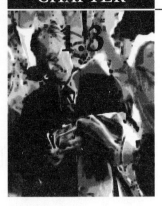

CHAPTER 13

PRIMARY CARE AND THE GENERAL PRACTITIONER

Simon A. Smail

KEY ISSUES

- The development of British general practice
- Evolution of primary health care philosophies; the Alma-Ata declaration
- Common features of primary health care (PHC)
- Key development trends in UK PHC

INTRODUCTION

'Primary health care' is the phrase often used to describe medical and nursing care in the community. Yet the concepts encompassed by this phraseology have been changing over the past few years and are often misunderstood. Furthermore, there is often confusion about terminology; different usage applies in different countries. In the UK, it is usual to refer to 'general practice' as the key element of the primary care system. This chapter explores the relationship between primary health care and general practice.

The organization of primary care services in the UK is, at the time of writing, in considerable flux. Nevertheless, some principles of terminology still hold good. 'General Medical Services' are those obligatory services that are provided by a general practitioner (GP) by virtue of his or her contract with a Family Health Services Authority, and can be described as 'core' services. These have been defined as 'reactive services provided to patients who are or believe themselves to be ill, including the reactive management of chronic diseases' (General Medical Services Committee, 1994). General practitioners do also provide certain other 'non-core' services, such as health promotion, pro-active management of disease etc., which are additional to the core contractual obligation of a GP, and governed by supplementary contracts. However, GPs are customarily involved in the provision of a wide range of other services including many of the activities of a primary care team. The term 'general practice' is usually used to refer to all those services provided directly by the general practitioner and the staff immediately associated with the GP, including the general practice nurse. Some members of the primary care team may be in the employ of a GP, although others may be employed by other authorities. However, the recent trend has been for GPs to hold and manage budgets for the purchase of a broad range of services for the benefit of patients registered with the practice. 'Fundholding' GPs hold budgets to commission a defined range of non-urgent secondary care (specialist) medical services, but may also purchase certain elements of primary care provision, such as community nursing services.

Historical Development of General Practice in the UK

The earliest identifiable forerunner of the modern GP was the apothecary – known to have been practising in the sixteenth century. In 1858, with the establishment of the Medical Register, apothecaries were listed separately from physicians and surgeons, allowing members of these distinct professions to be identified by the public.

The origins of the British general practitioners' *registered list* can be traced to the development in the nineteenth century of the system of 'Club Doctors'. Friendly Societies were cooperatives ('clubs') formed by groups of working men, who employed doctors on a salaried basis to look after their members. In 1911, the state took over the medical functions of the Friendly Societies, the National Health Insurance Act provided general practice care for all manual workers and those non-manual workers with low incomes who were able to register on a doctors' *panel* (Jarman, 1988). After the First World War, a visionary report by Lord Dawson set out for the first time the concept of primary care teams working from a central unit, or health centre (Ministry of Health, 1920).

The next landmark in the development of primary care in the UK was the enactment of the National Health Services Act in 1948. This extended the provision of the 'panel system' to all the population. However, by 1965 government funding of primary care had dropped to such a considerable extent that many doctors felt the system was starting to fail. In 1966 radical improvements in the system of remuneration of general practitioners were introduced in a negotiated settlement that became known as the 'Family Doctors' Charter'. The next decade or so was marked by the increasing attachment of nursing staff to general practice and a number of other minor alterations. The next major change to UK general practice came in 1990, when the government imposed a new contract for GPs, which was neither negotiated nor agreed with the profession. This contract not only included a number of new controls over the activities of GPs, but also widened the services expected of GPs to include certain 'health promotion and illness prevention' services. Between 1990 and 1995, the number of nurses employed as general practice nurses has risen considerably, to the point where virtually every practice employs one or more such nurses.

Elements of 'Primary Health Care'

First-level care

Put at its simplest, primary care has been contrasted with secondary (specialist) care in the following WHO definitions, published in the early 1970s (Hogarth, 1975):

Primary care:
. . . frontline medical care; as a rule not limited to patients in specific age groups; the field of practice where the patient usually makes his first contact with the physician and has direct access to him or her.

Secondary care:
. . . care requiring attention of a special nature, usually more sophisticated and complicated than could be handled by the general practitioner.

These simple definitions emphasize the fact that primary care is the *first level* of care, but do not explain in any detail the underlying philosophy of primary care.

General Practice

Over the last few decades, both in the UK and in many other parts of Europe, primary care has developed around those services historically provided by the general practitioner. In 1977, a number of medical academic bodies from Europe collaborated to produce a definition of the work of the general practitioner (Box 1.3.1), which was subsequently adopted in its entirety as a policy of the UK Royal College of General Practitioners (RCGP, 1977). This statement was presented at a conference at Leeuwenhorst, and has since usually been referred to as the 'Leeuwenhorst definition'. (The definition is quoted here verbatim, *he* should be taken to include *she*.)

A useful revision of the Leeuwenhorst definition may be found in the report of a Welsh working group (Welsh Council RCGP and Welsh GMSC, 1994). This definition emphasizes the importance of the 'core team' in the delivery of services.

Implicit in the use of the phrase 'general practitioner' is the notion of the doctor having a *generalist function*. Pellegrino (1978) describes this function succinctly as follows:

> The generalist function . . . subsumes intellectual and practical components that culminate in the process whereby a patient's condition is evaluated, his or her needs identified and placed in some priority, and a plan of management developed efficiently and optimally to satisfy the identified needs. The generalist is differentiated from the specialist by the types of clinical situations with which he or she is confronted. The generalist deals with patients in three categories: (1) those who have not yet been classified into some organ- or technique-oriented specialty, (2) patients in whom, having been so categorized, new signs and symptoms develop that may or may not be related to the previous category, (3) patients with problems simultaneously in more than one organ system.

Unfortunately, the role of the generalist is still misunderstood by many – both within and outside medicine. McWhinney points out (1989) that any organization (including health care organizations) must have generalists and specialists to remain viable. In organizational terms, generalists have special functions in relating to all

Box 1.3.1. The Leeuwenhorst definition

The general practitioner is a licensed medical graduate who gives personal, primary and continuing care to individuals, families and a practice population, irrespective of age, sex and illness. It is the synthesis of these functions which is unique. He will attend his patients in his consulting room and in their homes and sometimes in a clinic or a hospital. His aim is to make early diagnosis. He will include and integrate physical, psychological and social factors in his considerations about health and illness. This will be expressed in the care of his patients. He will make an initial decision about every problem which is presented to him as a doctor. He will undertake the continuing management of his patients with chronic, recurrent or terminal illness. Prolonged contact means that he can use repeated opportunities to gather information at a pace appropriate to each patient, and build up a relationship of trust which he can use professionally. He will practise in co-operation with other colleagues, medical and non-medical. He will know how and when to intervene, through treatment, prevention and education, to promote the health of his patients and their families. He will recognise that he also has a professional responsibility to the community.

parts of the organization. They operate as communication centres, and identify problems that can be presented to specialists for solution.

In medicine, generalists become knowledgeable about a wide range of conditions that do not reach specialists. General practice is *not* a summation of the whole range of specialist practice – rather it has special features and attributes of its own, and complements specialist practice. The knowledge of a specialist relates to the detail of those diseases experienced by a *small proportion* of patients with medical or surgical conditions within his or her specialty. The general practitioner's expertise relates to the breadth of experiences gained from dealing with the vast majority of patients presenting in primary care with conditions that never reach secondary care. The same is true of general practice nursing. The knowledge, skills and attitudes required in general practice are different from those required of specialists.

Indeed, health professionals in general practice are sometimes called upon to provide initial assessments of problems that may not have an underlying medical cause at all. Undifferentiated malaise may have roots in social or spiritual distress. Yet the GP or general practice nurse must maintain a respect for the determinants of health in his or her dealings with patients.

Family Practice

Although the European model of primary medical care has tended to emphasize the importance of first contact ('primary' care) and of generalism ('general' practice), American and Canadian practice emphasizes the *family* context of care. In North America it is not uncommon for paediatricians, gynaecologists and some other specialists to offer direct access care to patients, i.e. they are providing primary, first contact *specialist* care. The term 'generalist' is not acceptable in North America as it apparently has a pejorative connotation. Hence the terms 'family practice' or 'family health care' are commonly used to distinguish primary generalist services from those of specialists (Rakel, 1990; McWhinney, 1989; Sawa, 1992). The American Academy of Family Practice offers the following definition:

> Family Practice is the medical specialty which provides continuing and comprehensive health care for the individual and the family. It is the specialty in breadth which integrates the biological, clinical and behavioural sciences. The scope of family practice encompasses all ages. Family practice is the continuing and current expression of the historical medical practitioner and is uniquely defined within the family context.

The importance of the family context of care, and the need for family physicians to take this context into account when making assessments and management plans has been emphasized by a number of researchers and commentators (Huygen, 1990; Rakel, 1990). Therefore family practitioners value family diagnosis and family management plans, and may organize their notes and charts to allow the family perspective to be taken into account in clinical management.

Despite the research evidence that a 'family diagnosis' can aid management, UK general practitioners have been somewhat reticent to coordinate records and systems around family structures. There are important considerations of confidentiality in the dealings with individual members of families (both ethical and legal) that may militate against taking a 'family' perspective when managing the problems of adults or older children.

Primary Health Care

One of the most important and seminal documents in developing thinking about primary health care over the last few decades has been the 'Alma-Ata declaration'

Box 1.3.2. Articles V, VI, and VII from the Alma-Ata declaration

V   Governments have a responsibility for the health of their people which can be fulfilled only by the provision of adequate health and social measures. A main social target of governments, international organizations, and the whole world community in the coming decades should be the attainment of all peoples of the world by the year 2000 of a level of health that will permit them to lead a socially and economically productive life. Primary health care is the key to attaining this target as part of development in the spirit of social justice.

VI   Primary health care is essential health care based on practical, scientifically sound, and socially acceptable methods and technology made universally accessible to individuals and families in the community through their full participation and at a cost that the community and country can afford to maintain at every stage of their development in the spirit of self-reliance and self-determination. It forms an integral part both of the country's health system, of which it is the central function and main focus, and of the overall social and economic development of the community. It is the first level of contact of individuals, the family, and community with the national health system bringing health care as close as possible to where people live and work, and constitutes the first element of a continuing health care process.

VII   Primary health care:

1.   reflects and evolves from the economic conditions and socio-cultural and political characteristics of the country and its communities and is based on the application of the relevant results of social, biomedical, and health-service research and public-health experience;

2.   addresses the main health problems in the community, providing promotive, preventive, curative, and rehabilitative services accordingly;

3.   includes at least: education concerning prevailing health problems and the methods of preventing and controlling them; promotion of food supply and proper nutrition; an adequate supply of safe water and basic sanitation; maternal and child health care, including family planning; immunization against the major infectious diseases; prevention and control of locally endemic diseases and injuries; and provision of essential drugs;

4.   involves, in addition to the health sector, all related sectors and aspects of national and community development, in particular agriculture, animal husbandry, food industry, education, housing, public works, communications, and other sectors; and demands the co-ordinated efforts of all those sectors;

Box 1.3.2. (contd.)

> 5. requires and promotes maximum community and individual self-reliance and participation in the planning, organization, operation, and control of primary health care, making fullest use of local, national and other available resources; and to this end develops through appropriate education the ability of communities to participate;
>
> 6. should be sustained by integrated, functional, and mutually supportive referral systems, leading to the progressive improvement of comprehensive health care for all, and giving priority to those most in need;
>
> 7. relies, at local and referral levels, on health workers, including physicians, nurses, midwives, auxiliaries, and community workers as applicable, as well as traditional practitioners as needed, suitably trained socially and technically to work as a health team and to respond to the expressed health needs of the community.

(Box 1.3.2) (WHO, 1978) which deals with the overall framework in which primary care practitioners should work.

The declaration takes its name from an international conference held under the auspices of the World Health Organization (WHO) in 1978 at the town of Alma-Ata in Kazakh SSR. This conference was preceded by a large number of national and regional meetings sponsored by the WHO. The main conference was attended by governmental delegations from no less than 134 member states together with representatives from 67 United Nations organizations. The immediate outcome of the conference was a declaration setting out, in ten numbered paragraphs, the key concepts of a universal health care system based on primary health care. The first paragraph sets out the importance of health as a fundamental human right. Every paragraph deserves special study and carries an important message. Paragraph V introduces the concept of 'Health for All'. Paragraph VI is a succinct definition of primary health care, whilst paragraph VII describes in detail the essential components of such care. Other paragraphs emphasize the need for governments to be committed to developing infrastructures for primary health care.

Since the Alma-Ata declaration, the definition of 'primary health care' used in the declaration has been adopted by many commentators. However, it will be obvious that the concept is extremely broad and much broader than the customary usage in the UK. One should perhaps reserve the usage of the term 'primary health care' to the overarching concept, and utilize the term 'general practice' or 'family practice' to refer to the generalist medical services provided. Some authors have used the term 'primary *medical* care' to refer to the services provided by doctors, nurses, health visitors and other staff of the health care professions. In the UK, the term 'primary health care team' has taken on a meaning of its own, and in effect refers to the core services provided by medical and nursing staff, ignoring the wider ideas proposed in the WHO definition.

A Primary Health Care Team is an interdependent group of general medical practitioners and secretaries and/or receptionists, health visitors, district nurses and midwives who share a common purpose and responsibility, each member clearly understanding his or her own function and those of the other team members, so that they all pool skills and knowledge to provide an effective primary health care service (Standing Medical Advisory Committee (SMAC), 1981)

Hasler (1994) argues for the continued development of the 'primary health care team', emphasizing the increasing role of the practice manager as a key component of the post-1990 team, and also emphasizing the concept of team-working and cooperation in team work which is implicit in the final sentence of the SMAC definition of the primary health care team. The definition quoted here also ignores the role of the general practice nurse who has become a key member of the team since this definition was set out in the 'Harding report' (Standing Medical Advisory Committee, 1981).

International
Perspectives

Since the Alma-Ata declaration, primary care systems in many countries have progressed and often changed dramatically (Fry and Hasler, 1986; Fry and Bouchier-Hayes, 1993). Perhaps the most notable recent developments have occurred in some of the developed countries. In the USA, the uncontrollable increases in the cost of the health care system and the increasing inequity of provision has led the Clinton administration to undertake a major review of health care. A fundamental feature of the review has been a re-examination of the place of primary health care (PHC), and proposals for a re-orientation of health care provision towards PHC, with an anticipated reduction in overall health care costs and improved equity of health care provision.

The place of primary health care in Europe varies from one country to another (Evans, 1993), but recently the EC has recommended a uniform system of basic postgraduate training for all general practitioners throughout the EC. In some countries (e.g. in Spain and Portugal) this has meant that a number of general practitioners will need to be retrained in accordance with modern principles of general practice. The Scandinavian countries and Holland have systems of primary health care based on general practice that are very similar to the UK model. However, in some European countries – in particular Finland – the public health aspects of primary health care have been emphasized for a number of years (Kekki, 1986), with the provision of a range of proactive services. Another interesting feature of the Finnish health care system has been an agreement at national level to apply all growth moneys to PHC developments, rather than to specialist medical services.

Recent political upheavals in Eastern Europe have been accompanied by a simultaneous upheaval in the provision of primary health care. Under the previous regime, most countries in the Eastern bloc had a system of primary health care based on the 'polyclinic'. Virtually all doctors were specialists, and indeed were trained in a single specialty from a very early stage of medical undergraduate training. The system was inefficient and provided poor quality of first-contact care. The importance of the generalist has been rediscovered, and many doctors in Eastern Europe are being retrained as generalists. Many medical schools (e.g. in Estonia) have reoriented their curricula so that medial students follow a broadly based curriculum, and can later undertake higher training for general practice.

Primary health care in the developing world has tended to concentrate on preventive measures, and on community programmes. The involvement of whole communities in health projects has often had significant impact (Streefland and Chabot, 1990). Such initiatives have often had a sense of urgency that many commentators would like to see in those preventive programmes in the developed countries which have set out to address the 'lifestyle' diseases of the West.

One feature of primary health care that does vary from country to country is the existence of the 'gatekeeper role'. In many countries (the UK and some other countries with socialized medical care systems) it is not possible for patients to consult specialists directly, except in clearly defined emergency situations. The general practitioner has to refer the patient for specialist care and can exert some control over specialist referral, acting as a 'gatekeeper'. The practitioner can ensure that the most appropriate specialist is chosen and can coordinate specialist care to the benefit of the patient. Furthermore, this system has considerable benefits in containment of health care costs.

Key Philosophies of PHC

Although different aspects of primary health care are emphasized in the various health care delivery systems around the world, there are nevertheless a number of features that emerge as key components or underlying philosophies.

Valuing Self-Care

It is an obvious but neglected truism that self-care is the largest part of the whole health care system (Williamson and Danaher, 1978). Self-care is universally practised; individual self-care practices vary widely and are deeply rooted in the culture of all societies (Helman, 1990). Studies in the UK have shown that around four-fifths of the population self-medicate within any two-week period (Dunnell and Cartwright, 1972). Elliott-Binns (1973, 1986), a Northampton general practitioner, found that 96% of his patients had taken some advice about their problem prior to consulting him – from a relative, a friend, or from a reference source such as a self-care manual. Practitioners in primary care need to accept the importance of self-care (Smail, 1983), and give appropriate advice to ensure appropriate self-care in the future, and to enhance 'help-seeking behaviour' (Stott and Davis, 1979).

Personal Care

The personal nature of primary care is one of its undoubted strengths. Not only do many professional organizations recognize this, but patient surveys show that the nature of the professional relationship between patient and primary care professional (doctor or nurse) is of considerable importance. The relationship provides a basis not just for treatment of patients, but *care of people*.

Primary, First-Contact Care

The point has already been made in an earlier section of this chapter that primary care is the first point of contact of patients with the caring professions. It is important to recognize that primary care professionals have to make an initial decision on any problem that is presented, if the patient *believes* that the problem is one that legitimately may be presented to that professional – in other words if they are ill, or believe themselves to be ill. Both Stott and Davis (1979) and Helman (1990) emphasize the importance of 'help-seeking behaviour' in determining the work of a primary care professional.

Continuing Care

In the UK, registration of patients according to the 'list' system emphasizes the continuing nature of the contract between doctor and patient. Ritchie *et al.* (1981) reported that 19% of patients had been registered with their GP for 10–20 years, and as many as 42% for 20 years or more. Continuing care has much to commend it: the practitioner can build up a long-term professional relationship with the patient, and use prior knowledge of the patient in making assessments and formulating management plans. In the UK, patients consult their doctor on average five times per year, although the rates vary with age. The highest rates are for small children (average seven times a year for children 0–4 years) and the elderly (six times a year for those over 65). Women consult more than men overall; in the 16–44 age group the average consultation rate for men is three consultations per year, whilst for women it is five per year (OPCS, 1993). An average household of four people (two adults, two children) will therefore consult their doctor around 20 times per year. Given that the average consultation time is reported to be 8 minutes (GMSC, 1992) this represents some 160 minutes of face-to-face consultations between members of a typical family and the doctor per year – ample opportunity to provide planned continuity of care.

Integration and Coordination of Care

Generalists are at the centre of the health care system and therefore have a major role in integrating and coordinating care provided to patients and their families. They must be aware of the strengths and weaknesses of the health care system and be able to utilize this knowledge in ensuring the patient has appropriate care. The practitioner may act as a source of information and advice about other forms of health provision. However, in referring patients to other practitioners, the primary care practitioner has an ethical duty (and in some cases a legal duty) to ensure that the care provided by the other practitioner is appropriate. For example, if the general practitioner is aware that the patient no longer has confidence in the care provided by a secondary care practitioner, he or she should intervene to remedy the difficulty, or to refer the patient to another specialist.

Consultation Based Care

The consultation is often seen as the major focus of primary care practice. The value of the consultation in building relationships with patients, in providing the key element in diagnosis and in management of patients has been emphasized by many and been the subject of wide research (Balint, 1964; Pendleton et al., 1984; Neighbour, 1987). One of Balint's special contributions was to emphasize the role that the doctor himself or herself can play in a therapeutic sense: the doctor can be considered as a therapeutic tool which can be just as important as a drug or a surgical procedure. Interpersonal skills of a high order are required of primary care practitioners, combining the qualities of compassion, empathy and personalized concern.

Population Based Care

The Leeuwenhorst definition mentions the general practitioner's obligation to care for the practice population. Over the past decade, this concept has been developed further. Tudor Hart (1988) has proposed that there should be 'a new kind of doctor', who will develop a role in caring for the health of the community. Some practitioners find that there are nevertheless some conflicts in day-to-day practice between adopting a community perspective of care on the one hand and responding to the expressed needs of individual patients on the other.

Team Based Care

For many years, since the earliest experiments of attachment of nurses and health visitors to general practice, and indeed since the Dawson report (Ministry of Health) of 1920, the importance of team care in primary care has long been accepted. However, continual arguments rage about who should be considered as being within the team, and how the team should be managed or led. Many commentators emphasize the need for a team to have common objectives in order to call itself a team. Some emphasize the need for a common geographical base, and regular contact between staff members in the team. If one accepts that the PHC team consists of doctors, nurses (practice and district nurses, health visitors), midwives, practice manager and secretaries/receptionists, it may then be useful to consider other linked services as part of the *Primary Health Care Network* (e.g. social services, pharmacists, dentists, opticians, professions supplementary to medicine, and perhaps some of the voluntary organizations).

Prevention and Anticipatory Care

The WHO has pointed out that primary health care is one of the key factors in achieving the *European Targets for Health for All* (WHO, 1985). Primary health care is in a unique position to integrate preventive and curative care, and to apply the principles of health promotion on a one-to-one basis (Smail, 1992). However, there is nevertheless a limit to what can be achieved in PHC. Governmental action through the development of healthy public policy and community action is required to support PHC initiatives. For example, government food policy should work in tandem with national objectives to improve the national diet, fiscal measures and subsidies can be used to drive the production and marketing of healthier food. Primary care teams will have an uphill struggle in advising on healthier diets if such a diet is inevitably more expensive than an unhealthy diet.

Trends in UK General Practice

Changes in administration

Full discussion of the terms of service of general practitioners and the method of payment is beyond the scope of this chapter, but details may be found in a number of publications (e.g. Chisholm, 1990). Suffice it to say that the principle of the doctor's contract is that he or she is responsible for rendering 'to his patients all necessary and appropriate personal medical services of the type usually provided by general medical practitioners'. The terms of service then describe in some detail the types of service to be provided. Doctors also hold certain responsibilities for the acts and omissions of the staff employed by them within the practice. Although nursing staff are personally accountable for their professional practice, an employer (whether a health authority or a general practitioner) also carries certain legal responsibilities for the acts of employed staff, particularly in relation to civil liability.

GPs are self-employed; their remuneration for the services they provide is made up of a range of individual payments for specific activities described within the contract. The total payments made to doctors in the UK are calculated to achieve a 'target net remuneration' worked out from year to year by the doctors' review body, plus various allowances for certain (but not all) expenses. Each year, the payments made to doctors for the various services provided are set at a rate to ensure an *average* overall payment to the GPs in the UK of the target net remuneration. The payments that are made to GPs include sums payable for each patient registered on the doctor's list, plus various payments for 'items of service', each of which has to be claimed individually. Over the years, the government has varied the weighting of the different payments in order to encourage the provision of certain types of service; however, payments for new services (such as health promotion) have, in general, not been funded by new money, simply by a redistribution of funding. Hence, for example, payments made for 'health promotion' were funded by reductions in payments under other headings.

The new contract for general practitioners imposed by the government in 1990 introduced a number of new features. Some new management controls over general practitioners were introduced, and some of the principles of the Family Doctors' Charter were overturned. For example, cash limits were introduced for the direct reimbursement of GPs' staff. Two key features were to make more specific the services that GPs were expected to provide, and secondly to improve the flow of information to family health services authorities. In addition, the 1990 contract stipulates that GPs must provide health promotion and disease prevention advice. Such services were originally to be based on health promotion 'clinics' and general practitioners had an obligation to send for patients who had not been seen in the previous three years for a regular check-up. Although the new services were introduced as a result of political pressure, this was against a background of considerable international effort to evaluate such preventive services and concentrate on those of proven effectiveness (US Preventive Services Task Force, 1989).

Health Promotion

Many commentators had doubts about the merit of the original proposals for health promotion services which were expected under the 1990 contract (Smail, 1990). The contract did not appear to be based on research evidence. Furthermore, many of the key concepts developed by the WHO to underpin health promotion programmes in primary care were noticeably lacking in the proposals. Both *Targets for Health for All* (WHO, 1985) and the *Ottawa Charter for Health Promotion* (WHO, 1987) set out a number of such concepts and in particular emphasize community participation and inter-sectoral collaboration to achieve 'Health for All'.

The system of 'health promotion clinics' rapidly fell into disrepute. Not only were many of the recommended procedures untested and unevaluated, but some of the screening tests recommended (for example a requirement to carry out routine urinalysis on healthy people) had been shown to be valueless. In 1993, the contract was yet again amended, to allow practices to develop health promotion programmes to suit their own circumstances, and the needs of the population. Three 'bands' were introduced, to reward practices with additional income for achieving targets in health promotion and disease prevention activity at three levels of increasing activity. Practices are expected not only to collect information on lifestyle practices and health risks of the registered population, but also to carry out intervention programmes, working with other agencies in the area.

Fundholding

Another concept introduced at the same time as the 1990 contract was that of 'fundholding' for GPs. The concept is that practices who choose to do so are provided with a notional 'fund' to purchase secondary care for the patients registered with them, up to certain limits. General practitioners thus become 'purchasers' or 'commissioners' of care for their patients. The advantages claimed for the system are that GPs as purchasers can 'drive hard bargains' for the benefit of their patients, and improve the quality of secondary care provision. Critics suggest, however, that fundholding introduces an ethical dilemma for GPs who are now expected to take decisions about how overall resources are to be managed within a cash limit whilst at the same time acting as the advocate for the patient for whom he or she should be seeking optimal care. Critics also point to evidence of a two-tier service to the benefit of the patients of fundholders, and the detriment of others. Nevertheless, by April 1993, 1.2 thousand practices in the UK were fundholding, covering 25% of the population (OCPS, 1994). At the time of writing, the government is anticipating that the majority of the population will soon be served by fundholding GPs. General practitioners will then hold key responsibility for commissioning non-urgent health care provision for the community.

Information Systems

Over the past decade, computer systems have increasingly been introduced into general practice in the UK. Well over 80% of practices now use computers that hold patient data of varying complexity. The new contract of 1990 required practices to provide routine health data on the aggregated population of the practice. Increasingly, practice computers are being used to provide such population data, and in many practices are also providing data about health needs which can assist the primary care team to manage its day-to-day work and prioritize services. Future developments in information systems are likely to occur rapidly, as GPs become linked via computers to hospitals, and perhaps more importantly to information resources which can assist in clinical decision-making.

CONCLUSION

Concepts of primary health care implicit in the Alma-Ata declaration emphasize the breadth of the activity which can be considered as contributing to the achievement of 'Health for All'. The WHO itself regards the development of PHC as one of the key elements in achieving 'Health for All', but the systems of community medical care in different countries vary, and the scope for inter-professional cooperation also varies. In the UK, general practice has tended to be the key component of primary health care, although within the last few decades there is a perceptible change. The primary health care team is now accepted as a crucial element in the delivery of community based medical care, and the services offered have developed. Perhaps the next challenge is to seek to strengthen relationships between the PHC team and the other health networks within the community so that the vision of PHC embodied within the Alma-Ata declaration can be achieved.

SUMMARY

- Landmarks have been considered in the historic development of general practice in the UK, beginning with the register of apothecaries in the mid nineteenth century and ending with more recent influences such as fundholding and information technology.
- The concepts of generalist, family care, first contact and gatekeeping have been explored and, where appropriate, compared with aspects of primary care in Europe and America.
- Common features of primary health care have been identified and discussed in relation to change and development in the NHS, with special reference to the Alma-Ata declaration.

DISCUSSION QUESTIONS

- ◆ Discuss the impact that the different elements of the primary health care system can have on the health of the community.

- ◆ What is the evidence that routine consultations in PHC can have an impact on health behaviour of individuals?

- ◆ What part do complementary practitioners play in the primary health care system?

- ◆ How might fundholding for general practitioners influence the future development of primary care services?

- ◆ How might the application of information technology affect the use of records within the primary care team?

FURTHER READING

Fry J and Hasler JC (Eds.) (1986) *Primary Health Care 2000*. Edinburgh: Churchill Livingstone.
Provides an international perspective of the development of the concepts of PHC in countries around the world.

Hart CR and Burke P (1992) *Screening and Surveillance in General Practice*. London: Churchill Livingstone.
A multi-author book which examines the current state of preventive care and health promotion in UK general practice.

Hicks D (1976) *Primary Health Care: A review*. London: HMSO.
An extremely thorough review of UK general prac-

tice in the 1970s. The author has included in his review practically every published paper of importance which refers to UK PHC up to the date of publication. Massive bibliography.

McWhinney I.R. (1984) *A Textbook of Family Medicine*. New York: Oxford University Press.

Rakel RE (Ed) (1990) *Textbook of Family Medicine*, 4th Edn. Philadelphia: WB Saunders.
Two of the key textbooks from North America explaining the scientific basis of family practice. McWhinney is Canadian; Rakel is professor at Houston, Texas. His is a large multi-author textbook of family practice.

REFERENCES

Balint M (1964) *The Doctor, his Patient and the Illness*, 2nd Edn. London: Pitman Medical.

Chisholm J (1990) *Making Sense of the New Contract*. Oxford: Radcliffe Medical Press.

Dunnell K and Cartwright A (1972) *Medicine Takers, Prescribers and Hoarders*. London: Routledge & Kegan Paul.

Elliott-Binns CP (1973) An analysis of lay medicine. *Journal of the Royal College of General Practitioners* **23:** 255.

Elliott-Binns CP (1986) An analysis of lay medicine – fifteen years later. *Journal of the Royal College of General Practitioners* **36:** 542.

Evans PR (1993) General practice in Europe. In J Fry and T Bouchier-Hayes (Eds) *The Medical Annual 1993/4*. Nailsea: David Kingham.

Fry J and Bouchier-Hayes T (Eds) (1993) *The Medical Annual 1993/4*. Nailsea: David Kingham.

Fry J and Hasler JC (Eds) (1986) *Primary Health Care 2000*. Edinburgh: Churchill Livingstone.

General Medical Services Committee *Your Choices for the Future. A Survey of GP Opinion. UK Report*. London: Electoral Reform Ballot Services, 1992.

General Medical Services Committee (1994) *Core medical services and the classification of general practitioner activity. A discussion paper*. (mimeo) London: General Medical Services Committee, BMA House.

Hasler JC (1994) *The Primary Health Care Team*. London: Royal Society of Medicine Press.

Helman CG (1990) *Culture, Health and Illness*, 2nd Edn. London: John Wright and Sons.

Hogarth J (1975) *Glossary of Health Care Terminology*. Copenhagen: WHO Regional Office for Europe.

Huygen FJA. (1990) *Family Medicine – the Medical Life History of Families*. London: Royal College of General Practitioners.

Jarman B (1988) *Student Reviews – Primary Care*. Oxford: Heinemann Professional Publishing.

Kekki P (1986) National perspectives – Finland. In JC Hasler J Fry and (Eds) *Primary Health Care 2000*. Edinburgh: Churchill Livingstone.

McWhinney IR (1989) *A Textbook of Family Medicine*. New York: Oxford University Press.

Ministry of Health (1920) *Interim Report on the future provision of medical and allied services: by the Consultative Council on Medial and Allied Services*. (Dawson Committee) (Cmd 693). London: HMSO.

Neighbour R (1987) *The Inner Consultation*. Lancaster: MTP Press.

OPCS (1993) *General Household Survey, No. 22, 1991*. London: HMSO.

OPCS (1994) *Social Trends 24*. London: HMSO.

Pellegrino E (1978) The academic viability of family medicine. *Journal of the American Medical Association* **240:** 132.

Pendleton D, Schofield T, Tate P and Havelock P (1984) *The Consultation – an approach to Learning and Teaching*. Oxford: Oxford University Press.

Rakel RE (1990) *Textbook of Family Medicine*, 4th Edn. Philadelphia: WB Saunders.

Ritchie J, Jacoby A and Bone M (1981) *Access to Primary Health Care*. London: King's Fund.

Royal College of General Practitioners (1977) The work of the general practitioner: Statement by a working party of the Second European Conference on the Teaching of General Practice. *Journal of the Royal College of General Practitioners* Feb., 117.

Sawa JS (1992) *Family Health Care*. California: Sage Publications.

Smail SA (1983) Patient Education in General Practice. In JAM Gray and GH Fowler (Eds) *Preventive Medicine in General Practice*. Oxford: Oxford University Press.

Smail SA (1990) Health Promotion and the new GP Contract (Editorial). *Practice Nurse* 391.

Smail SA (1992) Health Promotion in General Practice. In P Burke and CR Hart *Screening and Surveillance in General Practice*. London: Churchill Livingstone.

Standing Medical Advisory Committee (1981) *The Primary Health Care Team: report of a Joint Working Group (Harding report)*. London, Dept of Health.

Stott NCH and Davis RH (1979) The exceptional potential in each primary care consultation. *Journal of the Royal College of General Practitioners* **21:** 201.

Streefland P and Chabot J (Eds) (1990) *Implementing Primary Health Care - Experiences since Alma-Ata*. Amsterdam: Royal Tropical Institute.

Tudor Hart J (1988) *A New Kind of Doctor*. London: Merlin Press.

US Preventive Services Taskforce (1989) *Guide to Clinical Preventive Services; an Assessment of the Effectiveness of 169 Interventions*. Williams and Wilkins, Baltimore.

WHO (1978) *Alma-Ata 1978: Primary Health Care*. Geneva: World Health Organization.

WHO (1985) *Targets for Health For All*. Copenhagen: WHO Regional Office for Europe.

WHO (1987) Ottawa Charter for Health Promotion. *Health Promotion* **1**(4):183.

Welsh Council of the Royal College of General Practitioners and the Welsh General Medical Services Committee (1994) Patient Care and the General Practitioner. *British Medical Journal.* **309:** 1144–1147.

Williamson JD and Danaher K (1978) *Self-Care in Health*. London: Croom Helm.

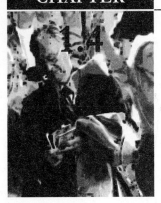

EPIDEMIOLOGY I: CORONARY HEART DISEASE

Michael L. Burr

Michael L. Burr

KEY ISSUES

- Coronary heart disease (CHD) provides a good example of the influence of epidemiology on the practice of community health.

- Research studies show the importance and feasibility of prevention.

- Community health workers are particularly well placed to promote preventive measures in the general population

KEY TERMS

Risk factor. A factor that is associated with an increased risk of a particular disease; for example, smoking, high blood pressure and high serum cholesterol are risk factors for coronary heart disease.

Case–control study. A comparison between people who have a certain disease and people without that disease, looking for associations (positive or negative) between the disease and factors which may cause or prevent it.

Cohort study. A follow-up study of a group of people about whom information is obtained at the start, in order to see what aspects of their initial condition predict their subsequent experience.

INTRODUCTION

There can be few people in Britain today who do not have a relative or friend suffering from CHD. There is therefore great public interest in the topic. During recent decades it has become evident that the disease is to an appreciable extent preventable, but its prevention requires changes in people's lifestyles which to some extent depend upon themselves. Community nurses have an important part to play in providing the public with the information which it increasingly demands.

This chapter will summarize the evidence with which health professionals should be familiar so that they can make the best use of their opportunities. Nurses who work in the community should be aware of the real impact they can have on reducing the amount of death and suffering caused by this disease.

Epidemiology

Death rates

CHD is the commonest single cause of death for both men and women in Britain and many Western countries. During the past two decades the death rate in Britain has gradually declined, but the disease is still the major cause of premature death.

Important geographical variations occur. CHD death rates are higher in northern and eastern Europe than in Mediterranean countries. To a lesser extent there are differences within countries also. Thus in Britain the rates are higher in Scotland and northern England than in the south and east. There is a clear gradient in relationship to social class, the death rates being lowest in the upper socioeconomic groups and highest in the lowest groups. To some extent this can be explained by differences in risk factors such as smoking, but there may be more complex factors which have not been fully accounted for. Certain ethnic groups are at particularly high risk, notably those from the Indian subcontinent; people of Afro-Caribbean stock have somewhat lower death rates than the general population.

Survey Data

Much more precise information about the risks of CHD in different people can be obtained by means of surveys. The most useful type of survey is the prospective cohort study. This involves collecting information about possible determinants of CHD (such as diet, smoking habit, blood cholesterol level, and blood pressure) from large numbers of healthy people, who are then followed up for several years. It eventually becomes possible to see to what extent the original characteristics of the subjects predict their risk of death or disease. For example, a large number of British doctors completed a questionnaire about their smoking habits in 1951 and have been followed up since, so that their risk of death from various causes can be related to their smoking history (Doll *et al.*, 1994a). Such studies have shown the substantial effect of cigarette smoking in increasing the risk of death from heart disease. Other studies have shown the risk associated with raised blood pressure and serum cholesterol levels.

This kind of information can be obtained more quickly by means of case-control studies, in which people with CHD are compared with healthy people in respect of their past history of various potential risk factors. The main weakness of this approach is that it may be difficult to ensure that the history really relates to the period before the onset of the disease; people with early symptoms may modify their lifestyle, and if they are questioned at a later stage their answers may not truly reflect their previous habits.

Randomized Trials

The effect of changing a risk factor can be studied by means of randomized trials. Trials designed to prevent (rather than treat) disease include studies of dietary intervention, control of blood pressure, and anti-smoking advice. The difficulty about such studies is they have to be very large and compliance is liable to be imperfect. The absence of a positive finding may be attributable to insufficient numbers or poor compliance rather than ineffectiveness of the intervention. Nevertheless important information has arisen from randomized trials showing the effects on CHD mortality of reducing blood pressure, blood cholesterol and smoking, particularly in people whose risk is already high.

The drug treatment of acute myocardial infarction (MI) has been revolutionized by the results of several randomized trials, which have shown the value of early administration of thrombolytic therapy and aspirin. The implications of these findings will be further considered below.

Prevention

General considerations

Acute myocardial infarction carries a high mortality – about 40% die before they can receive medical treatment (Colling *et al.*, 1976). It is therefore important to consider how the disease can be prevented, and this is where the community approach becomes essential. To some extent the risk factors are under the control of the individuals concerned, so that good health education is called for. Community nurses and other health professionals are well placed to influence members of the general public, and they should ensure that they are adequately informed about the relevant evidence and keep themselves up to date.

Childhood and adolescence are formative periods in relation to lifestyle factors such as diet, smoking and exercise. The school nurse is in a unique position to reduce the risk of disease in later life. It is much easier not to acquire the habit of smoking than to give it up after becoming 'hooked' on it. Health professionals should also remember the importance of example – we cannot expect our advice to carry much weight if we do not follow it ourselves.

Prevention may be better than cure, but in some ways it is less straightforward for the health professional. If a man suffers from angina, he may reasonably expect his doctor to give him the best available treatment. If a woman has a heart attack, she has the right to the best hospital treatment. But people who feel perfectly well do not necessarily want to be told to change their eating habits or take tablets for their blood pressure, so as to prevent an illness which may never happen anyway. The onus is on the health professional to show why such actions are advisable and to be sure that they are likely to do more good than harm.

Even if we are agreed on the advisability of a preventive measure, it is not necessarily clear as to how it should be carried out in practice. There are several ways in which it can be applied to the general population. Firstly, we can carry out a *systematic screening* programme. This entails inviting people in suitable age groups to attend clinics where various tests are carried out, such as height, weight, blood pressure, serum cholesterol and urine analysis. Those with adverse risk factors are then given appropriate advice and treatment. This approach is being taken by practice nurses in general practices which have computerized age–sex registers; people of various age groups are given appointments at 'well person clinics' and followed up as necessary. Another type of opportunity is provided by the occupational health service of a large organization, where the nurse can invite the workforce to be tested in this way.

Secondly, *opportunistic screening* can be carried out on middle-aged and older people who attend their doctors' surgeries for any reason. Patients can be referred to the practice nurse for the tests to be performed. Since most people have occasion to visit their general practitioners at some time, this approach ensures that most of the population at risk is screened in a particularly inexpensive way.

Thirdly, a *high-risk strategy* can be employed. This involves targeting those individuals or groups who are already known to be at higher risk of CHD. Such people include patients already known to have hypertension or diabetes, those with a family history of heart disease, and possibly certain ethnic groups. Practices with computerized records can readily identify such people and invite them to visit the doctor or practice nurse for this purpose. The advent of genetic screening may make possible the identification of people at particularly high risk amongst those with a family history.

Fourthly, a *population strategy* addresses the subject in broad public health terms. Here the objective is not to deal with selected individuals but rather to alter the population norms. Thus we may endeavour to reduce the overall consumption of saturated fat, or to encourage people to walk rather than ride, or to promote a non-smoking policy in public places. All community nurses should be aware of their opportunities to influence the public health.

These various approaches will be considered in relation to various risk factors and interventions.

Smoking

All health professionals and particularly those who work in the community should be well informed about the effects of smoking and be acquainted with some of the relevant studies. The classic study by Doll and Hill on 34 439 British male doctors, recently updated, is perhaps the best, in view of its exceptionally long follow-up period of 40 years (Doll *et al.*, 1994a). This study shows the effects of cigarette smoking on a wide range of diseases. The CHD death rate of heavy smokers (25 or more cigarettes daily) was about twice that of non-smokers; although the proportional effect was small in comparison with that for lung cancer, the much larger number of CHD deaths means that smoking causes far more CHD deaths than lung cancer deaths.

There have been fewer prospective studies of CHD in women. One example is the Walnut Creek Contraceptive Drug Study of 16 759 women in America. Among the factors considered, cigarette smoking was overwhelmingly the most important risk factor for vascular disease, and seemed to act synergistically with oral contraceptive use in increasing the risk of subarachnoid haemorrhage, haemorrhagic strokes and MI. The authors concluded that smoking should be considered a contraindication to oral contraception, or, at very least, women wishing to use oral contraceptives should be strongly urged to stop smoking (Petitti *et al.*, 1979).

Giving up smoking is well worthwhile, even in people who have smoked for many years. The risk of CHD attributable to smoking decreases rapidly after smoking cessation, and after several years it approaches that of people who have never smoked. MI patients who stop smoking have a lower risk of death and reinfarction than those who continue to smoke (Burr *et al.*, 1992). This fact can be used as a powerful incentive in motivating MI patients not to resume smoking after their involuntary cessation on entering the coronary care unit. There is no need for them to be fatalistic about their risk of further MIs, which they are particularly well placed to reduce.

During recent years it has become increasingly clear that exposure to other people's tobacco smoke, or 'passive smoking', carries a measurably increased risk of CHD. It is estimated that the risk of death due to heart disease is increased by about 30% among those exposed to environmental tobacco smoke at home (Taylor *et al.*, 1992). Passive smoking at work could be more dangerous in this regard owing to the high concentrations that may occur. This is obviously an area in which community health workers, particularly nurses working in industry and large organizations, can be influential in affecting policy.

Blood Pressure

The relationship between blood pressure and risk of CHD is well documented. People with clinical hypertension are at very high risk of CHD, but it has been increasingly realized that the relationship extends across the whole range of blood pressure in the population, i.e. there does not seem to a threshold at which the risk begins to appear. An overview of the evidence suggests that a prolonged difference of 5 mmHg in diastolic blood pressure is associated with 21% less CHD, and a difference of 10 mmHg is associated with 37% less CHD (MacMahon *et al.*, 1990).

What has been unclear is whether the treatment of blood pressure reduces the risk of CHD to a corresponding degree. A review of randomized trials of hypotensive therapy suggested that a reduction of 5–6 mmHg produces a 14% reduction in CHD mortality within five years, and a much greater reduction in stroke (Collins *et al.*,

1990). In view of the side effects of antihypertensive drugs it is difficult to specify a threshold above which blood pressure should be treated, but there is no doubt that it can be beneficial. The detection of raised blood pressure is probably best carried out by opportunistic screening of people who attend doctors' surgeries and see practice or district nurses for any reason.

Salt intake may also be relevant to blood pressure control. It has been estimated that a moderate reduction in dietary salt (of about 3 g daily) would reduce the incidence of CHD in Western countries by 16% – more than could be achieved by fully implementing the recommended policy of treating high blood pressure by drugs – and that a further effect would be obtained by reducing the amount of salt added to processed foods (Law *et al.*, 1991).

Blood Cholesterol and Fat Intake

It has long been known that the risk of CHD morbidity and mortality is related to the serum cholesterol level, which is partly determined by the intake of saturated fat. Several randomized trials have investigated the effects of reducing serum cholesterol levels (by dietary changes or drug treatment) on CHD incidence and mortality. Some of these trials have been hampered by poor compliance, but in general there seems little doubt that a reduction in serum cholesterol produces a lower death rate from CHD. The evidence has recently been reviewed by Law *et al.* (1994), who conclude that a 10% reduction in serum cholesterol (achievable by moderate dietary change) would reduce the risk of CHD by 50% at age 40 years and by 20% at 70 years, and that this benefit takes place within five years. They advocate a population approach, involving health education, food labelling, and new policies on food subsidies, rather than screening programmes, since many CHD deaths occur in people whose cholesterol levels are not particularly high and there is no threshold below which cholesterol reduction is of no value.

Fish

CHD is rare in populations (such as Japanese and Eskimos) who eat a lot of fish. This observation led to investigations into the likely component of fish that is protective; certain long-chain fatty acids characteristic of oily fish were identified as having antithrombotic actions. The relationship between fish intake and subsequent MI was then examined in cohorts of people in populations with a lower average intake, so that those who eat fish could be compared with those who do not. Several studies of this kind have shown that people who eat fish regularly have a lower risk of CHD than those who eat no fish (e.g. Kromhout *et al.*, 1985). A randomized controlled trial of men who had recently recovered from MI showed a 29% reduction in two-year mortality in those who were advised to eat moderate amounts (300 g weekly) of fatty fish (Burr *et al.*, 1989).

It therefore seems reasonable to encourage people – particularly those at high risk of CHD – to eat fatty fish such as herring, mackerel, salmon, pilchard and trout. The same protective effect can probably be obtained by taking fish oil capsules, but most people will feel that a fish meal is more enjoyable.

Fruit, Vegetables and Antioxidants

Heart disease mortality tends to be lower in countries with a high intake of fruit and vegetables and high mean plasma levels of vitamins C and E. A study in Italian women showed that MI patients tended to have eaten less fruit and vegetables than women admitted to hospital for other reasons (Gramenzi, 1990); cohort studies have shown negative relationships between CHD incidence and vitamin E (Rimm *et al.*, 1993), and between CHD mortality and certain dietary antioxidants (flavonoids) present in tea, onions, and apples (Hertog *et al.*, 1993).

The antioxidants (including vitamins C and E and β carotene) in fruit and vegetables may confer some protection against CHD, perhaps by acting as scavengers of oxygen-derived free radicals which seem to be implicated in atherogenesis. This protection could explain the low CHD death rates of vegetarians in comparison with other people.

Some confirmation of this protective effect is supplied by intervention studies. Two randomized trials have shown that a diet rich in fruit and vegetables reduced mortality in patients who had recently recovered from MI (Singh *et al.*, 1992; de Lorgeril *et al.*, 1994). In each case the increases in fruit and vegetables formed part of a 'package' which included other dietary changes, so the effects cannot be ascribed to one element of the diet with any certainty. But together with evidence of other health benefits, these studies suggest that the eating of fruit and vegetables should be encouraged in the general population.

Alcohol

Alcohol has a paradoxical relationship with CHD. On the one hand, it constitutes an obvious danger to health, particularly when taken in excess, and even in moderate amounts it can adversely affect body weight, serum triglyceride concentrations, and blood pressure. On the other hand, there is a substantial body of evidence to show that a moderate intake confers protection against CHD, in that moderate drinkers have a lower incidence and mortality rates from the disease than total abstainers. The relationship between alcohol intake and all-cause mortality is U-shaped, particularly in men – i.e. moderate drinkers have a lower mortality than total abstainers and heavy drinkers. This relationship still exists if ex-drinkers are excluded, so it cannot be explained by the presence of unhealthy ex-drinkers among the abstainers. It has been shown in numerous studies and the evidence is remarkably consistent; the most recent is the 40-year follow-up of British doctors by Doll *et al.* (1994b).

It is obviously desirable to know what is the optimum intake of alcohol. In middle-aged men, one or two drinks on average daily confer the greatest overall benefit; above three drinks a day, progressively greater levels of consumption are associated with progressively higher all-cause mortality. It does not seem to matter in what form the alcohol is taken.

Health workers accustomed to emphasizing the dangers of alcohol may find it difficult to know how to view these findings in public health terms. Anything that encourages excessive drinking is to be deprecated. But there seems little doubt that moderate drinking confers protection against CHD which is not offset by other hazards to health, and this effect is particularly important in middle-aged men whose risk of CHD is high.

Exercise

Several cohort studies (e.g. Morris *et al.*, 1980) have shown that people who take regular exercise are less likely to acquire CHD than those who do not. It is of course difficult to be sure that this represents a truly causal relationship; people who take exercise differ from those who do not in a wide variety of ways and may be more healthy for other reasons. But the weight of evidence suggests that exercise really does confer some protection. Some experimental confirmation of this protection was obtained in a randomized controlled trial which showed a favourable effect of exercise on the progression of coronary lesions as shown by angiography (Schuler *et al.*, 1992).

Other Factors

Gender is an obvious risk factor in that men have higher incidence and mortality rates than women. It is, however, misleading to regard CHD as a disease of men, since it is also the leading cause of death among women in developed countries, although its onset is delayed by 10–20 years in comparison with men. The incidence rises abruptly at the menopause and becomes equal with that in men after the age of 60 years. Oestrogen replacement therapy seems to confer some protection in post-menopausal women; the reduction in risk may have been overestimated. Modern low-dose oral contraceptives do not affect the risk of CHD in healthy non-smoking women (Brezinka and Padmos, 1994).

Social and psychological factors seem to play a part in CHD, although it is difficult to separate them from the other major risk factors. The effect of low social class is even greater in women than in men; tension, anxiety and other adverse emotions seem to increase the risk (Brezinka and Padmos, 1994).

Obesity has long been recognized as conferring an extra risk of CHD. To some extent this is dependent on its association with other risk factors such as blood pressure and serum cholesterol. But there is a distinct risk attached to 'central obesity' (i.e. that form of obesity characterized by a high waist : hip ratio) in both men (Donahue *et al.*, 1987) and women (Bengtsson *et al.*, 1993). Community nurses should be aware of this risk so that dietary advice can be targeted to those who will benefit most by weight reduction.

Management of Myocardial Infarction

Cardiopulmonary Resuscitation

The period of greatest risk of death from MI is the time immediately after it begins. In one epidemiological survey, 43% of MI patients died rapidly, before receiving medical treatment (Colling *et al.*, 1976). A high proportion of these deaths are presumably attributable to cardiac arrest. No amount of improvement in hospital treatment can reduce mortality during this critical period. One approach is the training of ambulance staff in cardiopulmonary resuscitation (CPR) so that it can be applied in the patient's home or wherever the MI occurs. The use of defibrillators by mobile teams has led to the saving of many lives in this way.

There are, however, inevitable delays in contacting the ambulance service and in its journey to the patient. During this interval some lives will be lost and other patients will suffer irreversible brain damage unless some form of CPR can be provided by people who are already at hand. There is good evidence that ordinary members of the public can administer effective CPR without the use of any equipment. This possibility obviously requires large-scale public education on the use of simple CPR. Community programmes of CPR training have been put into effect in various American and European cities. The results of several such studies show that victims of cardiac arrest are more likely to survive if they receive CPR from a bystander than if they do not (Cummins *et al.*, 1991).

This is an area in which community health workers such as health visitors and occupational nurses can play an important part. They can encourage various groups of people to undergo mass training; such groups can include workers in large firms, clubs, societies, and churches. Particular attention should be paid to the lower social classes, in which MI most often occurs.

In view of the fact that most MI deaths occur before admission to hospital, the potential benefits of community CPR are likely to exceed those of further advances in hospital management.

Hospital Treatment

Recent advances in treatment with thrombolysis and aspirin have produced notable reductions in the case fatality of MI patients who are admitted to hospital.

Although this form of treatment is not in the realm of community health, it is relevant to it in that cases need to be recognized and referred rapidly to hospital in order for the treatment to be most effective. One byproduct of community CPR training is that it raises the general level of awareness of the signs and symptoms of acute MI, leading to quicker notification of ambulance services and earlier hospital treatment.

Rehabilitation

Rehabilitation after MI needs to be tailored to the individual patient's requirements. Health workers in the community are in a good position to assess the patient's needs for detailed explanation and advice regarding his or her lifestyle. Although the rehabilitation programme may be conducted initially by the hospital team, nurses who work in the primary care sector can give more detailed and specific help in the light of the patient's progress and their knowledge of the particular circumstances. They can ensure that there is a sound transfer of care from hospital, and that patients with particular problems (e.g. depression) are detected and counselled appropriately.

Referral to Hospital

Referral of patients for revascularization procedures (coronary artery bypass grafting and angioplasty) is obviously dependent in part on the attitude and activities of various community health workers. There is some geographical variation in the rates of referral for no very obvious reason, and female patients seem to be less likely to receive coronary artery surgery than males. It is important that patients with chronic CHD should be made aware of interventions that could prolong their lives or reduce their symptoms. Community nurses are in a good position to discuss these possibilities with patients so that they can make informed decisions about whether to seek further treatment.

CONCLUSION

Community nurses are well placed to help to reduce the mortality and morbidity of CHD in the population. They need to keep themselves up-to-date on the current state of evidence, and should always be ready to explain relevant issues to patients and members of the public. They are likely to have a particularly important impact in the areas of prevention and health education.

SUMMARY

■ CHD is the major cause of death and disability in men and women in most developed countries. All community nurses should be aware of the impact they could make on its mortality and morbidity.

■ All health professionals should be well informed about the evidence relating smoking to CHD risk and should be able to explain why smoking is inadvisable. School nurses can play a particularly important part here.

■ Practice nurses, district nurses and occupational nurses should take the opportunity to measure the blood pressure of members of the public so as to detect those in whom it may need treatment.

■ Health education and other public health measures should be employed to encourage the general public to eat a healthy diet and take more exercise. Health visitors and other community nurses should regard health promotion as an important part of their work.

■ CPR training should be promoted in all sections of the public; community nurses should participate in setting up and maintaining this approach.

■ Community nurses should be ready to counsel individual patients according to their needs, particularly in relation to post-infarct rehabilitation and possible referral for revascularization.

DISCUSSION QUESTIONS

◆ How would you reply to a young man who said 'My grandfather smoked like a chimney and lived to be 83'?

◆ Should we positively encourage middle-aged men to take one or two alcoholic drinks every day if they do not already do so?

◆ People in the lower socioeconomic groups are less likely than others to come forward for training in community CPR. Yet it is this group which has the highest incidence of MI. How would you recruit them for a local training programme?

◆ How could the general population be encouraged to eat a more healthy diet?

FURTHER READING

Jacobson B, Smith A and Whitehead M (Eds) (1991) *The Nation's Health: a Strategy for the 1990s. Revised edition*. London: King Edwards Hospital Fund for London.
This book contains a chapter on circulatory diseases, which summarizes the evidence on the risk factors for CHD. It presents a strategy for improving circulatory health; other chapters deal with lifestyles for health and preventive services. It is a very readable text with excellent illustrations.

Rose G (1992) *The Strategy of Preventive Medicine*. Oxford: Oxford Medical Publications.
This book explains why the prevention of many diseases requires change in the behaviour of the general population rather than attention only to those who are at particularly high risk. These issues are presented mainly with reference to CHD, about which the author was an acknowledged epidemiological expert.

REFERENCES

Bengtsson C, Björkelund C, Lapidus L and Lissner L (1993) Associations of serum lipid concentrations and obesity with mortality in women: 20 year follow up of participants in prospective population study in Gothenburg, Sweden. *British Medical Journal* **307:** 1385-1388.

Brezinka V and Padmos I (1994) Coronary heart disease risk factors in women. *European Heart Journal* **15:** 1571-1584.

Burr ML, Fehily AM, Gilbert JF *et al.* (1989) Effects of changes in fat, fish, and fibre intakes on death and myocardial reinfarction: diet and reinfarction trial (DART). *Lancet* **ii:**757-761.

Burr ML, Holliday RM, Fehily AM and Whitehead PJ (1992) Haematological prognostic indices after myocardial infarc-tion: evidence from the diet and reinfarction trial (DART). *European Heart Journal* **13:** 166-170.

Colling A, Dellipiani AW, Donaldson RJ and MacCormack P (1976) Teesside coronary survey: an epidemiological study of acute attacks of myocardial infarction. *British Medical Journal* **2:** 1169-1172.

Collins R, Peto R, MacMahon S *et al.* (1990) Blood pressure, stroke, and coronary heart disease. *Lancet* **335:** 827-838.

Cummins RO, Ornato JP, Thies WH and Pepe PE (1991) Improving survival from sudden cardiac arrest: the 'chain of survival' concept. *Circulation* **83:** 1832-1847.

de Lorgeril M, Renaud S, Mamelle N *et al.* (1994) Mediterranean alpha-linolenic acid-rich diet in secondary prevention of coronary heart disease. *Lancet* **343:** 1454-1459.

Doll R, Peto R, Wheatley K, Gray R and Sutherland I (1994a) Mortality in relation to smoking: 40 years' observations on male British doctors. *British Medical Journal* **309:** 901-911.

Doll R, Peto R, Hall E, Wheatley K and Gray R (1994b) Mortality in relation to consumption of alcohol: 13 years' observations on male British doctors. *British Medical Journal* **309:** 911-918.

Donahue RP, Abbott RD, Bloom E, Reed DM and Yano K. (1987) Central obesity and coronary heart disease in men. *Lancet* **i:** 821-824.

Gramenzi A, Gentile A, Fasoli M, Negri E, Parazzini F and La Vecchia C (1990) Association between certain foods and risk of acute myocardial infarction in women. *British Medical Journal* **300:** 771-773.

Hertog MGL, Feskens EJM, Hollman PCH, Katan MB and Kromhout D (1993) Dietary antioxidant flavonoids and risk of coronary heart disease: the Zutphen Elderly Study. *Lancet* **342:** 1007-1011.

Kromhout D, Bosschieter EB and Coulander C de L (1985) The inverse relation between fish consumption and 20-year mortality from coronary heart disease. *New England Journal of Medicine* **312:** 1205-1209.

Law MR, Frost CD and Wald NJ (1991) Analysis of data from trials of salt reduction. *British Medical Journal* **302:** 819-824.

Law MR, Wald NJ and Thompson SG (1994) By how much and how quickly does reduction in serum cholesterol concen-tration lower risk of ischaemic heart disease? *British Medical Journal* **308:** 367-373.

MacMahon S, Peto R, Cutler J *et al.* (1990) Blood pressure, stroke and coronary heart disease. Part 1, prolonged differences in blood pressure: prospective observational studies corrected for the regression dilution bias. *Lancet* **335:** 765-774.

Morris JN, Everitt MG, Pollard R and Chave SPW (1980) Vigorous exercise in leisure-time: protection against coronary heart disease. *Lancet* **ii:** 1207-1210.

Petitti DB, Wingerd J, Pellegrin F and Ramcharan S (1979) Risk of vascular disease in women. Smoking, oral contraceptives, noncontraceptive estrogens, and other factors. *Journal of the American Medical Association* **242:** 1150-1154.

Rimm EB, Stampfer MJ, Ascherio A, Giovannucci E, Colditz GA and Willett WC (1993) Vitamin E consumption and the risk of coronary heart disease in men. *New England Journal of Medicine* **328:** 1450-1456.

Schuler G, Hambrecht R, Schlierf G *et al.* (1992) Regular physical exercise and low-fat diet. Effects on progression of coronary artery disease. *Circulation* **86:** 1-11.

Singh RB, Rastogi S, Verma R *et al.* (1992) Randomized controlled trial of cardioprotective diet in patients with recent acute myocardial infarction: results of one year follow up. *British Medical Journal* **304:** 1015-1019.

Taylor AE, Johnson DC and Kazemi H (1992) Environmental tobacco smoke and cardiovascular disease. A position paper from the Council on cardiopulmonary and critical care, American Heart Association. *Circulation* **86:** 699-702.

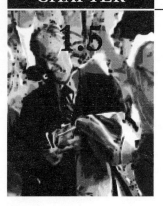

EPIDEMIOLOGY II: CARE OF OLDER PEOPLE IN COMMUNITY HEALTH

Dee Jones

KEY ISSUES

- Demographic changes
- Health of older people
- Medication
- Contact with primary care team
- Contact with health and social services
- Housing
- Informal care system

KEY TERMS

Impairment. Any loss or abnormality of psychological, physiological or anatomical structure or function.

Disability. Any restriction or lack of ability resulting from an impairment to perform an activity in a manner or within the range considered normal for a human being.

Handicap. Any disadvantage for a given individual resulting from an impairment or disability that limits or prevents the fulfilment of a role that is normal for that individual.

Informal carers. Those relatives, friends or neighbours who provide regular support and assistance to an older person who is unable to carry out all activities of daily living unaided.

Older people. Those who are beyond usual retirement age – 60 for women and 65 for men.

Epidemiology of Ageing

Demography

The numbers of older people aged 60/65 years and over have been growing in this country, and indeed throughout the world, in absolute and proportional terms and this trend will continue well into the next century. Since the turn of the last century we have, in Britain, moved from a situation in which 6% of the population was aged 60/65 years or over to one where in 1991 the proportion was 18% (OPCS, 1991). In absolute terms the numbers, during this period, rose from 2.2 million to 10.5 million, an increase of almost 400%. During the same period, however, the proportion of those aged less than 16 years fell from 35% to 20% of the total population.

It is often erroneously assumed that the dramatic increase in the population of older people is a consequence of reduced mortality rates and longer life expectancy, that is people living longer. But it is the level of fertility (the number of children born) and their early mortality rates which, in general, dictates the age profile of a population. Improved survival in the upper age groups can also have a significant effect on the population profile. The term 'elderly population' covers a range of some 40 years and in recent times the age profile of this group has changed significantly and will continue so to do well into the next century. The number of people in the younger age band (60–74) has levelled off but the rate of increase of the older age group (75 plus) has increased dramatically. In particular, the number of people aged 85 years or more has shown, and will continue to show, a very marked increase – from 8% of the elderly population to 13% by the end of the century (OPCS, 1991). Another feature of demographic change in this age group has been the increase of the proportion of women to men: in 1981 the proportion of women to men aged 85 or over was 3.26 (OPCS, 1991).

The most significant feature of the age profile over the next three decades will therefore be the increase in the numbers of those aged over 85 years. This factor has caused great concern and anxiety to policy-makers and government departments who perceive it not as a challenge but a burden. Since disability and ill-health increases with age, particularly among the over 75 year old age group, older people use more health and social services than do younger people. Also a higher proportion of over 75 year olds are cared for in residential or nursing homes. Hence, the changes in the population structure have enormous implications for the planning and organization of the health and social care systems.

Health Status

At all ages most people report their health as being good or fairly good. However a higher proportion of older people report their health as being not good, with 27% of men and 33% of women aged 85 years and over reporting their health as not good. Ill health can be caused by acute, long-term or chronic health problems. Rate of long-standing or chronic conditions which restrict levels of normal activity increase with age and are higher among women of all ages. Sixty-two per cent of those aged 75 years and over reported a long-standing illness, in particular musculoskeletal problems and hearing and vision difficulties show a marked increase with age (Jones and Cranton, 1993). In addition to an increase in prevalence of long-standing illness with age, there is also an increase in the number of chronic health problems experienced, with women experiencing, on average, a greater number of problems. Although this trend with age exists, that is not to say that all older people are ill and disabled, almost half of those aged 75 years and over report no such problems. However, long-standing, limiting disability is not equally distributed among the social classes; those from professional classes are less likely (37%) to experience long-standing illness than those in the semi-skilled or unskilled occupational groups (47%) (Victor and Evandrou, 1986).

Functional Capacity

Health professionals are increasingly adopting a functional approach to health of older people, that is the ability to perform key activities of daily living and dependency or the need for assistance. Evidence indicates that, contrary to common stereotypes, the majority of older people are able to undertake most self-care and house-care activities unaided. Those activities with which they most frequently require assistance are: shopping (24%), cutting toenails (19%) and heavy housework (17%). Such measures or assessments do not indicate the nature of chronic illness but rather indicate the impact of ill health upon ability to maintain independence and therefore may enable professionals to assess needs for services. Difficulty with personal care indicates a higher level of dependency.

Three of the more significant issues with implications for community nursing services, are incontinence, psychological health and health related behaviour and each will be considered separately.

Incontinence

Incontinence, though a common problem, has until recently, received very little attention from health professionals. Eighteen per cent of older people report being incontinent to varying degrees – 9% of men and 24% of women – and 8% report being frequently incontinent of urine (at least daily), again more women than men (Jones *et al.*, 1981; Jones, 1994). Incontinence can markedly affect the quality of life of older people and also their carers. Incontinent people tend to have poorer health profiles, are more depressed and more often report feelings of loneliness. In spite of this many sufferers have never discussed the problem with any health professional and have therefore not been assessed, treated or enabled to manage their problem optimally. Evidence would indicate that many could be cured of their incontinence and the remaining sufferers enabled to cope more effectively with their problem. Major benefits would result from raising awareness of incontinence among the general public as well as health and social care professionals and developing effective case-finding and management strategies (Jones, 1994).

Psychological Health

The principal mental disorders of later life are the dementias and affective disorders. As with physical impairments, cognitive impairment increases exponentially with age, doubling every five years (Jorm, 1990), and current evidence indicates that approximately 10% of older people living in the community have some degree of organic disorder (Bond and Carstairs, 1982; Milne, 1985). Approximately one in three of those aged 85 years and over have an identifiable organic disorder. Though the overall prevalence of dementia is the same in men and women, Alzheimer's disease is more common among women, independent of age. People living in nursing homes have a much higher prevalence, rates vary from 25% to 75% of all residents. This indicates the need to ensure that appropriately trained staff are available and that the environment is appropriately designed for their needs.

Affective disorders include anxiety, depression and mood disturbances and approximately a quarter of older people have an affective disorder, the prevalence being higher among men than women (Bond and Carstairs, 1982).

Owing to the increasing interest in dementia in elderly people the issue of depression among older people has been relatively neglected. Only a small proportion of sufferers tend to be identified and treated despite the fact that they are high users of health and social services, and even fewer are treated by hospital specialists despite the evidence that treatment has been shown to be effective among older people. Some of the symptoms of depression may be attributed erroneously to ageing and considered inevitable by health professionals and also sufferers themselves.

Despite popular stereotypes and the fact that older people have major losses to cope with (bereavement, loss of paid employment, ill health) elderly people do not have an excess of depressive disorders but they may have more depressive symptoms. The absence of a close supportive relationship has been found to be a risk factor for depression and older people living alone are especially at risk of depression (Henderson, 1992).

Depression is strongly associated with feelings of loneliness; approximately a quarter of older people report ever feeling lonely and only 7% often or always (Jones *et al.*, 1985). There is a trend of increasing prevalence of reported loneliness with age and more women than men report experiencing some degree of loneliness. Loneliness tends to be associated with widowhood, household composition (living alone) and disability (Jones *et al.*, 1985). Not surprisingly feelings of loneliness are high amongst those who have suffered a recent bereavement. A high proportion (over a quarter) of successful suicides are aged 65 years and over (OPCS, 1991).

Health Behaviours

Although a smaller proportion of people aged 60 years and over smoke than do younger adults, a significant minority (24% of men and 20% of women) continue to do so, male smokers averaging 100 cigarettes a week and women over 80 per week (DOH, 1992; Jones and Cranton, 1993). Despite the evidence that the health of older people can benefit from cessation of smoking and can be enabled within the primary care setting, to quit smoking, few such opportunities exist for them.

Fewer older people consume alcohol than younger adults and fewer drink to excess. Fewer than one in ten men and one in twenty women are exceeding the 'sensible drinking' levels.

Despite the evidence of benefit to older men and women, only a minority appear to be taking regular exercise and fewer women take exercise than men. Leisure facilities and exercise classes are mostly oriented towards younger people and the specific needs of older people are not often catered for.

Primary Care

The fact of a rapidly increasing number of frail elderly people with complex needs living in the community, presents an unprecedented challenge to health and social services in general and in particular to those involved in primary and community health care.

Since the late 1980s the central role of the primary care team in achieving the goals of the NHS, has been increasingly acknowledged. The new arrangements for supporting people in the community – particularly older people – has provided a new impetus to the further development of a comprehensive primary health care service.

Primary health care has traditionally been the first point of contact with health services for the whole population, including older people. It provides health care as close as possible to where people live and provides promotive, curative and rehabilitative services (NHS/ME, 1993). Indeed general practitioners have been considered and referred to as 'gatekeepers of health and social services' because of their assessing and referring function. The primary health care team members are therefore key players in the health and social care of older people living in the community and primary health care is most effective when it works collaboratively with other health and social care agencies.

In 1990 a new contract for GPs was introduced which substantially altered their existing terms of service (DOH, 1989). The new contract was more specific in its requirements and the fees and allowances were amended to reward performance and quality of service, reflecting the general philosophy of the NHS reforms (Secretaries of State, 1989). GPs were encouraged to become more accessible to their patients and to develop their services according to the 'needs of the consumer'. Two specific requirements of the new contract were that GPs should provide practice leaflets giving information on surgery times and services provided by the health centre, and offer annual health checks to patients aged 75 years and over.

Contact with GP

By far the majority (85%) of older people see their GP at least once a year and a third see their GP (either at home or in the surgery) in any one month. Those aged over 75 years see the GP more frequently and receive more home visits than those aged under 75 years (Jones *et al.*, in press). In recent years there has been an increase in the number of home visits made by GPs; this reflects the increased number of very elderly people and the small proportion of these living in residential nursing homes.

Nurses in Primary Care

Currently about 50 000 whole time equivalent (WTE) nurses are working in primary and community health care. Most of these are district nurses, practice nurses, health visitors, school nurses and community psychiatric nurses (NHS/ME, 1993) and for some, the lion's share of their workload is with older people. While there is an organizational line between practice nursing services and others, it is envisaged that general practice will, in the future, provide a full range of nursing services. More nurses will be based with GP fundholders or in commissioning groups of GPs, working closely in teams with other health professionals such as chiropodists, physiotherapists, occupational therapists, clinical psychologists, etc. A proportion of nurses involved in primary health care will be employed directly by GPs and others will be linked through contracts with provider units (and trusts) (NHS/ME, 1993).

There has been an increase in recent years of the number of practice nurses working in primary health care, though as yet, not all older people are aware of their role. Since the introduction of the NHS reforms and the new contract an increasing proportion of older people are consulting practice nurses – in 1992 it was reported that half of older people had consulted a practice nurse in a 12 month period, whereas before the introduction of the reforms it was a third (Jones *et al.*, in press). The most frequent reasons for practice nurse consultations include: blood pressure measurement, flu injections, blood tests, ear syringing and health checks. In the same study, half of the sample of older people, when asked, reported that in their practice they were able to consult the practice nurse directly. It seems, then, since the reforms that the role of practice nurse has expanded greatly. It is, however, interesting to note that older people did not report attending any health promotion clinics although these have developed in some areas. In some practices, practice nurses run well-women and well-men clinics, smoking clinics, exercise classes, etc. The role of the practice nurse is obviously still expanding but many clinics seem to be oriented towards younger people, reflecting the link with contractual requirements for health promotion activity directed towards those between the ages of 15 and 74 years. There is an opportunity, however, for the development of innovative health promotion clinics that potentially are of benefit to older people.

Changes in both demography and in clinical practice (20% of surgery is on a day case basis; length of hospital stay has significantly reduced) have led to changes in the role of community nurses. The new contract and the NHS and community care reforms have also added impetus to the development of these services. Community nurses have historically worked within the homes of older frail people and responded mostly to GP referrals. In recent years much of their previous routine work which required lower levels of skills (e.g. bathing, getting people out of bed and putting to bed) has been redefined as social care and is undertaken by home carers, enabling community nurses to undertake those activities which require various levels of clinical nursing skill and which cannot be 'substituted'.

Health Checks

The GP contract requires those aged 75 years and over to be offered an annual assessment and to include in that assessment: mobility and functioning, sensory function, physical health, mental health, social aspects and medication use. Instruments or strategies for carrying out this policy effectively were not provided. Current policies and practice therefore vary greatly between primary care teams; some practices send one letter with no follow-up to those failing to respond and other practices follow up all their patients (Brown *et al.*, 1992). Letters to patients vary considerably in tone, from encouraging invitations to formal notifications that do not encourage attendance (Chew *et al.*, 1993). Some GPs carry out the health checks themselves while in other practices the practice nurses or health visitors organize and carry out the health check strategy. In some practices, assessments are organized in special clinics and in others GPs assess or 'case find' opportunistically (Wells and Freer, 1988). Such varying levels of commitment to assessing older people reflects general practitioners' ambivalent views on the effectiveness and efficiency of such assessments. Many studies have been undertaken to evaluate such a policy (Vetter *et al.*, 1985; Pathy *et al.*, 1992) but the findings have, as yet, not been consistent. Some studies have reported benefits in mortality, quality of life and institutionalization (Tulloch and Moore, 1979; Vetter *et al.*, 1985; Pathy *et al.*, 1992). A large national study is currently being undertaken by the author and colleagues to evaluate different methods and models of assessing and treating older people in the community.

Medication

Multiple pathology, which is characteristic of old age, is often accompanied by polypharmacy; three-quarters of older people take one or more prescribed medications in any 24 hour period and, on average, they are on two drugs per person (Jones *et al.*, in press). Since the NHS reforms, the average number of drugs prescribed has risen and this may be a consequence of identifying (at health checks) new problems which are treatable (Jones *et al.*, 1994). As older people are more prone to side effects and iatrogenic disease, their medication requires careful monitoring. Many elderly people inevitably will have difficulty taking their multiple medications correctly and could benefit from written advice, information, training and other aids to compliance.

The changes and increasing focus on primary health care will enable primary health care nurses to develop their role in innovative areas using their unique skills most effectively: developing continence services, introducing effective models of assessment and screening, case management, health promotion, provision of advice and liaising with hospitals and community hospitals. There is increasing evidence of the health benefit to older people of smoking cessation, regular exercise, flu injections and treatment of hypertension, for example (Jones, 1996).

The public health aspects of primary health care will require collaboration, not only with users and carers, but with statutory, voluntary and private agencies in order to provide the most effective health and social care to older people.

Community Care

The role of informal carers For many years it has been the philosophy and policy of the health departments that older people should be enabled to live in the community rather than in institutions

(DOH, 1981), a policy which has recently been reinforced by the Community Care Act (Secretaries of State, 1990). This policy has implications not only for health and social services, voluntary organizations and the private sector but also for friends and relatives who provide support to frail older people. The lion's share of the care given to older people in the community is provided by friends and relatives, and the successful functioning of care in the community depends upon their continuing to provide that level of support (Jones, 1992; Jones and Peters, 1992). They play a crucial role in enabling people to remain in the community rather than be admitted to nursing or residential homes.

There have been significant changes in the nature of society which have implications for the informal care system. In the last twenty years the average number of children per family has reduced from 2.2 to 1.8, and the proportion of families having only one child has increased (OPCS, 1987). This, coupled with the rising divorce rate, has altered the nature of the traditional family considerably. Changes in employment patterns have also affected the family and hence the informal care system. Over the last four decades there has been a consistent increase in the proportion of working women, 66% of adult women of working age are currently in paid employment (CSO, 1992). Also for employment purposes a larger number of children move away from their parents. Together these sociodemographic changes have a significant impact on the availability and accessibility of informal carers.

Currently, the main source of informal care in the community is family, where there are elderly couples the spouses are the main source of support, but where elderly people are widowed, daughters are the main source of support. Friends and neighbours tend only to care for the less frail elderly people in the community. For most older people there is no extensive network of care. Rather, responsibility for caregiving tends to fall upon one person. Those carers who are totally unrelated to the recipient of care, or who are not resident, are more likely to be part of a larger network or team. Many carers are themselves not in good health and inevitably many of the carers who are spouses, and themselves elderly, will have disabilities; more than half of carers have health problems that make it difficult to care (Jones and Vetter, 1984). Nevertheless, evidence consistently demonstrates that families wish to care for their elderly relatives and to enable them to remain in the community for as long as possible. The view that families generally neglect their elderly relatives is a myth that is unsubstantiated.

Effects of Caring

Relatives report that many aspects of their life are detrimentally affected by their caring role, including: health, social life, family life and employment. Heavy nursing care is required by some care recipients, such as assisting up and down stairs, transferring in and out of bed, in and out of baths and chairs. Inevitably this has an impact on the health of carers: more than a quarter report negative effects on their health. A breakdown in the health of carers can often be a reason for seeking institutional care for their older relative.

A quarter of carers also report their social life being affected by their care giving; resident carers are more likely to be affected in this way than are non-resident carers. Regular involvement in social activities is difficult if carers are unable to leave the home, apart from short periods. A quarter of carers also report that the lack of privacy and personal freedom has detrimental effects upon their family life. For carers who are not partners, but sons or daughters, one of the main problems is that of conflict of responsibilities and conflict of interests. Daughters more often report negative effects on family life than do other carers (Jones, 1986). Sons and daughters are the carers most likely to report an effect on their paid employment, either leaving employment altogether or, more commonly, reducing their hours. Women, particularly daughters, are more likely to reduce their working hours as a consequence of their caregiving role (Jones, 1986).

Prolonged care for elderly people can cause emotional distress to many relatives; a fifth seem to report a moderate or unbearable amount of stress experienced as a consequence of their caring role. Daughters, particularly co-resident daughters, report more stress than others. The greater the frailty of the older person the greater the degree of stress experienced by these carers. Characteristics of recipients of care that tend to be associated with distress among carers include: incontinence, night disturbance, inability to communicate and dangerous behaviour. Of all the aspects of quality of life upon which caring has an impact it seems to be consistently demonstrated that detrimental effects on social and family life are most likely to lead to perceived stress and significant anxiety (Levin *et al.*, 1989; Gilleard *et al.*, 1984, Jones and Peters, 1992).

Support of Carers

Time apart from dependants seems to be one of the most important factors in the alleviation of carer stress, whether this respite is a consequence of the carer being able to leave home for paid employment or to participate in social and leisure activities. Studies have shown that carers who receive support and assistance from domiciliary services experience less stress than those who do not.

If families are to continue providing substantial support to the frail older population in order to maintain them in the community, they will need limited support from community services. Care in the community can enable frail older people to have a better quality of life, but this should not be at unreasonable cost to relatives. Regular and reliable respite or relief from their caring role is necessary to enable them to maintain fulfilling social and family lives and hence to continue to support older people in the community.

Contact with Services

Elderly people living in the community are cared for by a network of health and social services, voluntary organizations and the private sector. Chiropody is the service most often utilized by older people, apart from the general practitioner, and within any month 8% of older people have seen a chiropodist (but 22% within a three month period); 4% have seen a community nurse, less than 1% a health visitor, less than 1% a bath attendant and less than 1% have attended a day hospital (Jones, unpublished).

By far the most frequent contact with social services is with home helps (15%), who are in many ways the mainstay of community care. Other contact with social services includes meals on wheels (4%), social services (3%), day centre (3%) and lunch club (2%). Contact with health and social services is much more prevalent among those aged 75 years or older, for example contact with chiropody, home help and meals on wheels is at least twice as prevalent in the older age group, that is people aged 75 years or over.

When all the health and social services are combined, only a quarter (28%) of older people are assisted by one or more services each month, and only 10% receive more than one service (Jones, unpublished). In terms of packages of care, those aged 75 years or older are much more likely to be receiving two or more services a month. The nature of these packages varies greatly geographically, depending on the provision of services and their roles, in particular home helps. In some areas home helps are increasingly undertaking personal tasks that were previously the remit of community nurses. Similarly, authorities vary in their response to needs for provision of meals.

Opinions of Services

In general older people tend to be very grateful for any support or assistance required. Satisfaction surveys have repeatedly reported very high satisfaction levels, which perhaps indicates more the inadequacy of basic satisfaction studies than the needs and wishes of older people or how to improve services. Critical comments that can be operationalized have been documented, a significant minority of users report that the chiropody service (29%) is not provided as often as it is needed, and the same is so of the home help service (34%).

When older people's unmet needs are investigated they consistently report the need for cutting toenails, for regular baths and aids and adaptions. With ever increasing demands being made on community services and the changing structures, they have responded by targeting their services to those most in need (those who are very frail, living alone and without informal carers) and redefining their roles. This can leave gaps between and within services – as perceived by elderly people – whose priorities do not necessarily match those of service providers; and some roles can be shed without ensuring that another service provider is taking them on, for example cutting toenails, bathing and household care.

Care is needed when priorities are redefined so that new roles and practices are developed in collaboration with the other service providers. This may also require negotiation and transfer of budgets to follow changes in roles. Targeting services at the very frail may eventually be ineffective and inefficient, it may be more cost efficient to invest services in people with moderate disability who have carers – these people may thus be enabled to remain permanently in the community whereas the admission of the very frail without informal carers may only be postponed by a substantial input of community services.

Housing

For many years the association between health and housing has been acknowledged. According to *Florence Nightingale*, for example, 'the connection between health and the dwelling of population is one of the most important that exists'. More recently the centrality of suitable good quality housing to enable people to remain in their own home has been reiterated as a policy statement (Secretaries of State, 1990). There are many aspects of ill-health that have been associated over the years with poor housing (Box 1.5.1).

A disproportionate number of elderly people live in older, poor quality housing with fewer modern amenities. In particular, those in the lower social classes or with disabilities live in poor quality homes (Victor *et al.*, 1986). Many older people, on limited incomes, are unable to afford to modernize, adapt or maintain their homes. Others lack the information required to apply for relevant grants, thus older

Box 1.5.1. Ill health associated with poor housing

- Mortality
- Respiratory problems –
  infections, chronic bronchitis,
  asthma, pneumonia
- Cold/hypothermia
- Loneliness
- Heart disease/stroke
- Falls and fractures

- Depression
- Creation of dependency
- Accidents

people are more likely to live in homes that are damp, cold, contain mould and without central heating – all conditions which create ill health. Twelve per cent of deaths in this age group are cold related; a rate twice that of most Western societies. The median temperature of non-centrally heated bedrooms in the UK is 10°C below WHO recommendations (Welsh Office, 1993a). Increasingly, older people are being made aware of alarm systems, but as yet only a minority of older people have means of summoning help in an emergency, apart from telephones. There is therefore a need, particularly in some areas, to provide elderly owner-occupiers with specialist advice and support, such as that provided by Care and Repair and Staying Put projects, developed by voluntary organizations and supported by health and social services.

Housing is often seen as part of social care and hence not within the orbit of health care professionals, but there are health gains to be made in investing in higher quality more appropriate housing for older people: preventing ill health, preventing admission to hospital, preventing accidents, maintaining independence and enabling people to live in their own homes. There is a need to disseminate information to older people, their carers and health and social service professionals and to raise their awareness regarding the role of housing in health maintenance. It is also desirable to include a review of housing conditions and amenities in assessments (including health checks) and when necessary, to make appropriate referrals to statutory services and voluntary organizations.

CONCLUSION

The rapid increase in the number of 'old old' people living in the community and the recent changes in the structure of health and social services provides primary health care nurses with the opportunities to develop innovative and creative strategies to meet the health needs of this client group and their carers. Primary care nurses will need to further develop their alliances with health and social care professionals and to work in partnership with older people and their carers. Commissioners, users and carers will require high quality health care to be provided efficiently and effectively. These requirements will necessitate good information systems, and monitoring and evaluation strategies.

SUMMARY

- The most significant feature of the age profile of the population is the rapidly increasing number of those aged 85 years and over.
- The expected changes in demography will have significant implications for the planning and organization of the health and social care systems.
- Old age, for many, is characterized by multiple pathology and consequently polypharmacy.
- The prevalence of long-standing illness increases with age, as does the number of chronic health problems.
- Despite the evidence of the benefits, particularly for women, only a minority of older people participate in regular exercise; a lower proportion of women than men take exercise.
- Most older people are in contact with the primary health care team at least once a year.
- The lion's share of care provided in the community is provided by family members, and the maintenance of older people within the community depends upon their continuing to provide such support.

■ If families are to be enabled to provide support to frail older people they require appropriate support from health and social services.

■ Recently there have been substantial policy changes in health and social services which affect older people particularly.

■ Health and social services in the community need to be innovative, appropriate, and flexible in order to meet the needs of frail older people without creating dependency.

DISCUSSION QUESTIONS

♦ Consider how best to profile the health and social care needs of those over 75 years in a practice population. How does this compare with the methods currently used in your practice?

♦ What are the implications of maintaining frail elderly people in the community – for health and social services, for voluntary organizations and for relatives and friends?

♦ What are the main opportunities for health professionals to promote the health of older people?

♦ Is ageism apparent in policy or practice in health and social services?

♦ In what circumstances might it not be the better option for older people to remain in their own homes in the community? When are there likely to be conflicts of interests between carers and those for whom they care?

♦ To what degree is there equity and equality for older people in health and social services?

FURTHER READING

Epidemiology of ageing

Bond J, Coleman P and Peace S (1993) *Ageing in Society: an Introduction to Social Gerontology*. London: Sage.

This is a valuable textbook in social gerontology and is a set book for a new undergraduate level Open University course.

Grimley Evans J and Williams JF (1992) *Oxford Textbook of Geriatric Medicine*. Oxford: Oxford Medical Publications.

This textbook is a thorough overview of geriatric medicine with an international authorship and serves as an excellent reference on all medical aspects of old age medicine.

Kane R, Grimley Evans J and Macfayden C. (1990) *Improving the Health of Older People: A World View*. Oxford University Press.

This text examines the worldwide growth of elderly populations and its consequences for future care. It discusses the health of older people, specific diseases, health care and social policy from an international perspective.

Welsh Health Planning Forum (1994) *Health and Social Gain for Older People*. Welsh Office, Wales.

This document highlights health and social gain issues that are of particular relevance to older people and outlines the principles that should underpin future care of older people.

Primary Care

Wells N and Freer C (1988) *The Ageing Population: Burden or Challenge*. London: Macmillan.

Community Care

Levin E, Sinclair I and Gorbach P. (1989) *Families, Services and Confusion in Old Age*. Avebury.

Philipson C and Walker A. (1986) *Ageing and Social Policy: a Critical Assessment*. Gower.
The editors, with other social gerontologists and social policy analysts, have sought to examine the relationship between old age and social policy. They describe social structures and processes that create dependency and ageism.

Robinson R and Le Grand J. (1994) *Evaluating the NHS Reforms*. London: King's Fund Institute.
King's Fund funded several studies to examine the impact of the NHS reforms and this book covers such topics as older people, GP fundholding, primary care and audit.

Wilson G. *Community Care: Asking the Users*. London: Chapman & Hall (in press).
This book explores the notion of consumer opinion and examines methodological issues and presents findings of several studies which have examined user and carer opinions of services.

REFERENCES

Bond J and Carstairs V (1982) Services for the elderly: Scottish Health Service Studies No 42. Scottish Home and Health Department, Edinburgh.

Brown K, Williams EI and Groom L (1992) Health checks on patients 75 years and over in Nottinghamshire after the new GP contract. *British Medical Journal* **305:** 619-712.

Central Statistical Office (1986) *Social Trends*. London: HMSO.

Central Statistical Office (1992) *Social Trends 21*. London: HMSO.

Chew C, Glendenning C and Wilkin D (1993) GP assessments of patients aged 75 and over, GP/nurse survey. Centre for Primary Health Care Research, University of Manchester, Manchester.

Department of Health and Social Security (1981) *Growing Older*, Cmnd 8173 London: HMSO.

Department of Health (1989) *Terms of service for doctors in general practice*. London: HMSO.

Department of Health (1992) *The health of elderly people. An epidemiological overview*, Volume 1. London: HMSO.

Gilleard CJ, Bedford H, Gilleard E *et al.* (1984) Emotional distress amongst the supporters of the elderly mentally infirm. *British Journal of Psychiatry*, **145:** 172-177.

Henderson A. (1992) The epidemiology of mental disorders in elderly people. In: JG Evans and JF Williams (Eds) *Oxford Textbook of Geriatric Medicine*. Oxford: Oxford Medical Publications.

Jones D (1986) *A Survey of Carers of Elderly Dependents Living in the Community*. Report to the Department of Health, Cardiff.

Jones D (1990/91) Weaning elderly patients off psychotropic medication in general practice: a randomized controlled trial. *Health Trends* **22:** 164.

Jones D (1992) Problems of carers; the United Kingdom view. In JG Evans and JF Williams (Eds) *Oxford Textbook of Geriatric Medicine*. Oxford: Oxford Medical Publications.

Jones D (1994) Quality of life and service use in a random sample of elderly people with urinary incontinence living in the community. Paper presented at the Society for Social Medicine, 38th Annual Scientific Meeting, Leeds.

Jones D (1996) Health maintenance for frail elderly people. In: Detels R and Omenn G (Eds) *Oxford Textbook of Public Health*, 3rd edn. Oxford: Oxford Medical Publications.

Jones D and Cranton S (1993) Health and wellbeing of a random sample of older people. Research Team for the Care of Elderly People, Cardiff.

Jones D and Peters T (1992) Caring for elderly dependents - effects on the carers quality of life. *Age and Ageing* **21:** 421-428.

Jones D and Vetter NJ (1984) A survey of those who care for the elderly at home: their problems and their needs. *Social Science and Medicine* **19:** 511-514.

Jones D, Lester C and West R (1994) Monitoring changes in health services for older people. In R Robinson and J Le Grand (Eds) *Evaluating the NHS Reforms*. London: King's Fund Institute.

Jones D, Lester C and West R. Changes in primary health care as reported by a random sample of older people (in press).

Jorm AF (1990) *The Epidemiology of Alzheimer's Disease and Related Disorders*. London: Chapman and Hall.

Levin E, Sinclair I and Gorbach P (1989) *Families, Services and Confusion in Old Age*. Aldershot: Gomer.

Milne JS (1985) *Clinical Effects of Ageing*. London: Croom Helm.

NHS/ME (1993) *Nursing in Primary Health Care. New World New Opportunities*. Leeds: NHS.

Office of Population Censuses and Surveys (1987) *General Household Survey*. London: HMSO.

Office of Population Censuses and Surveys (1991) *National population projections, 1989 based series PP2 No. 17*. London: HMSO.

Pathy J, Bayer A, Harding K and Dibble A (1992) Randomized

trial of case-finding and surveillance of elderly people at home. *Lancet* **340:** 890–893.

Secretaries of State (1989) *Working for Patients*. London: HMSO.

Secretaries of State (1990) *Caring for People – Community Care in the next Decade and Beyond*. London: HMSO.

Sinclair I, (1988) Residential care for elderly people. In: I Sinclair (Ed) *Residential Care: the Research Reviewed* (Vol 2 of the Wagner Report). London: HMSO.

Tulloch AJ and Moore V (1979) Randomised controlled trial of geriatric screening and surveillance in general practice. *Journal of the Royal College of General Practitioners* **29:** 355–359.

Vetter NJ (1989) Why persuading the elderly to give up smoking is worthwhile. *Pulse* **49:** 76.

Vetter NJ, Jones DA and Victor CR (1985) Effect of health visitors working with elderly patients in general practice: a randomised controlled trial. *British Medical Journal* **288:** 369–372.

Victor CR and Evandrou M (1986) Social class and the elderly: analysis of the 1980 General Household Survey, Paper presented at the British Sociological Association Annual Conference, University of Loughborough, Loughborough.

Victor CR, Jones DA and Vetter NJ (1986) The housing of the disabled and non-disabled elderly in Wales. *Archives of Gerontology and Geriatrics* **3:** 109–113.

Wells N and Freer C (1988) *The Ageing Population Burden or Challenge*. London: The Macmillan Press.

Welsh Office, (1993a) *Protocol for Investment and Health Gain: Healthy environments*. Welsh Health Planning Forum, Cardiff.

Welsh Office, (1993b) *Health and Social Gain for Older People*. Welsh Health Planning Forum, Cardiff.

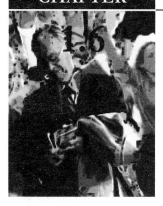
MENTAL HEALTH: POLICY AND PRACTICE

Judy Boxer and Gary McCulloch

KEY ISSUES

- Policy – a vehicle for change and diversity
- Policy – maintaining status quo
- Policy – implications which detract from the initial focus
- Policy – relating to primary care and practice
- Policy – influences on future practice

INTRODUCTION

This chapter seeks to examine critically recent changes in mental health policy and practice. These issues will be considered in relation to the opportunities and limitations for change outlined in government strategies such as England's *The Health of the Nation* (DOH, 1992). Other sections of the book also highlight the move from secondary to primary care and how that affects individuals across the spectrum of health and social care needs. Defining practice relates as much to individual skill and competence within a community setting, as it does to linking practice to current changes in policy. As this is an overview of current issues and practice, key aspects to be addressed are supported by current up-to-date references and essential reading.

Against a background of change in mental health service planning and provision, there is unsubstantiated evidence that the service is moving in the right direction. This chapter is therefore inevitably selective but considers the themes within both government policy and our perceptions of the diversity of service organization throughout the United Kingdom.

Mental Health in Context – Prevalence

Most people with mental illness are not treated in hospital. For every 1000 people, 230 attend their general practitioner each year with symptoms of mental illness, with only 21 of this number ever being referred to hospital. Over six times as many people see consultant psychiatrists as outpatients, as opposed to inpatients (*The Health of the Nation*, DOH, 1992) England. In terms of health service use, the UPA-8 (under privileged) score is frequently used as a simple predictor of need for inpatient psychiatric admissions in England. The relationship between sociodemographic characteristics and service use, including admission rate is well-established. The Jarman 8 under-privileged area score was developed to indicate workload in general practice (Jarman *et al.*, 1992). The score is derived from eight census variables including the percentages of unemployed people living in overcrowded households and one-parent families.

The prevalence of psychiatric morbidity appears to have increased (Lewis and Wilkinson, 1993). This may be due to unemployment, adverse life events and poor social support. This is a contentious area with research on the one hand which suggests that psychosocial factors are not significant in influencing the outcome in mental illness (Andrew *et al.*, 1993). On the other, there are numerous counter claims which suggest that socioeconomic inequality is the basic cause of persistent ill health (Carroll *et al.*, 1993).

In relation to the Health of the Nation target for mental illness and people from ethnic communities, the Department of Health has produced a guide for the NHS which raises three areas of concern (Balarajan and Raleigh, 1993) (Box 1.6.1).

This guide on mental illness suggests possible reasons for the higher incidence of psychiatric morbidity in these groups including economic deprivation, racism and discrimination, diagnostic accuracy and the way services are provided. It concludes with a series of questions which purchasers and providers of mental health services need to address. These include questions about how services respond to the particular needs of black and ethnic communities, liaison with voluntary agencies and equity health service provision.

Policies and Mental Health

Prior to the *Health of the Nation* document, three previous white papers have markedly influenced practice and the potential for modifying practice by secondary and primary care staff in the field of nursing and mental health.

Promoting Better Health (DOH, 1987)

This White Paper had as its focus primary health care services and emphasized prevention and preventative health care. It also aimed to introduce a new contract for general practitioners and dentists with annual targets, including health checks. These contracts were introduced in 1990.

Working for Patients (DOH, 1989b)

This White Paper was intended to alter radically the management of health care in the UK. It set out purchaser and provider functions and created a business culture in the NHS via trust hospital status and general practitioner fundholding.

Caring for People (DOH, 1989a)

This White Paper highlighted the need to integrate the health provision of social and health care. Its aims are broadly to promote home care, assess need and clarify the roles and responsibilities of agencies, as well as to provide value for money. The lead role for these initiatives is taken by local authorities, and is currently having a major effect on the health and social care for those experiencing mental health problems.

A review of the policy changes and their implementation is given by Butler (1993).

The culmination of the changes in policy and practice came together with the

Box 1.6.1. Areas of concern

1. The African-Caribbean population has high admission rates to psychiatric hospitals.
2. The diagnostic rates for schizophrenia are relatively high in African-Caribbeans, and are raised in the Asian population.
3. Suicide rates are relatively high among young Asian women.

NHS/Community Care Act (DOH, 1990) which is discussed in more detail in Chapter 5.1.

Another key document with the potential to influence mental health policy and practice is the Department of Health and Home Office Review of Health and Social Services for Mentally Disordered Offenders and Others requiring similar Services. This review is frequently referred to as the Reed Report (1992) which highlighted the need for the treatment and care of mentally disordered offenders. This report was partly in response to the significant numbers of the prison population with identifiable mental illness (Gunn *et al.*, 1991). The report and subsequent documents emphasized the need for inter-agency working, and for an increase in medium secure provision at local level. Nursing involvement in this area includes the increasing development of court diversion schemes as an aspect of implementing the Reed Report recommendations (Backer-Holst, 1994). In terms of current provision it is recommended that the role of mental health social workers and probation officers are included in any detailed analysis of multidisciplinary roles, and function (Brown, 1994).

The Reed Report (1992) includes five guiding principles on the care and treatment of patients. (Box 1.6.2).

Putting these principles into practice suggests the need for pre- and post-registration training and education for specialist roles in forensic psychiatry and creative and collaborative working with a view to keeping the mentally ill out of gaol.

The most contemporary documents which link previous policy to major initiatives affecting primary health care include England's *The Health of the Nation* (DOH, 1992). In this strategy mental illness is prioritized as one of the key areas for achieving health gain. As well as setting specific targets in relation to mental illness and suicide, it also highlights several areas for action.

These include the development of a comprehensive system of services, information of prevalence and outcomes, and identifying good practice.

The key objective for mental illness is to reduce ill health and death caused by mental illness.

Examples of targets include:

- To improve significantly the health and social functioning of mentally ill people.
- To reduce the overall suicide rate by at least 15% by the year 2000 (baseline 1990).
- To reduce the suicide rate of severely mentally ill people by at least 33% by the year 2000 (baseline 1990).

In each of the key areas of its strategy, handbooks have been produced, designed as practical guides for developing local strategies for reducing mortality and morbidity. In the context of mental health the *Key Area Handbook Mental Illness*

Box 1.6.2. The Reed Report's five guiding principles

1. Proper attention to the needs of individuals.
2. Care in the community rather than in institutional settings.
3. No greater security than is justified by the degree of danger they present to themselves or others.
4. Maximize rehabilitation and the chances of sustaining an independent life.
5. As near as possible to their own homes or families.

(DOH, 1992) is addressed at both the National Health Service and Social Service Departments.

Themes for action highlighted in this publication are:

- Working with a range of agencies to promote mental health and reduce stigma around mental illness.
- Assessing need and reviewing existing service provision.
- Taking account of user and carer views.
- Joint planning, cooperative working and developing health alliances.

Staff development is also highlighted and it recommends that training on mental health issues be developed for all staff in hospital and community settings. The emphasis should be on improving the recognition and assessment of suicidal risk, depression and anxiety. Joint training is proposed across disciplines and specialties in order to maximize the skills of the whole primary health care team.

Since the publication of the 'Health of the Nation' strategy the Department of Health (England) has produced a report on its progress – *One Year On* (DOH, 1993). This reports that the major challenge during the first year of the strategy has been to gain its wide ownership and integration into strategic planning processes. The need for action at all levels is highlighted. It defines the 'Health of the Nation' strategy as more than just setting targets to improve health – rather it places the onus on professionals, organizations and others to improve (mental) health. This includes governments, the National Health Service, local authorities, the voluntary and private sector, families and individuals. In other words (mental) health is everybody's business.

The response in *One Year On* to an increase in the number of suicides has been to forge broad alliances with a range of agencies. *One Year On* acknowledges the lack of quality information on the prevalence of mental illness but suggests various initiatives to improve matters, such as brief standardized assessment procedures (quantifiable measures).

Under the heading of 'Raising Awareness of Mental Health and Suicide' a range of initiatives are described, including a survey of public attitudes to mental illness, a public information strategy and the creation of a Mental Health Task Force. A ten-point plan to reinforce community care for people when they leave hospital is also described.

The implications of this for community practitioners is clear; achieving the targets in mental illness requires improved understanding, raised awareness and the development of good practice.

This document specifies three ways of achieving mental illness targets.

1. *Improving information and understanding*. Government action cited within the report includes the undertaking of a national psychiatric morbidity survey, and the establishment of a public information strategy.
2. *Developing comprehensive services*. The Mental Health Task Force aims to ensure the transfer of services away from large hospitals to locally based services.
3. *The continuing development of good practice*. In relation to this the Department of Health is evaluating different approaches in delivering mental health care in primary settings. Other examples include. The Defeat Depression campaign run by the Royal Colleges of Psychiatrists and General Practitioners and the funding by The Gatsby Trust, of a senior General Practitioner Fellow to work with general practitioner tutors and course organizers on mental health.

The role of the nursing profession in achieving the targets in the key areas is made more explicit in *Targeting Practice: The Contribution of Nurses, Midwives and Health Visitors* (DOH, 1993). This sees the nursing contribution as assisting in changing the behaviour of individuals, enabling people to make healthy choices, and improving public understanding of mental illness especially in relation to managing stress.

The Mental Health Nursing Review

The report of the Mental Health Nursing Review Team *Working in Partnership; a Collaborative Approach to Care* (DOH, 1994a). This committee was chaired by Professor Butterworth. Its terms of reference were to identify the future requirements for skilled nursing care in the light of developments in the provision of services for people with mental illness. It describes as its common theme the profession's responsibilities to people who use mental health services. In this sense it is in line with much of the policy formulation and implementation over recent years which places a focus on putting patients and clients first.

The review makes a total of 42 recommendations in six key areas:

1. Building relationships with service users.
2. The practice of nursing.
3. The delivery of services.
4. Issues that are challenging.
5. Research in mental health nursing.
6. Pre- and post-registered education.

The recommendations range from a focus of attention on the needs of people with an enduring mental illness to the importance of providing information to service users and carers. It highlights new roles for mental health nurses, including psychosocial interventions and liaison nursing with general medical and primary care services.

A suggested framework for collaborative working by nurses, midwives and health visitors in mental health care is proposed. The Report outlines a preventative model of care aimed at reducing the incidence of mental illness. It suggests that this can be achieved by working with vulnerable groups and developing early detection and intervention approaches.

The review recognizes that the increase in general practitioner fundholding will result in an increase in demand for mental health nurses. Equally, community care initiatives mean people with enduring mental health problems are coming under the wing of primary care. In order for their mental as well as physical health needs to be met, mental health nurses need to act as a consistent point of contact for users, carers and other professionals. As part of the care programme approach mental health nurses act as key workers to coordinate packages of care for users admitted to hospital and those about to be discharged. Therefore, their role, especially with and within the primary health care team is crucial.

Alongside these recommendations the review team considered it essential to retain mental health nursing as a specialty. It stressed that mental health nurses should share their special skills with users and primary health care teams.

At the present time it is not clear how best this can be effected. As with most policy review recommendations implementation rests at a local level and it is becoming clear that the positive and diverse projects being developed are not cohesive at national level. Hence, the role of community psychiatric nurses within primary care is dependent on local health need, purchaser and provider priorities, and there would appear to be a real need for a national and strategic framework for research and skill development (White, 1992).

The Mental Health Nursing Review cites training as a key issue. The final recommendation of the Review is that the United Kingdom Central Council for Nursing, Midwifery and Health Visiting considers the accreditation of appropriate prior learning for entrants to pre-registration of appropriate prior learning for entrants to pre-registration programmes. The development of National Vocational Qualifications (NVQs) within the health and social care sector should be welcomed, but it has implications for future nursing practice.

The core competencies and skill base of specialist community mental health nurses need to be affirmed and marketed within the business culture of the reformed National Health Service. This is especially true in the area of general practitioner fundholding. Issues of service quality and effectiveness need to be demonstrated and the particular expertise of mental health nursing to the practice population, and the Primary Health Care Team highlighted.

A concern is that the skill mix of mental health teams may become biased in favour of unqualified staff. In a cost-driven market there is the potential for fundholding practices to purchase the cheapest, as opposed to the most effective, option. Fundholders are also responsible for their *whole* practice population with mental health issues, ranging from emotional distress to acute and enduring mental ill health. Much government policy recognizes the needs of the mentally ill and for the skills of specialist practitioners to be shared with other agencies. This is the key point of recent policy, reports and reviews in the area of mental health. *The Health of the Nation* and subsequent documents, the Reed report and the Butterworth review all talk about the expansion of the role and skills of specialist mental health nurses and their support for other health professionals. Yet, set alongside other policy implementation, such as fundholding, the contract culture and the assessment of need is an acknowledgement and reorientation of services to the needs of the severely mentally ill. Mental health nurses within this framework are expected to give power back to the users. They are also expected to share skills and workload with other non-specialist nurses, especially in the primary care arena and, at the same time, respond to those with enduring mental health problems.

There is further tension in that much government policy places a focus on behaviour change and healthy lifestyles, minimizing the social context of health. Without significant structural change it is difficult to see how nursing can respond to issues such as the management of stress which can have its roots in poverty, discrimination and powerlessness.

Against this backdrop there are clear training and cost implications which will not be solved by improved inter-agency dialogue and the development of health alliances. Whilst mental health is everybody's business, good business requires appropriate investment.

Roles of Non-specialist

The prevalence of mental illness and distress is such that it would be impossible for specialist mental health services to meet all the demand. The role of primary carers, namely, family and social support networks, is well-documented in *Caring for People* (DOH, 1989a), and is still the front-line response to the care and support of those experiencing the whole gamut of what is termed 'mental health problems or illness'.

However, much distress in the community presents to the general practitioner and primary health care team (Dowrick, 1992) and this provides opportunities for planning service development.

Whilst all community nurses have a part to play, two groups involved in detecting and managing mental health in the community are health visitors and practice nurses.

With over 1800 (Thomas, 1993) practice nurses currently in post and their numbers increasing, there is potential for this professional group to become more proactive in mental health work. Health visitors frequently provide social and emotional support to families and increasingly have a key role to play in relation to the statutory requirements of the Children Act (DOH, 1989c). They are also in a unique position to access community based information as part of their public health function (Peckham and Spanton, 1994).

The Primary Care Team

A recent scheme implemented by Northamptonshire, for example, intends to link training and audit schemes to primary care, by making funds available for all primary care team members to support or contribute to counselling services throughout general practitioner practices. However welcome, this does not really solve the issue of accessing primary health care for those with enduring mental health problems. And, general practitioners cannot avoid their need for training by equating, 'improving the mental health of a community' by merely providing a counselling service (Patmore, 1994).

In nursing's pursuit and concern to provide a response to emotional distress, nurses may inadvertently be implementing policy which decontextualizes people and makes victim-blaming and collective responsibility on issues such as poverty, crime, unemployment and dependence problems, the norm (Caraker, 1994). In appraising the *Strategy for Health*, Ranade (1994), as with many other critics, observes a failure to acknowledge an absence of poverty and deprivation as significant causes of ill health. Indeed, the *Key Handbook for Mental Illness* even uses the word 'disemployment' as opposed to unemployed (Thomas, 1993).

Counter Policy

The debate in relation to the National Health Service reforms, the *Strategy for Health* and other related publications should be examined in the light of the UK's leading mental health charity, MIND.

In terms of the policy statement on primary care, MIND wants an improvement in information for patients, including information on local statutory and voluntary services. This should include a choice of general practitioner, including a 'respectful response', choice of services and service monitoring.

The principles which guide MIND's approach to care and those which also guide the development of a comprehensive community nursing service are summarized in Box 1.6.3.

Good Practice

The Community Care Act (DOH, 1990) emphasized the role of carers and social networks. Further policy and the NHS reforms have placed needs-led services and the importance of consultation and partnership with users and carers high on the government's and therefore purchaser's and provider's agenda.

The shift in mental health service provision from hospital to community settings

Box 1.6.3. MIND's eight principles

- A local comprehensive service is one which:
- Values the client as a full citizen with rights and responsibilities, entitled to be consulted and to have an active opportunity to shape and influence relevant services, no matter how severe his or her disability.
- Aims to promote the greatest self-determination of the individual on the basis of informed and realistic choice.
- Aims to provide and evaluate a programme of treatment, care and support, based on the unique needs of the individual, regardless of age or severity of disability.
- Aims to minimize the dependence of the client on professional resources.
- Is easily accessible locally and delivered, wherever possible, to the client's usual environment.
- Plans actively for those in institutions and to reintegrate them into society if they so wish.
- Aims to enhance the individual or collective capacity to cope with or alleviate distress.

also requires an awareness by those services of the social context within which people operate. For good practice it is essential that all community mental health nurses include the assessment of a person's social network and social support system regularly (Simmons, 1994).

Targeting Practice (DOH, 1993) describes a range of good practice interventions by nurses. It identifies a range of themes which reflect good practice including multidisciplinary working, involving service users, service accessibility and continuity of care. Again, there is a focus on individual needs in relation to health and there are few examples of good practice which highlight community wide strategies aimed at the comprehensive support of all (Baldwin, and Spencer, 1993).

Primary care staff and locally based mental health teams have workers with extensive knowledge of, and contact with, the communities in which they provide care. Good practice could include community development approaches by nurses in an attempt to redress inequality and discrimination.

The authors are based in the Trent Region and the present failure to disseminate good practice makes it is impossible to highlight all developments in mental health nursing. What constitutes 'good practice' is usually locally determined, but key themes would include:

- user involvement,
- support for self-help,
- mental health promotion,
- examples of positive anti-oppressive strategies

Evaluation of any project is also locally determined and some developments are still to be evaluated.

Examples of good practice

The Hanover project

This is a primary health care initiative for the homeless and rootless, based on a two-surgery general practice in inner city Sheffield. It aims to improve both the quality of primary care for this group and to deliver care in an integrated way. The project team is multidisciplinary in form and practice, including a community psychiatric nurse and a social worker. The community psychiatric nurse can respond quickly to the specific needs of this client group and has established links with residents and staff of local hostels. There is close liaison with health visitors working on women's health needs. There is also work involvement with issues to do with male sexual abuse. The project provides a mixture of individual work, training, counselling, welfare advice and facilitating group work.

The project relates to the good practice pointers in *Targeting Practice* (DOH, 1993) in so far as its general objective is to improve the health and social functioning of mentally ill people.

Nottingham Group Therapy

A therapeutic group for clients with acute mental health problems has been run by nurses in a community mental health centre in Nottingham. It provides support and structured social therapy to people resolving a crisis. The project has been evaluated with users who identified their involvement with the group as a positive experience. The group has also improved communication with other community mental health workers and the local hospital. The project is particularly aimed at improving social functioning. It takes place in a more normative setting than a hospital.

Mental Health Promotion

A recent development is an increasing interest in and appointment of mental health promotion staff working specifically in this field. The majority of these posts are based within health promotion departments, but there are also moves by providers of mental health services to incorporate mental health promotion into practitioner's roles. In addition, specific projects in relation to mental health are being established.

The role of mental health promotion as part of the purchasing function of health authorities is also recognized.

At the time of writing only a small section of the mental health strategy is devoted to mental health promotion. This accepts that it is a long-term strategy to increase awareness about mental illness, shape public opinion and produce a range of preventive programmes.

Mental health promotion is about facilitating a process whereby agencies and communities develop structures and environments which enable people to create local support and assistance. It is essentially about giving power and control to people in order to maintain or improve their mental health regardless of their health status. As such, it inevitably touches on issues of poverty, discrimination and environments. In this sense it includes issues within government policy but goes beyond the individual to the collective experience.

In summary there have been a range of policy changes with both positive and negative implications. The dilemmas for community nurses have been considered and the potential for good practice explored.

CONCLUSION

Government policy is potentially a vehicle for change. It can provide opportunities to respond creatively to a range of agendas, such as community participation. A negative aspect of policy is that it can act as a constraining framework, one that works within rather than beyond; that is, it can lull purchasers, planners and statutory providers of mental health services into an uninspiring mind set. Good practice should become part of the nursing culture, as well as part of the value base and activity of purchasers and providers. This means involving a wide range of professionals, communities, service users, carers and the public in shaping mental health services.

It is considered essential that the nursing profession should be an integral part of this process. Recent developments have highlighted the emerging role of the 'mental health worker', as some kind of generic 'specialist', but it is considered crucial that specialism be retained for improving clinical effectiveness.

Government policies emphasize a reconfiguration of services and resources from hospital to community settings. Yet, at the same time, there is increasing pressure on hospitals to provide more and more treatment. The forecasted shift of finances and staff from hospital beds to community budgets has yet to take place.

A lot and a little could best sum up the UK experience in policy and practice in the last five years. For the future, whilst the debate and discourse continues, actions will speak louder than words.

SUMMARY

- The dilemma and the challenge for nurses in the mental health field is that they are expected to be specialized, different, and focus on the needs of the severely mentally ill. At the same time the focus toward empowerment, incorporating a shift in power to the client in terms of individual and collective involvement, might create fundamental ideological differences, not just in care per se, but in genuine collaborative planning and implementation of care.

- What is required for front-line workers, such as community psychiatric nurses, when both changes in policy and education and training are still not clear-cut, might never be, and care in a primary health care setting has perhaps only transferred the dynamics of power balance amongst professionals.

- Autonomous practice in mental health nursing is considered a vital function in the past and in the future. Increasingly, in terms of accountability, as with social work role and function, this is now not only determined by economic constraints, but also by statutory duties (CPA (Care Programme Approach) risk assessment).

- The impact of policy on the task and practice of community mental health nursing includes them being gatekeepers for primary, secondary and tertiary care, but also as resource coordinators for a range of non-statutory service and support.

- The recent policy changes have put the service user (client) into the role of a consumer as opposed to the traditional role of a dependent person (patient). Purchasers are not users, so there is a fundamental difference in how the free market philosophy matches up with the needs and experiences of users.

- The dilemma is that even if the mental health specialist in a community setting focuses on enduring mental illness, the needs of this care group are more around social than medical needs, including housing, poverty and discrimination. Perhaps this has always been the case?

DISCUSSION QUESTIONS

◆ What are the advantages and disadvantages of people without an established mental illness engaging with primary care and community mental health teams?

◆ How can the problematization of emotional distress be resolved?

(a) If the general practitioner practice is forward thinking and offers a variety of clinics and self-help initiatives. This is further complicated if they are fundholders or not.

(b) Despite a wide array of resources in more forward thinking areas of the country, the cry still tends to be 'I wish the general practitioner had more time to talk with me and then I wouldn't need to be told I require counselling intervention'.

◆ How can people fully utilize the resources available within primary care if there are barriers in terms of ethnic background, class and cultural difference, gender, age and disability?

◆ How can the non-specialist be supported in order to broaden their practice, enabling positive social change with the people they work with?

◆ When working with clients who have mental health problems, discuss the shift from seeing clients in terms of risk-taking rather than dangerousness.

FURTHER READING

Health Promotion

Badura B and Kickbusch I (Eds) (1991) *Health Promotion Research: Towards a New Social Epidemiology.* WHO Regional Publications No. 37, Copenhagen.

Downie RS, Fyfe C and Tannerhill A, (1991) *Health Promotion: Models and Values.* Oxford: Oxford University Press.

Trent Regional Health Authority and Centre for Mental Health Services Development (1994) *Focus on Promoting Mental Health at Work in the National Health Service: an aid to contracting.*

Newton J (1990) *Preventing Mental Illness.* London: Routledge.
The texts highlight issues around promoting mental health.

Community Mental Health Services

Brooker C (1990) *Community Psychiatric Nursing: a Research Perspective.* London: Chapman & Hall.

Johnson WA (1992) *A cry for change: an Asian perspective on developing quality mental health care* 2nd edn. Confederation of Indian Organizations, UK.

Prior L (1993) *The Social Organization of Mental Illness.* London: Sage Publications.

Thompson A and Mathias P (Eds) (1994) *Lyttle's Mental Health and Disorder*, 2nd edn. London: Baillière Tindall.
Contained in these resources is a varied but balanced perspective relating to current issues around community mental health practice.

User Perspectives

Barham P (1992) *Closing the Asylum: The mental patient in modern society.* London: Penguin.

Rodgers A, Pilgrim D and Lacey R (1993) *Experiencing Psychiatry: User's views of services.* MIND in association with Macmillan. London.

Harding C and Sherlock J (1994) *Women and Mental Health. Good Practices in Mental Health*. London. Critical appraisal of the prevailing medical approaches to mental health practice.

MIND (1992) *From Anger to Action Video* plus resource book. This publication examines the role of survivors of mental illness and challenges the assumption that ex-users have nothing to offer.

REFERENCES

Andrew B, Hawton K, Fagg J and Westbrook D (1993) Do psychosocial factors influence outcome in severely depressed female psychiatric patients? *British Journal of Psychiatry* **163:** 747-754.

Armstrong E (1993) Promoting mental health. In A Dines and A Cribb (Eds) *Health Promotion: Concepts and Practice*. London. Blackwell Scientific Publications.

Backer-Holst A (1994) A New Window of Opportunity; the implications of the Reed Report for psychiatric care. *Psychiatric Care* **1:** 1.

Balarajan R and Raleigh VS (1993) *Ethnicity and Health: A Guide for the NHS*. London: HMSO.

Baldwin N and Spencer N (1993) Deprivation and Child Abuse: Implications for Strategic Planning in Childrens' Services. *Children and Society* **7:** 4, 357-375.

Brown J (1994) The Hybrid Worker: Lessons based upon a study of employers involved in two pioneer joint qualifying training courses. CCETSW Department of Social Policy and Social Work. University of York.

Butler T (1993) *Changing Mental Health Services: The Politics and Policy*. London: Chapman & Hall.

Butterworth T (1994) Working in Partnership, A Collaborative Approach to Care. *Report of Mental Health Nursing Review Team*. London: HMSO.

Caraker M (1994) Nursing and Health Promotion Practice; the creation of victims and winners in a political context. *Journal of Advanced Nursing* **19:** 465.

Carroll D, Bennett P and Smith GD (1993) Socio-economic health inequalities: their origins and implications. *Psychology and Health* **8:** 295-316.

Department of Health (1987) *Promoting Better Health*. London: HMSO.

Department of Health (1989a) *Caring for People: Community Care in the Next Decade and Beyond*. London: HMSO.

Department of Health (1989b) *Working for Patients*. London: HMSO.

Department of Health (1990) *National Health Service and Community Care Act*. London: HMSO.

Department of Health (1992) *The Health of the Nation* London: HMSO.

Department of Health (1993a) *One Year On: A Report on the Progress of the Health of the Nation*. London: HMSO.

Department of Health (1993b) *Targeting Practice: The Contribution of Nurses, Midwives and Health Visitors*. London: HMSO.

Department of Health (1994a) *The report of the Mental Health Nursing Review Team. Working in Partnership: A Collaborative Approach to Care*. London: HMSO.

Dowrick C (1992) Improving Mental Health through Primary Care. *British Journal of General Practice* **42:** 382-386.

Gunn J, Maden A and Swinton M (1991) Treatment needs of prisoners with psychiatric disorders. *British Medical Journal* **303:** 338-341.

Healthy Sheffield Support Team (1993) *Community Development and Health: The Way Forward in Sheffield*.

HMSO (1994) *The report of the Inquiry into the Care and Treatment of Christopher Clunis*. February.

Jarman B, Hirsch S, White P and Driscoll R (1992) Predicting psychiatric admission rates. *British Medical Journal* **304:** 1146.

Lewis G and Wilkinson G (1993) Another British Disease? A recent increase in the prevalence of psychiatric morbidity. *Journal of Epidemiology and Community Health* **47:** 358.

Lindow V (1994) *Self-Help Alternatives to Mental Health Services*. London: MIND Publications.

MIND (1993) *Mind Policy 1*. Mind Publications: London.

Patmore C (1994) A problem shared. Mental health section. *Health Service Journal*, August.

Peckham S and Spanton J (1994) Community development approaches to health needs assessment. *Health Visitor* 4.

Punmaki RL and Aschan H (1994) Self-care and mastery among primary health care patients. *Social Science and Medicine* **39:** 733.

Ranado W (1994) *A Future for the National Health Service? Health Care in the 1990s*. Essex: Longman.

Reed J (1992) *Review of Health and Social Services for Mentally Disordered Offenders and Others Requiring Similar Services*. London: HMSO.

Thomas C (1993) Public health strategies in Sheffield and England; a comparison of conceptual foundations. *Health Promotion International*.

White E (1992) *The Future of Nursing by the year 2000: A Delphi Study*. University of Manchester, Department of Nursing Studies.

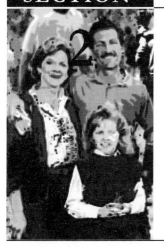
THE FAMILY AS A FRAMEWORK FOR PRACTICE

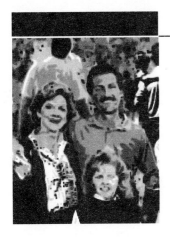

INTRODUCTION

This section introduces the reader to the family as a focus for practice. The opening chapters remind the reader of various concepts and perspectives in relation to the study of families and in this context, the first chapter considers 'families' from the sociological perspective. Readers are challenged to consider whether or not there is such a thing as a relevant family perspective! Factors influencing family health are explored along with a consideration of changing statistics, re-marriage and divorce.

The second chapter adopts a psychological perspective to explore family issues. Family dynamics, including conflict and conflict management are discussed together with a consideration of factors such as the impact of children on the quality of marriage or partnership. A linking chapter builds on this discussion by exploring aspects of violence within families and the potential need for risk assessment and child protection.

The closing chapters centre around family nursing, family policy and families with special needs. The reader's attention is drawn to theoretical perspectives and research findings where they are relevant and these underpin discussions concerning their implications for practice. Chapter five in this section takes a rather different and perhaps provocative stance by exploring the politics of lifestyle and the impact of behaviour on the health of those living in relative poverty. Tessa Davies confronts the nurse by forcing the profession to consider the impact of the socio-economic climate and to question the degree to which nurses are being urged to collude with government strategies 'born of political expediency'.

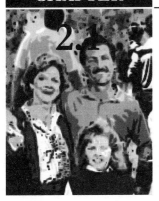

THE FAMILY: A SOCIOLOGICAL PERSPECTIVE

Graham Allan and Graham Crow

KEY ISSUES

- Continuities and changes in households and families
- Diversity in people's experiences of families
- Influence of factors outside the domestic sphere on dominant patterns of family life

INTRODUCTION

While we all talk about 'the family' as though it were obvious and unproblematic, in a very real sense 'the family' as such does not exist. Rather what we have are many different forms of family, each of which gets modified and changed, over time, generally slowly, but sometimes more radically. This point is not as banal as it might seem. Indeed arguably the key to understanding the nature of family life lies in recognizing the interplay between continuity and change which characterizes all aspects of family relationships. It is this notion of the family as dynamic rather than static, variable rather than uniform, which will provide the framework for much of what follows in this chapter.

We can recognize that change occurs within families at a variety of levels. Clearly individual relationships within families change over time. Think here about your own relationships with your parents. Whether or not they are still married, the ways they have treated you, their expectations about your behaviour, and the forms of control they have exercised over you, have all altered as you have grown older. In adulthood, your relationship with them is likely to continue but not in anything like the same form as when you were a child. So too relationships between husbands and wives, between brothers and sisters, or any other family members also alter as people age and take on different responsibilities. Most of the time this change is considered routine and normal, though there are occasions, such as divorce or the onset of severe infirmity, when it is more traumatic and requires more rapid adjustment.

But just as relationships between family members alter over time, so too the patterns of family living within a society are liable to change as wider social and economic conditions alter. Traditionally within sociology, a great deal of attention has been paid to the impact that industrialization had on family relationships. For example, there has been much debate around whether industrialization led to the decline of extended family relationships or, in contrast, actually generated the conditions necessary for greater solidarity between extended family members. Such debates are echoed in much popular discourse, though this tends to emphasize the pathological character of contemporary family life and the decline of family values. Thus, we often hear claims that family life has become more insular and less community oriented, or that elderly people do not receive sufficient support from their families. Recently too there has been much emphasis placed on shifts occurring within marriage, though here there are more conflicting views as to how this should be interpreted. Some argue that in comparison to the past – though exactly how far back in the past is often left unspecified – marriage is now a much more equal relationship, a far more genuine partnership than it used to be. Others point to the rising levels of divorce as an indicator that many no longer regard marriage with the sanctity it deserves.

So what has been happening to family life and family relationships? How different are our experiences from those of our grandparents? How much change has there been and how much continuity? In order to examine these issues, this chapter will focus on key aspects of the social organization of family and domestic life pertinent to community nursing. These include marriage, divorce, lone parent households, and the family circumstances of elderly people. We will begin by examining the contemporary patterning and social organization of marriage.

Marriage

Throughout the first two-thirds of the twentieth century marriage became a more common experience. By the late 1960s approximately 95% of men and women were or had been married by the time they were in their mid-forties. Marriage age also decreased over this period, with the average age of first marriage for men being 23 and for women 21 in the late 1960s. Since the early 1970s though, demographic aspects of marriage have altered quite noticeably. To begin with, age at first marriage has shown a steady increase since the mid 1970s. By 1991 the average age had risen to 26.5 for men and 24.5 for women. In part this reflects the increased levels of cohabitation now occurring. While there have been few studies of cohabitation as a specific form of relationship, what is clear is that since the late 1980s the majority of marrying couples now live together prior to their marriage, typically for a period of about a year. Whereas such actions would have brought a good deal of censure a generation ago, in the light of high divorce rates, this is now seen socially as an appropriate form of courtship.

Along with these changes in the demography of marriage, there is also a widely-held belief that the basis of marriage has been altering. Contemporary ideology, or what Cancian (1987) rather usefully calls 'blueprints' of marriage, emphasize the idea of marriage as much more of a partnership between equals than it was in the past. It is now seen as an emotionally closer relationship, based on developing conceptions of personal compatibility, commitment and love. It consequently carries with it a heightened range of expectations, including a greater belief that personal expression and mutual satisfaction provide the central rationale for the relationship. It is this which people getting married seek. More than their grandparents or even their parents, they want their marriages to encompass a mutual sharing, a union between equals, premised on contemporary images of romantic love as a means to personal fulfilment.

However, despite these ideologies, the basic organization of marriage has remained relatively constant. While cohabitation appears sometimes to entail a more symmetrical and equal relationship, once married, couples tend to revert to more traditional patterns. Mansfield and Collard's (1988) study of the early months of marriage is particularly relevant here. They found that even early in the marriage husbands and wives tended to assume quite distinct 'marital careers' with, for example, husbands' jobs being prioritized over their wives'. Thus some two-thirds of the new wives changed their job around the time of their marriage, usually to a less well-paid and less secure one, whereas fewer than a third of new husbands had changed jobs, usually without any detrimental occupational consequences. At the heart of these decisions lay the notion that the couple would soon have children, and that it would be the female 'partner' who left employment to provide the necessary care. Similarly, while many couples devoted much of their energy, time and resources to decorating and refurbishing their home, the mundane tasks of cooking, cleaning and other domestic work fell disproportionately to wives.

What is important about this is that comparatively early in a marriage it gives rise to a traditional domestic division of labour. Men are accepted as continuing to have the major commitment to the job market and to the securing of household finances, with women being more responsible for domestic labour and household management. The patterns here of course are not identical to those occurring in the past. There has undoubtedly been important change, particularly with respect to wives' employment. For example, in 1961 less than 40% of wives aged 16–59 were in employment. By 1991 this figure was nearly 70%, with a third being in full-time employment. There have also been important changes in the speed with which women return to employment after childbirth. Currently 42% of those with children under five years are employed (11% full-time and 31% part-time) compared with 25% twenty years ago.

The division of labour and domestic responsibilities within a marriage, and consequently the division of opportunities and constraints affecting each spouse, becomes most marked if the couple have children, as some 90% of married couples do. In particular where mothers leave employment, as the large majority do at least for some period after the birth of children, they typically assume major responsibility for most of the domestic and child care tasks. As various studies have shown (Graham, 1993), the workloads involved in this can be very high, with husbands generally giving only limited help, despite myths to the contrary. As children age, as wives return to employment and as the couple develop different commitments outside the home, we might expect that some aspects of their division of work are renegotiated. Yet, while there are modifications over time, rarely does such renegotiation appear to lead to radical change (Brannen and Moss, 1991). Husbands and older children may help somewhat more in household tasks, but the primary responsibilities for domestic management and familial care seem to remain as before. Even following major changes in household circumstances, for example with male unemployment, the renegotiation of responsibilities appears to be limited. In general, the household division of labour continues to be patterned in the ways established early in the marriage.

The continuation of a high division of labour within marriage is linked very strongly to the inequalities which flourish within the job market. Notwithstanding recent equal opportunities legislation, occupations still tend to be highly gendered. For example, the majority of women employees work in a few female-dominated occupations, e.g. as secretaries, nurses, teachers, sales staff and cleaners. Importantly too, the jobs women are in typically pay significantly less than male occupations. For the last twenty years, and with very little variation between years, full-time women employees have received approximately 70% of the wages male employees receive, with this relationship being broadly consistent across different skill levels. Part-time employees, the vast majority of whom are married women, usually receive even lower proportional pay (Crompton and Sanderson, 1990).

Thus for most couples, it is not really surprising that a conventional division of labour continues to be 'negotiated'. As well as husbands earning more than wives, women are socialized into being more accomplished at domestic activities than men and tend to have child care and other relationship responsibility built more into the construction of their personal and social identities. Of course, in principle a division of labour need not be associated with an unequal distribution of resources within the marriage, nor with the dominance of one spouse over the other. Yet research has regularly shown that within most marriages, though not all, this is the outcome. Despite the prevalence of ideologies of coupledom, men have greater control of financial resources, more freedom for leisure and more control over key decisions than their wives do (Allan, 1985). So notwithstanding modifications in employment patterns, marital ideology, domestic standards, child care practices and the like, the point remains that individual couples construct their marriages within an economic and social context which remains structurally unequal and usually provides men with more options and a greater access to resources than women.

Divorce

Divorce is one aspect of family life where there has been a clear change in the last thirty years. Whereas in the late 1960s there were only 45 000 divorces each year, throughout the late 1980s and early 1990s there have been over 150 000. This is a rise in the annual rate from 4 per 1000 marriages to nearly 14 per 1000. Each year approximately 150 000 children under the age of 16 experience their parents' divorce, almost a doubling since 1971. Alongside this there has been an expansion in the number of lone-parent families, not all of which arise through divorce of course, and a large increase in the number of step-families. This has resulted in much more diversity in family patterns compared to even a short while ago. It also means that many individuals now experience different forms of family life at first hand, moving say from a two-parent family to a lone-parent one, and then later forming a step-family.

It is difficult to be precise about the reasons for the rise in divorce. Divorce, like marriage, is a legal procedure, so at one level the heightened rate of divorce merely reflects changes in the law, especially with the 1969 Divorce Reform Act. However, the law itself reflects changed marital ideologies, and moreover the fact that divorce is made more available does not of itself explain why people have increasingly chosen it as an option. Three factors seem particularly important. First, as we have already noted, there have been changes in marital 'blueprints'. Increasingly people are expecting continued personal satisfaction from marriage and not just a convenient domestic, sexual and economic arrangement. This change is reflected clearly in the 1969 Divorce Reform Act. Until then the law specified marriage as a contract between two people which could only be terminated if broken, for example by adultery or desertion, and then only through the injured party seeking a divorce. With the 1969 Act, the emphasis moved to viewing marriage as an essentially personal arrangement which could be terminated if it had 'irretrievably broken down', no matter what the cause of this or the respective behaviour of the two spouses.

Second, increasing divorce rates are only feasible if both spouses normally have access to sufficient material resources to sustain themselves. Of particular importance here are the changes over the last fifty years allowing separated women to maintain a sufficient standard of living independently of their (ex)husbands. The creation of increased employment opportunities for married women has been important in this, as has the availability of social security payments and the protection given in divorce settlements to the housing needs of those caring for children. Third, divorce is now far less stigmatized than it once was. It is seen as undesirable, but as an event which has a personal rather than a social significance. Divorce is no longer treated as a moral issue to the same extent as it once was, nor as indicative of questionable character. As divorce becomes accepted as an unfortunate but not unusual occurrence, so it comes also to be seen as a solution to marital difficulties that in a previous era would have been tolerated. It is this 'normalization' of divorce in both legal and social terms which lies at the heart of the currently high levels of divorce.

In understanding the impact which divorce has on those involved, it is crucial that it is viewed as a process occurring over time, rather than as a specific legal event. The factors that lead up to the breakdown of the marriage, and the understandings each spouse has of these, will have an impact on the way in which the divorce and its aftermath are handled. This is particularly important when there are children, for as is now better recognized, divorce represents the ending of a marriage but not the ending of parenting. Legislation governing the Child Support Agency has brought the economic implications of this to the fore, but it also applies to the personal relationship each child maintains with the non-residential parent. American research has indicated the importance for children of maintaining an active relationship with both parents (Heatherington and Arasteh, 1988). Moreover, it is in the child's interests that the two parents develop a consistent and cooperative relationship with one another with respect to parenting. This is rarely easy, given the history of hostility and conflict characterizing much pre- and post-divorce behaviour. When parents continue to be in conflict over, say, financial arrangements or childcare responsibilities, or indeed when recrimination, jealousy and other strong emotions are still being experienced, it is difficult to develop a mutually consistent and supportive stance in relation to children. Given the tensions and problems which can be generated, it is perhaps not surprising that up to 50% of non-residential fathers cease to have regular contact with their child(ren) (Bradshaw and Millar, 1991).

Lone-parent Households

In 1977 Chester argued that the single-parent family was becoming recognized as a *variant*, rather than a *deviant*, family form. Since that time, the number of lone-parent households has continued to increase, both as a result of high levels of divorce and because more children are being born outside marriage. As these numbers have grown, the range and diversity of experiences of those living in such households has also increased. Undoubtedly the majority of lone-parent households have much in common, especially with respect to their poverty and material deprivation. Yet variations in the living conditions, family histories and economic opportunities of different lone-parent households should not be ignored. Just as the routes into, and indeed out of, lone parenthood have become more complex, so too the social, economic and domestic circumstances of those involved have become more diverse (Hardey and Crow, 1991).

Currently it is estimated that there are over 1.3 million lone-parent households in Britain, containing approximately 2.2 million children – nearly one in five of all dependent children. Of these, only 110 000 are headed by men. While this is not an insignificant number in itself, the predominance of female-headed lone-parent households warrants emphasizing as it plays a major part in shaping the experience of lone parenthood. Of the 1.2 million female-headed lone-parent households there are, nearly 60% stem from divorce or marital separation, with only 80 000 being the result of widowhood. Over a third are headed by single (i.e. never married) women (Haskey, 1993). This represents a quite remarkable demographic change since the mid 1970s. Then only some 10% of children were born 'out of wedlock'. Now the figure is over 30%, with four-fifths of mothers aged under 20 unmarried. However, it is worth noting that approximately half of all mothers recorded as being unmarried on their child's birth certificate are cohabiting with the father when the birth is registered.

The route into lone parenthood has implications for the material well-being of lone-parent households. In the majority of instances, lone fathers and widowed mothers tend to be better off than other lone parents. Both these groups tend to have older children than other lone parents, and as a result fewer problems with the coordination and costs of child care. They are also more likely to have employment or pensions which make them less dependent on state benefits and to be in owner occupation. In contrast, divorced, separated and single mothers – collectively some 85% of all lone parents – are frequently in poverty. For example, over 70% of all lone mothers are now in receipt of income support and thus living on the minimum officially considered viable (Millar, 1992).

The reasons for so many lone mothers being at the poverty level are various. Clearly women's disadvantaged position in employment is one factor. The relatively low pay of many female jobs, especially for women without significant qualifications, means that many lone mothers having little prospect of enhancing their financial position. In addition, the need for flexibility over child care, given the acknowledged scarcity of affordable public or private provision, often makes it difficult to coordinate employment and parenting responsibilities. When children are at school, part-time employment may become feasible though the financial benefits of this, as distinct from its social and personal advantages, are generally quite limited as state support is consequently reduced.

As well as being in or on the fringes of poverty, lone mothers tend to be disadvantaged in other ways. For example, they have worse than average housing conditions, with a disproportionate number being in rented accommodation or sharing their home with other adults. Only 36% of lone-parent families are in owner occupation compared to 76% of all other households with dependent children living in them. Equally there is evidence that lone parents, especially lone mothers, suffer more health problems than those in two-parent families (Popay and Jones, 1990). This is not altogether surprising, given the relationship between material well-being and good health. Families in poverty and in poor housing, as so many lone-parent families are, generally experience worse health than those who have adequate resources (see Chapter 2.5).

Overall, then, there can be no doubt that a majority of lone-parent families are disadvantaged, especially those which are female-headed. Yet while poverty and material deprivation is the norm, various aspects of lone parenthood come to be valued by many. Simply in financial terms, some lone mothers are, in Hilary Graham's phrase, 'better off poorer' (Graham 1987: 59), because they now control all the household resources, whereas previously they only received from their husbands a small portion of the overall larger 'household' income. Equally, while many lone parents experience social isolation and a sense of having to cope with a wide range of demands alone, others value the freedom and autonomy over their use of time, domestic organization and social activities which lone parenthood offers. For some too, the curtailment of disharmony and marital violence more than compensates for poverty. The point here is not that these more positive aspects of lone parenthood necessarily counter its negative features, but rather that lone parenthood is often an ambiguous and diverse experience.

Step-families

Cohabitation and marriage represent major routes out of lone parenthood, though they are ones which are taken by some more readily than others. Ermisch (1989) has shown that single mothers form new unions quicker than those who have been married previously, with age, educational attainment and family size affecting the chances of remarriage for those who have divorced. But just as the levels of divorce, births outside marriage and lone parenthood have increased over the last twenty years, so has the number of step-families formed. Currently it is estimated that 8% of children live in step-families, though many more have a non-residential step-parent (Haskey, 1994). There has been surprisingly little research into step-families in Britain and also little official concern for them. The assumption has tended to be that step-families are essentially similar to other two-parent families.

However, the diversity and complexity of step-families makes this an over-simplified view. Aside from factors like the age of the children and how long they have known their step-parent, the social roles of step-father and step-mother are ill-defined. There are few guidelines about just how much of a parent a step-parent should be, for example, the extent of the step-parent's involvement, their rights to impose discipline, and the commitment expected between step-parent and child, are all much more open to negotiation than in natural families, so that the potential for disagreement and conflict is that much greater. Equally the 'boundaries' around step-families tend to be more permeable than in natural families, especially where contact is maintained with the non-residential parent and his or her kin.

In essence the symbolic 'unity' of a step-family cannot be assumed in the way it is in natural families. Given these structural dilemmas, it is hardly surprising that step-families appear particularly prone to friction, notwithstanding their efforts to present themselves as in essence no different from 'ordinary' families (Burgoyne and Clark, 1984).

Old Age

There is a strong belief that kinship ties outside the household have become less significant than they once were. In particular, the solidarities that exist across the generations are now seen to be weaker than in the past, with the result that many elderly people are left isolated, leading lonely and largely unfulfilling lives. This picture of contemporary old age is highly questionable. Certainly, as Dee Jones discusses in Chapter 1.5, the number of elderly people has increased very significantly in the twentieth century. There are now, for example, nearly four million people over the age of 75 compared to half a million in 1901, an increase which is 16 times that of the general population. Moreover nearly half of all women over 65 live alone. Along with these demographic shifts, there have been important changes in elderly people's social and economic circumstances. In particular, it is becoming increasingly inappropriate to treat the elderly population as homogeneous. The divisions within it are as important as the similarities. For example, the rise of private pension plans and of owner occupation since the mid twentieth century have exacerbated differences in income and wealth amongst those aged 65 and over. These factors, together with variations in life expectancy, have also led to very important gender differences in the experience of old age (Arber and Ginn, 1991).

On the surface, the fact that so many elderly women live alone appears to give credence to the claim that elderly people no longer receive the support they deserve and need. Undoubtedly some of these people are very isolated and receive inadequate social support; some will never have married or have no surviving children to whom they might turn. Yet there are other factors at work here too, which give a rather different picture. In particular, our kinship system gives a high priority to maintaining household independence. That is, while there is strong value placed on relationships between genealogically close adult kin being generally supportive, there is also much weight given to the idea that in adulthood personal and household autonomy takes priority. Kin, including parents and children, should not interfere too much in each other's lives. Here there can be a fine line between supporting and interfering, between assuming some responsibility and maintaining independence (Finch and Mason, 1993). Indeed, rather than neglecting their elderly parent(s), it would seem many adult children play a major role in helping them to sustain independent lives as infirmity encroaches.

Of course the nature of the relationship which elderly people have with their children varies a good deal. In part, this will be shaped by the past development of their bond, but it will also be influenced by a range of other personal factors such as geographical location, employment, other familial and domestic responsibilities, material resources and health. Here it is important to recognize that older age of itself does not have any necessary impact on family relationships. The great majority of older people are relatively fit and active, well able to manage their own lives, and have no reason for fuller involvement with their children than in preceding life stages. As in earlier times, the relationships are likely to be characterized by a degree of reciprocity with both sides providing support of different forms for one another, but without either being in a position of dependence.

It is not old age *per se* which alters the nature of these exchanges, but rather changes – sometimes gradual, sometimes radical – in older people's circumstances. However, such changes as reduced income, widowhood and poor health have a differential impact on the older population. Expressed simply, those with most resources, in particular those who have higher levels of private pension and significant investments, are in a better position to sustain their lifestyle and independence through purchasing services privately. Those with fewer resources, a position in which many older women find themselves especially after their husband's death, are likely to become more quickly dependent on kin for support. In nearly all cases though there is a desire to maintain some semblance of balance and reciprocity in these ties. This can often require careful and quite subtle 'negotiation' if the older individual's sense of self-worth is not to be undermined.

When extensive care is required, it tends to be provided by family members, though usually the responsibility falls most heavily on one particular person. This is typically the spouse where there is one, or another adult living in the same house

(Qureshi and Walker, 1989). Otherwise it is usually daughters or daughters-in-law who are most active in providing informal care. While this has now been much discussed in the research literature on caring (see, for example, Ungerson, 1994), it is still easy for health professionals and others to underestimate the actual level of work which such caring entails and its impact on the lifestyles and well-being of those who do it. With the growth of owner occupation, one of the intriguing questions for the future is whether those who provide care in later life will be rewarded through differential legacies. Previously this was a matter of little concern as so few people had property of much consequence to bequeath.

CONCLUSION

There has been little explicit focus in this chapter on issues directly concerned with health behaviour or practice. Other chapters in this section discuss these matters more directly. Its aim has been to provide an overall framework by analysing key aspects of contemporary family experience. However, the arguments made in this chapter certainly have relevance for health care provision and the work of community nurses. Three particular issues are worth highlighting in conclusion. First, there is much diversity in household and family patterns, both demographically, with recent increases in cohabitation, divorce and remarriage, and materially. In delivering health care, advice and support, the particular circumstances of individual families need to be recognized. Second, the family itself is not just a single entity or social unity. It comprises sets of relationships which change over time but which also typically entail a marked division of labour, resources and power. Recognizing these divisions and the impact they have on the experiences of different household members can be important in providing appropriate health services. Finally, it is important that all health workers recognize the extent to which health care continues to be delivered informally, principally by family members and predominantly by females responsible for the household's domestic organization. Despite the changes which are supposed to have occurred, most non-specialized nursing and health care is carried out by wives, mothers and daughters. At times the burden of such care can be extremely heavy, a fact which should not be downplayed even when those involved give the impression of 'coping'.

SUMMARY

■ Family life is characterized by both continuity and change, with change arising through life course transitions and altered social and economic conditions.

■ Recently there have been significant changes in patterns of family formation and dissolution, with far higher rates of cohabitation and divorce than a generation ago.

■ Despite changes in the ideology of marriage and partnership, the domestic division of labour typically remains highly gendered, as do employment patterns.

■ Increases in the divorce rate and in births outside marriage have led to a significant growth in the number of lone-parent households, 90% of which are female-headed. The majority of these lone-parent households are financially and materially disadvantaged.

■ There have also been increases in the numbers of step-families, a family form which is far more complex and diverse than is often assumed.

■ While the majority of elderly people remain fit and active, informal support for those who become infirm is generally provided by family members, especially spouses and daughters.

<table>
<tr><td>DISCUSSION QUESTIONS</td><td>

♦ What are the main changes to have affected family life in the last thirty years and why have these occurred?

♦ Why have cohabitation rates increased so much recently and what implications does this have for the organization of marriage?

♦ Are there ways of managing divorce that limit its negative consequences for children's development?

♦ What role can health professionals play in compensating for the disadvantages experienced by lone-parent families?

♦ Discuss whether and to what extent adult children feel a sense of responsibility towards their elderly parents.
</td></tr>
</table>

FURTHER READING

Crompton R and Sanderson K (1990) *Gendered Jobs and Social Change*. London: Unwin Hyman.
This book provides details of the differences between women's and men's employment experiences. Understanding the nature of these structural differences is central to a full understanding of why family relations are patterned as they are.

Finch J and Mason J (1993) *Negotiating Family Responsibilities*. London: Routledge.
This book provides a thorough discussion of the role of kinship in contemporary Britain. Based on a survey of kinship attitudes and behaviour, the authors highlight the negotiations which occur in assigning kinship responsibilities.

Gittins D (1993) *The Family in Question: Changing Households and Familiar Ideologies*, 2nd edn. Basingstoke: Macmillan.
This book draws on a range of different approaches to indicate how contemporary family patterns have emerged. The use of a feminist perspective to analyse the development of the family during this century adds an important dimension to common understandings of the processes of family transformations.

Graham H (1993) *Hardship and Health in Women's Lives*. Hemel Hempstead: Harvester-Wheatsheaf.
Although not only concerned with family matters, this book provides a very good overview of the range of factors which shape women's experiences. In focusing on women with few resources, it shows how family issues are intertwined with other aspects of women's social existence.

Hardey M and Crow G (Eds) (1991) *Lone Parenthood: Coping with Constraints and Making Opportunities*. Hemel Hempstead: Harvester-Wheatsheaf.
This edited collection of original papers provides a very useful review of the different circumstances of lone-parent families. Its strength is that it recognizes variation in people's experiences and ambitions, without losing sight of the common dilemmas facing many lone parents.

Mansfield P and Collard J (1988) *The Beginning of the Rest of Your Life? A Portrait of Newly-Wed Marriage*. Basingstoke: Macmillan.
This book provides an intriguing analysis of the ways in which a sample of newly married couples construct their relationship. By looking at the decisions made at this early phase about issues like employment, the domestic sphere and child care, the authors show very well how wider gender-based social and economic divisions influence the development of these personal ties.

Phoenix A, Woollett A and Lloyd E (Eds) (1991) *Motherhood: Meanings, Practices and Ideologies*. London: Sage.

This book contains a series of fascinating articles concerned with the social construction of motherhood. Some are concerned quite directly with the ways in which health professionals play their part in shaping the experience and meaning of motherhood.

REFERENCES

Allan G (1985) *Family Life: Domestic Roles and Social Organization*. Oxford: Basil Blackwell.

Arber S and Ginn J (1991) *Gender and Later Life*. London: Sage.

Bradshaw J and Millar J (1991) *Lone Parent Families in the UK*. London: HMSO.

Brannen J and Moss P (1991) *Managing Mothers: Dual Earner Households After Maternity Leave*. London: Unwin Hyman.

Burgoyne J and Clark D (1984) *Making a Go of It: A Study of Stepfamilies in Sheffield*. London: Routledge & Kegan Paul.

Cancian F (1987) *Love in America: Gender and Self-Development*. Cambridge: Cambridge University Press.

Chester R (1977) The one-parent family: Deviant or variant? In R Chester and J Peel (Eds) *Equalities and Inequalities in Family Life*. London: Academic Press.

Crompton R and Sanderson K (1990) *Gendered Jobs and Social Change*. London: Unwin Hyman.

Ermisch J (1989) Divorce: economic antecedents and aftermath. In H Joshi (Ed) *The Changing Population of Britain*. Oxford: Basil Blackwell.

Finch J and Mason J (1993) *Negotiating Family Responsibilities*. London: Routledge.

Graham H (1987) Being poor: perceptions and coping strategies of lone mothers. In J Brannen and G Wilson (Eds) *Give and Take in Families: Studies in Resource Distribution*. London: Allen & Unwin.

Graham H (1993) *Hardship and Health in Women's Lives*. Hemel Hempstead: Harvester-Wheatsheaf.

Hardey M and Crow G (1991) *Lone Parenthood: Coping with Constraints and Making Opportunities*. Hemel Hempstead: Harvester-Wheatsheaf.

Haskey J (1993) Trends in the numbers of one-parent families in Great Britain. *Population Trends* **71**: 26–33.

Haskey J (1994) Step-families and step-children in Great Britain. *Population Trends* **76**: 17–28.

Heatherington M and Arasteh J (1988) *Impact of Divorce, Single Parenting and Stepparenting on Children*. Hillsdale, NJ: Lawrence Erlbaum.

Mansfield P and Collard J (1988) *The Beginning of the Rest of Your Life? A Portrait of Newly-Wed Marriage*. Basingstoke: Macmillan.

Millar J (1992) Lone mothers and poverty. In C Glendinning and J Millar (Eds) *Women and Poverty in Britain: The Nineties*. Hemel Hempstead: Harvester-Wheatsheaf.

Popay J and Jones G (1990) Patterns of health and illness amongst lone parents. *Journal of Social Policy* **19**: 499–534.

Qureshi H and Walker A (1989) *The Caring Relationship: Elderly People and Their Families*. Basingstoke: Macmillan.

Ungerson C (1994) *Women and Social Policy: A Reader*. Basingstoke: Macmillan.

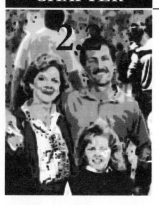

2.

THE FAMILY: A PSYCHOLOGICAL PERSPECTIVE

Neil Frude

KEY ISSUES

- The benefits of family relationships
- The family and health
- Differences between families
- Healthy and dysfunctional families

INTRODUCTION

The aim of the chapter is to provide a basic framework for thinking, psychologically, about families, rather than to summarize knowledge about the effects of particular events on families. An extensive review of the impact of illness, handicap, divorce, bereavement etc., on family life has been provided elsewhere (Frude, 1991). In the first part of this chapter the family as the background or context for the individual will be examined and family relationships will be shown to be important determinants of a person's physical health and psychological well-being. The second half of the chapter will focus on the family group or unit. The nature of 'healthy' and 'dysfunctional' families will be explored, and the way different types of families might respond when one of their number becomes ill, will be considered.

Medicine, as an applied biological science, has traditionally regarded the individual person (or, even, the individual body) as the principal unit of examination, diagnosis and treatment. In most cases attention usually narrows to one or more 'sub-systems' (the respiratory system, the cardiovascular system, etc.). Some physicians, and a majority of nurses, may have maintained a 'whole person' perspective, but traditionally relatively little attention has been paid to wider systems such as the family and the community. In the past few decades, however, there has been a growing acknowledgement of the important influences of wider systems, and 'family medicine', 'family nursing', 'family therapy', 'community medicine', and 'community nursing' have all become well-established disciplines.

In this chapter some of the ways of thinking about families from a psychological perspective will be examined. It needs to be acknowledged at the outset that there are many other ways of looking at family issues, including those offered by the political, ethical, legal and sociological perspectives. The various perspectives should not be regarded as competing or contradictory, but they do offer distinct analyses by virtue of the different issues they identify and the diverse ways in which they examine these issues. Thus whereas the sociologist is generally concerned with the family as an institution in society, and often emphasizes the relationship between the family and wider systems (the health service, for example, or the benefits system), psychologists are typically more concerned with the interactions and relationships within particular families and how these change as a result of the impact of events such as illness, death or the birth of a child.

The Family as the Context for the Individual

The Value of Family Relationships

Being part of a family brings a number of costs and benefits to an individual. If a person decides that the costs of family membership outweigh the benefits (so that family membership has a negative value), then he or she may decide to withdraw from the family. According to one influential psychological theory ('social exchange theory'), the decisions that people make about their lives, including their family life, reflect their own cost-benefit analyses (Nye, 1982). This kind of analysis has been used, for example, to explain why people choose to have (or not to have) children, why they may choose to separate, and why they may choose to engage in extramarital affairs. A good deal of research has been aimed at discovering what people want (i.e. the benefits they hope for) from relationships, and what they wish to avoid (i.e. the costs). Some adults who have had an unsatisfactory marital relationship in the past make the judgement that no such relationship in the future would be 'worth it'. The majority of people in this position, however, do look forward to a better relationship in the future and exert considerable effort to find 'the right person'. When interviewed, such people are able to say what they are looking for in a relationship – they are able to provide a list of hoped-for benefits.

In an age in which there is a very high rate of marital breakdown (some estimates suggest that around 50% of all those who are currently getting married will eventually divorce), in which there is a high rate of marital violence and child abuse, and in which few people would maintain that their family relationships are completely harmonious, it might be tempting to conclude that the family is a disaster area and that people would be better off without family ties. (For more detailed discussion of some of these issues, see Chapter 2.1.) Such a conclusion would not be warranted, however, because *on average* people value their relationships positively (despite acknowledging problems) and there is strong evidence that, on the whole, close relationships bring more benefits than they exact costs. Overall, an intimate relationship has a positive value for the individuals involved.

When people are asked what makes them happy, what provides them with satisfaction, and what gives meaning to their lives, they emphasize their close relationships much more than any other aspect of their lives, including their occupation, hobbies, health or money (Freedman, 1978). This is not to deny that many people blame a key relationship for their unhappiness, or that intimate relationships often provoke the most intense anger, anxiety and sadness, but – on the whole – people do assess the impact of their closest relationships in positive rather than in negative terms. Furthermore, in support of such subjective assessments, there is objective evidence suggesting that the effect of close relationships is more often favourable than unfavourable.

Relationships and Life Events

It is now well established that psychological and physical health is profoundly affected by life events such as divorce, the birth of a child, a bereavement, or moving house. Several lists (or 'inventories') of commonly experienced life events have been compiled (each item is given a score reflecting the relative strength or likely impact of the event), and these can be used to assess how much 'life change' an individual has experienced in the past six months, or the past year. The total life change score for an individual has been found to predict many aspects of the individual's health, including susceptibility to infection, and the risk of being involved in a serious accident. Generally speaking, those who have experienced several major changes are more vulnerable to physical and psychological illness than those whose life has recently been without such changes.

An examination of the various life event inventories (for example, those compiled by Holmes and Rahe, 1967, and by Paykel *et al.*, 1976) reveals that a very high proportion of the events which have critical implications for individuals are directly related to family life (such events include the illness of a family member, a bereavement, a child leaving home, marital separation and sexual problems).

Lists of positive events also show a preponderance of family-related items (Argyle and Henderson, 1985), and the same is true of minor positive and negative events (sometimes referred to as 'uplifts' and 'hassles', respectively). Those who live in a family setting have lives which are relatively full of incident. Compared with those who live in isolation, they experience more 'entrances' (such as the birth of a child) and more 'exits' (the death of a family member, marital separation, or a young adult leaving home). They experience more 'uplifts' (such as birthdays, anniversaries, and school successes) but they also experience more 'hassles' (such as minor illnesses of family members, or family rows). Those who live in isolation are often lonely, and many feel that their life lacks interest, excitement, or involvement. Whereas many early studies stressed the potential danger of exposure to 'excess life change', it is now appreciated that a modest degree of incident and transition may actually promote health.

Intimacy, Well-being and Health

It is possible to assess, at least roughly, how happy people are, how lonely they feel, and how stressed they feel, simply by asking them to rate their own levels of happiness, loneliness and stress on a fixed scale (say, from 'very happy' through to 'very unhappy'). Studies in this vein reveal a number of interesting findings. For example, Wood *et al.*, (1989) conducted a 'meta-analysis' whereby they re-analysed the findings from 93 previously published studies that had addressed the issue of happiness and positive well-being. They showed that, overall, women reported greater happiness and life satisfaction than men (despite the fact that women are twice as likely to be clinically depressed as men). They also showed that marriage was associated with higher levels of well-being both for women and for men (contradicting an earlier suggestion that marriage made men happier but women less happy; Bernard, 1973).

Other studies which have compared the self-reports of married people, single people, the widowed, and the divorced, concerning their happiness, loneliness and stress, also indicate that those who are currently married have fewer problems and have a greater sense of positive well-being than those in any of the other groups (Frude, 1991).

Objective indicators point in the same direction. Overall, married people have better physical health than those who have never married or are divorced or widowed. They are less likely, for example, to suffer from asthma, diabetes, ulcers, tuberculosis, cancer of the mouth and throat, hypertension, strokes and coronaries (Lynch, 1977; Reed *et al.*, 1983; Cohen and Syme, 1985). The association between health and being married is even apparent in mortality data. Compared with those who are single, widowed or divorced, few married people die young (Verbrugge, 1979; Berkman and Syme, 1979; Perlman and Rook, 1987). A broadly similar pattern emerges when we consider the statistics for mental health. When groups of people matched for age, sex and social class are compared in terms of their psychiatric history, morbidity rates are lowest for the married population (Bloom *et al.*, 1979; Gove, 1979). General community surveys also reveal that married people experience the fewest psychological symptoms, with an intermediate rate among widowed and never-married adults, and the highest rates among those who are divorced or separated.

Before we conclude that 'marriage is good for you', however, it does need to be stressed that the statistics merely show an average advantage for those who are married. We must not disregard the fact that many people find their marital relationship to be oppressive or violent, and that conflict and aggression can jeopardize health not only as a result of physical injury but also as a result of psychological distress. Some people, undoubtedly, would improve in their health if their current oppressive relationship were to end. Divorce is often a major stressor, but once a divorced person has adjusted to a new lifestyle, he or she may be healthier and better adjusted than many of those who have opted to remain in a conflictual or violent marital relationship (Frude, 1991).

Why Do Good Relationships Promote Health?

Several explanations are possible for the association between a stable, intimate relationship and an individual's health. One explanation is that a person with a secure relationship is likely to have a greater sense of well-being than someone who lacks a partner, and that as a result they may be less vulnerable to stress. Another suggestion is that a partner may be useful during critical periods, for example when the individual faces a major life change. One way in which a partner may help is by listening to the person's worries and providing informal therapy. In their study of the social origins of depression among women, Brown and Harris (1978) found that the presence of an intimate and confidante was associated with low vulnerability to stressful events. People often 'consult' their partners when under emotional strain, and many report that they derived great comfort from their partner's counsel and that it helped to see them through a crisis. Health and counselling professionals are often a 'last resort' for those who seek help for psychological problems. Relatives, friends, work colleagues, neighbours, volunteer helpers (for example, the Samaritans) and other professionals (for example, vicars, priests and rabbis) are frequently used as counsellors, advisers and 'sounding boards'. However, when people are asked whom they 'really depend on' when personal problems arise, they are more likely to cite their partner than anyone else (Griffith, 1985). Informal psychotherapy is a feature of the majority of marriages and it has been found that those who are satisfied with their partner's 'therapeutic' efforts are likely to be satisfied with the marriage as a whole (Nye and McLaughlin, 1982).

The presence of a partner may also contribute to health because of its regulatory effect. Partners, relatives and close friends often encourage a person to comply with certain 'rules' and help them to refrain from dangerous activities (Hughes and Gove, 1981). Thus a partner will often keep a watchful eye on an individual's smoking and drinking, encouraging them to eat well, to exercise regularly, to attend for medical checkups and to comply with medical advice. Those who are socially isolated are not able to benefit from such encouragement, and need not be concerned about their partner's censure. For this reason, and because they may be particularly distressed, those who are without a partner are more likely to lead disordered lives and to expose themselves to danger. Thus many of those who are newly divorced eat and sleep irregularly, smoke, and drink to excess.

The Family Unit

So far we have considered family relationships (especially marital relationships) in terms of their costs and benefits to the individual. In a sense then, we have maintained an individual perspective, considering the family as a 'context' or 'backdrop' which can help to explain variations in health and well-being. A somewhat different perspective on the family will now be taken. Families are not merely 'backdrops for individuals'. Neither are they simply collections of individual people. A family is, metaphorically, an organic unit in which 'the whole is greater than the sum of the parts'. A family unit, indeed, can be viewed as if it were an organism in which the individual family members are constituent elements. The organism metaphor can be a fruitful one, for it leads to a number of interesting questions. What are the anatomical features of this type of organism? What is known of its physiology? What is known of the life cycle? What variations are there between different organisms (families)? And what forms of pathology are found?

Like organisms, families pass through a developmental sequence or 'career'. They are 'formed', they undergo changes, and in the end they 'die'. Some analysts divide the 'family life cycle' into a number of stages. Duvall (1977), for example, formulated eight stages, starting with the married couple who have no children and ending with the ageing family – a stage that lasts from retirement until death. Such models are clearly oversimplified, but they can be useful in mapping broad patterns of change and identifying common problems at particular stages of development. Thus the pressures typically experienced by 'young families' are somewhat different from those faced by families with adolescent children. Families (like organisms) must adapt in response to both internal and external changes. The birth of a first child, for example, presents the couple with many new tasks and gives them new roles as parents. The family boundary becomes extended to include the infant, and there are marked changes in the nature of the couple's interactions. The original two-person ('dyadic') relationship (i.e. the couple) is replaced by three dyadic relationships (mother–father; mother–infant; and father–infant) and one 'triadic' relationship. Even with this simple arrangement we can begin to get some idea of the 'reverberations' that occur within families. For example, changes in the mother–infant relationship will affect the mother–father relationship and this in turn is likely to affect the mother–infant relationship (an example of what if referred to as 'circular causality'). The elements within a family system are not just the individual family members but also the relationships between them, and any change in one individual or one relationship will be likely to have effects on all other elements and on the 'tone' or 'atmosphere' of the family as a whole. Another metaphor which may be useful at this point is that of the family as a 'hanging mobile'. The elements of a mobile are the frame, the various suspended items, and the strings that link other elements together. Any change in one element will affect every other element as well as the position and movement of the mobile as a whole. It is impossible to move any element without having a global effect on the mobile. Furthermore, when any one element is moved the effect will be to move the other elements and these movements will then have a supplementary effect on the element which was originally moved.

Within a family system, any change such as an 'entrance' (a child being born; an elderly relative coming to live in the home) or an 'exit' (the death of a family member; an adolescent leaving) will have profound effects on individual family members and on the relationships between them and will sometimes completely transform the nature of the family interaction. Thus, in a family in which there is normally a good deal of hostility and open conflict, the knowledge that one family member is seriously ill may bring a period of apparent harmony and a cessation of hostilities. A family member who has previously appeared selfish and unhelpful may appear to change in his or her personality, suddenly becoming cooperative and helpful. Such personal changes will affect relationships between members and the overall 'family atmosphere', and this will have further effects on individuals. A crisis, such as that precipitated by a serious illness, can bring out the best in a family, although some are adversely affected and become unable to function effectively. Any family is likely to experience several 'entrances' and 'exits' throughout its life-time, and many other changes will also alter the pattern of family relationships. Over a thirty or forty year span there may be a complete reversal in roles, as the once-helpless infants grow towards middle-age and perhaps eventually take on the care of their aged parents. Thus even the normal processes of family development demand major changes in structure, while many families will also face more exceptional circumstances (the birth of a handicapped child, for example, or the sudden death of a young parent) that will require additional major adaptations.

Differences Between Families

Many different ways might be found to classify families. One obvious variation is that of structure. Some families are single parent units while others are two-parent families. Some families are childless, some have a single child, some have two children, etc. Families also differ in terms of their stage of development. Thus there are couples who have just formed a partnership and as yet have no children, there are families with young children, families with adolescent children, and 'empty nest' families in which all of the children have grown to adulthood and left home. It is easy to see some of the difficulties which might be involved in trying to classify families even in terms of their structure. Thus in the various lists given above, three-generational aspects have not been included. Step-families (or 'reconstituted families' as they are sometimes known), or families in which two partners of the same gender live with or without children, have also not been mentioned. Even when dealing with family membership (or 'family configuration'), the possibilities are almost endless.

Family Interaction Styles

It is sometimes useful to group families together in terms of a common structural characteristic; for example if we wish to understand (or to make policies for) single-parent families or, say, lesbian families. However, it soon becomes clear that families which may share a structural characteristic differ markedly in terms of the interactions between family members. Psychologists are typically less interested in structural characteristics than in interactional characteristics and therefore tend to identify families in terms of their 'interactive styles' or 'socio-emotional style'. Thus a psychologist might wish to differentiate between 'harmonious' and 'conflictual' families or, perhaps, 'happy families' and 'depressed families'. Of course there are many thousands of such characteristics, some of which are likely to be much more important than others. Of all the dimensions which can be used to differentiate between the interactive styles of families, two have been consistently identified as providing a useful basis for classification. These two dimensions, identified clinically by experienced therapists and also by means of research, are 'adaptability' and 'cohesion'. 'Adaptability' refers to the family's ability to change its structure, roles and rules when adjustment is called for. 'Cohesion' relates to the degree of emotional bonding between family members and to their independence and autonomy. According to the 'Circumplex Model' devised by Olson and his colleagues (Olson *et al.*, 1979), families can be classified into one of four 'types' on each of the two key dimensions which are identified in Box 2.2.1.

The labels used for the extremes of each dimension were chosen to convey the belief that all extreme positions are relatively 'unhealthy'. Thus families at either end of the adaptability dimension (i.e. both rigid and chaotic families) are likely to experience special problems, particularly when they face a need to change.

Families classified in terms of the middle positions on the adaptability dimensions (i.e. structured and flexible families) would be expected to respond to change more effectively.

In *'rigid' families* each member has established or has been assigned a number of specific roles and will rarely stray beyond his or her allotted position. The power structure within such families is inflexible, leadership is authoritarian, and discipline is managed in an autocratic way. 'Rules are rules' and compromise is rare. At the other extreme, *chaotic families* have few clear rules, so that without established patterns many things have to be negotiated 'from scratch'. If, for example, no chores are ever seen as 'belonging' to any individual then discussion (and, perhaps, conflict) will need to take place whenever something needs to be done. The power structure within such families is unstable, and support and permission are given in an irregular and arbitrary fashion. The lack of rules frequently leads to confusion, children lack guidance, and parental discipline is likely to be erratic and inconsistent.

The other dimension in the Circumplex Model is *'cohesion'*. Families that are very low in terms of cohesion are said to be 'disengaged' while those that have extremely high cohesion are described as 'enmeshed'. Families classified in positions between these extremes are described either as 'connected' or as 'separated', and such families are held to be well-placed in terms of cohesion, avoiding the lack of family unity and family feeling typical of disengaged families while also avoiding the suffocating closeness found in enmeshed families. Members of enmeshed families identify with the family very closely and the bonds between members are so tight that individuals have little sense of personal identity.

Dysfunctional Families

Many families can be identified as occupying an extreme position on one of the two dimensions of adaptability and cohesion. Some families, indeed, occupy extreme positions on both dimensions (they may be rigid–disengaged, rigid–enmeshed, chaotic–disengaged or chaotic–enmeshed). A family placed at one of the extremes

Box 2.2.1. The Circumplex Model (Olson *et al.*, 1979)

On the *'adaptability'dimension*, the classification proceeds from one extreme – *'rigid'* – through *'structured'* and then *'flexible'* to the other extreme – *'chaotic'*.

On the *'cohesion'* dimension, the classification proceeds from one extreme – *'enmeshed'* – through *'connected'* and then *'separated'* to the other extreme – *'disengaged'*.

on one or both dimensions is likely to have difficulty in maintaining a good level of functioning and in providing for the needs and personal growth of family members. Dysfunctional families are likely to develop problems even without external pressures, and their inadequacies are especially likely to become apparent when they are placed under severe stress. Thus whereas some families are able to work together, to be strong and supportive, and to avoid conflict when a family member has a serious accident, for example, or when a chronic disorder is diagnosed, dysfunctional families may be thrown into a crisis from which they cannot escape. The extreme stress generated by such a situation can then have adverse consequences for the health of other family members, and the family may 'break down' under the unbearable strain.

Dysfunctional families provide a major challenge for the health professional. Enmeshed families tend to be 'closed' to the outside world and are so used to keeping themselves to themselves that they are likely to regard all agencies and professionals with suspicion and disdain. The tight-knit nature of enmeshed families may mean that when one person becomes seriously ill every other family member feels personally stricken. At the other extreme, in a disengaged family, there is little family feeling. When one member becomes ill, the others will resent the inconvenience and will attempt to carry on their own lives regardless of their relative's illness or disability. The professional cannot rely on such families to offer significant emotional and practical support to the patient. Such families may avoid taking any share in patient care and expect professionals to 'do everything'. If a patient is hospitalized, for example, family members may try to insist that the patient should remain in hospital until she or he has completely recovered. They are likely to make high demands on community services, almost as if they are claiming that the patient's care is 'none of our business'. The two extremes on the adaptability dimension are labelled 'rigid' and 'chaotic'. Faced with the illness of one family member, a rigid family will find it difficult, or even impossible, to make appropriate adaptations. If the father is incapacitated, for example, his routine tasks will be left undone. No-one will attempt, temporarily, to 'step into his shoes'. The family will find it very demanding to make allowances for the new situation and to work out solutions to the new problems they face, and this may mean that family life becomes untenable. The challenge for the health professional is to help such a family to change its rules and interactional patterns sufficiently so that the patient is protected from undue pressure to 'carry on as normal' when she or he is unable to do so.

Finally, chaotic families have very few established patterns of interaction or problem-solving and are therefore very ineffective in dealing with a crisis such as a serious illness. Because they are unable to 'get their act together' even in normal circumstances they are likely to be completely thrown when a threatening situation arises. Such families may be willing to help the patient, but because they consult one another very little and engage in little forward planning, many of their attempts to adapt to a changed situation are doomed to failure. In providing such families with directions for patient care, it may be necessary to be highly specific in suggesting a timetable and allocating particular tasks to individuals. The normal assumption that a family will work out its own routines and devise strategies for handing over responsibility, etc., does not apply to families that are extremely chaotic in their organization.

Some families that manage to adapt fairly well to a patient's illness have difficulty in readjusting when the patient is recovering. In some of these families a person effectively maintains the patient role long after a return to health. In some cases an individual's recovery from a physical or psychiatric illness threatens to disturb a precarious and convenient equilibrium within the family, and the family as a whole may then have a 'vested interest' in the patient remaining unwell. Family therapists have long recognized the fact that an illness may be 'useful' to a family (for example, by postponing serious long-term arguments that threaten to destroy the family). Family therapy addresses such issues by dealing with the family system as a whole (Burnham, 1986).

All families maintain certain 'myths', most of which are harmless and some of which are constructive. When a family member is seriously ill, for example, many families develop positive myths about the quality of service they are receiving. They may regard their general practitioner as a leading authority in a highly specialized field, for instance, or imagine that the local clinic is internationally renowned for its treatment of the illness from which their relative is suffering. For the most part, such myths instil hope, alleviate anxiety, and contribute to good relations between the family and professionals. However, some families subscribe to a 'rescue myth' which can encourage passivity. According to such a myth, the family only has to wait and someone will come along who can provide all the help they need, rescue them from their predicament, and provide a perfect solution to all of their problems. Any likely professional may therefore be treated as a potential saviour, and family members may believe that there is no point in them actively seeking to improve the current situation without the help of such a person (Stierlin, 1973).

Other families, including many that are dysfunctional, will develop negative myths about the nature of the illness, about the professionals involved in the patient's care, and about the quality of service being provided. Such myths may jeopardize the patient's recovery in a number of ways (for example, they may lead a family to seek help from unqualified people or may reduce compliance with medical advice). It is important to identify negative myths about the nature of the illness, and it is also important to recognize that some families have well-established suspicions about all aspects of health care. In some cases this may lead to one or more professionals being unfairly 'scapegoated' by the family.

Healthy Families

Well-functioning, or 'healthy' families occupy the middle ground in terms of both adaptability and cohesion. They are neither rigid nor chaotic, neither disengaged nor enmeshed. Family members have reasonably warm and close relationships with one another, each identifying with the family as a whole and having some sense of 'family pride'. Within such families members share common goals. There is a general air of solidarity, but each person is also allowed to be an individual. Healthy families act as 'open' systems and are willing to accept help and advice from external sources. They interact with neighbours, they do not feel isolated from the community, and their interactions with other groups are generally positive.

Healthy families share power fairly, and everyone is encouraged to share their opinions and feelings. Such a sharing of power, however, does not mean that all members are treated as equals. The parents exercise control over the children and they work together to this end. Roles within the family are clearly differentiated and are complementary. Tasks are assigned fairly and appropriately to particular individuals, but some degree of flexibility is maintained so that when one person is unavailable another person is able to take on some of his or her responsibilities.

Family 'rules' are understood and supported by all family members, and infringements of these rules are confronted openly. Appropriate sanctions are applied firmly but without hostility or vindictiveness. Family rules are changed when necessary (for example, as children get older) and such changes are brought about through a process of negotiation.

Communication within healthy families is open and effective. Questions are clearly asked and plainly answered, and all transactions have a clear ending (Satir, 1972). Family members are able to disclose their opinions, hopes and fears without anxiety and there is also a healthy respect for an individual's (or the couple's) privacy. When conflicts arise they are usually resolved by negotiation and compromise. Healthy families are able to deal effectively with a wide range of challenges, for they have at their disposal a wide repertoire of effective coping strategies and are able to respond flexibly.

CONCLUSION

Although many families are devastated by serious troubles, in many cases both individuals and family units manage to endure the most formidable upsets and tragedies. Families often adapt to severe misfortune with remarkable resourcefulness. Thus despite the fact that family life often produces extreme anxiety, fear or depression, and despite the fact that many families break down in disarray, the majority show remarkable persistence and resilience. During times of change or crisis, however, a family's inner resources may not be sufficient to bring about effective coping, and support from other sources - from relatives, neighbours, community organizations and from professionals - can make a substantial contribution to the well-being of the family system and of the individuals who constitute the family group.

SUMMARY

- Increasingly, health professionals are coming to recognize that in order to provide the best medical care they must work not just with individuals patients but with the patient and his or her family.
- Psychologists study the interactions and relationships within families and the effects of events such as illness, death or the birth of a child.
- The family can be regarded either as the individual's 'intimate social context' or as a 'thing in itself' – the family system.
- Being part of a family brings numerous costs and benefits to the individual. In the majority of cases the benefits outweigh the costs (and thus the family has a positive value for the individual).
- On the whole, it seems that families are good for people's health. Thus those who are married have, on average, better physical health and better mental health than those who are single, divorced or widowed.
- 'The family' can be regarded as a dynamic and evolving system.
- Families differ in their interaction styles. Some can be regarded as 'healthy' and others as 'dysfunctional'.
- On the whole, families are resilient and resourceful. However, families sometimes need professional help in order to adapt successfully to change and to cope with the stressful impact of a crisis such as that induced by a major illness of a family member.

DISCUSSION
QUESTIONS

♦ Attempt to define the term 'family'. How does a family differ from another group such as a committee or a sports team?

♦ Overall, the available evidence suggests that family life brings many benefits to the individual. However, some family situations impose great hardship on the individual. Based on your personal and professional experience, discuss such 'costly' family situations (when referring to specific families, be sure to protect their anonymity).

♦ What effects might a patient's family have on the practice of nurses working (a) in a hospital setting, and (b) in a community setting.

♦ On the whole, married men and women are physically and psychologically healthier than divorced and widowed people of the same age. How can this be explained?

FURTHER READING

Burnham JB (1986) *Family Therapy: First Steps Towards a Systemic Approach*. London: Tavistock.
An excellent and easy-to-read introduction to family therapy theory and practice.

Dallos R and McLaughlin E (Eds) (1993) *Social Problems and the Family*. London: Sage.
Covers domestic violence, mental health, old age, poverty and homelessness. Clear and up-to-date.

Frude NJ (1991) *Understanding Family Problems: A Psychological Approach*. Chichester: Wiley.
An introduction to family psychology, and a detailed review of psychological research on illness, bereavement, violence and divorce.

Noller P and Callan VJ (1991) *The Adolescent in the Family*. London: Routledge.

Comprehensive psychological approach to family relationships when one or more children are at the adolescent stage.

Orford J (Ed) (1987) *Treating the Disorder, Treating the Family*. Baltimore: Johns Hopkins University Press.
Deals with a variety of psychiatric disorders, emphasizing the role played by social (and especially family) factors and the impact of the condition on the family.

Weber AL and Harvey JH (Eds) (1994) *Perspectives on Close Relationships*. Boston: Allyn and Bacon.
Introduces the ways in which psychologists have studied close relationships, and examines the state of knowledge on such topics as marital communication and social support.

REFERENCES

Argyle M and Henderson M (1985) *The Anatomy of Relationships*. Harmondsworth: Penguin.

Berkman LF and Syme SL (1979) Social networks, host resistance and mortality: A nine-year follow-up study of Almeda residents. *American Journal of Epidemiology* **109**: 186.

Bernard J (1973) *The Future of Marriage*. New York: Bantam.

Bloom BL, Asher SR and White SW (1979) Marital disruption as a stressor. *Psychological Bulletin* **85**: 867.

Brown GW and Harris T (1978) *The Social Origins of Depression*. London: Tavistock.

Burnham JB (1986) *Family Therapy: First Steps Towards a Systemic Approach*. London: Tavistock.

Cohen S and Syme SL (Eds) (1985) *Social Support and Health*. New York: Academic Press.

Duvall E (1977) *Marriage and Family Development*. Philadelphia: JB Lippincott.

Freedman JL (1978) *Happy People*. New York: Harcourt Brace Jovanovich.

Frude NJ (1991) *Understanding Family Problems: A Psychological Approach*. Chichester: Wiley.

Gove WR (1979) The relationship between sex roles, marital status and mental illness. *Social Forces* **51:** 34.

Griffith J (1985) Social support providers: Who are they? Where are they met? And the relationship of network characteristics to psychological distress. *Basic and Applied Social Psychology* **6:** 41.

Holmes TH and Rahe RH (1967) The Social Readjustment Rating Scales. *Journal of Psychosomatic Research* **11:** 213.

Hughes M and Gove WR (1981) Living alone, social integration and mental health. *American Journal of Community Psychology* **87:** 48.

Lynch JJ (1977) *The Broken Heart*. New York: Basic Books.

Nye FI (1982) *Family Relationships: Rewards and Costs*. Beverly Hills, CA: Sage.

Nye FI and McLaughlin S (1982) Role competence and marital satisfaction. In FI Nye *Family Relationships: Rewards and Costs*. Beverly Hills, CA: Sage.

Olson DH, Russell CS and Sprenkle DH (1979) Circumplex model of marital and family systems II: Empirical studies and clinical intervention. In LJ Vincent (Ed) *Advances in Family Intervention, Assessment and Theory*. Greenwich, CT: JAI.

Paykel ES, McGuinness B and Gomez J (1976) An Anglo-American comparison of the scaling of life-events. *British Journal of Medical Psychology* **49:** 237.

Perlman, D and Rook KS (1987) Social support, social deficits, and the family: Toward the enhancement of well-being. In S Oskamp (Ed) *Family Processes and Problems: Social Psychological Aspects*. Beverly Hills, CA: Sage.

Reed D, McGee D, Yano K and Feinleib M (1983) Social networks and coronary heart disease among Japanese men in Hawaii. *American Journal of Epidemiology* **115:** 384.

Satir V (1972) *Peoplemaking*. Palo Alto, CA: Science and Behaviour Books.

Stierlin H (1973) Group fantasies and family myths: Some theoretical and practical aspects. *Family Process* **12:** 111.

Verbrugge LM (1979) Marital status and health. *Journal of Marriage and the Family* **41:** 267.

Wood W, Rhodes N and Whelan M (1989) Sex differences in positive well-being: A consideration of emotional style and marital status. *Psychological Bulletin* **106:** 249.

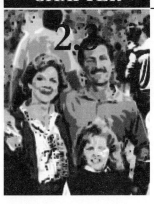

ABUSE WITHIN FAMILIES

Neil Frude

KEY ISSUES

- The widespread nature of family violence
- The interactional model of family violence
- Hostile and instrumental aggression
- Elder abuse and the 'burden of care'
- Sexual abuse as 'seduction'

INTRODUCTION

There are many forms of abuse within families, including physical (injurious) abuse, sexual abuse, emotional abuse and neglect. Abuse may take place between members of the same generation (marital abuse or sibling abuse) or between different generations (e.g. child abuse by parents, or elder abuse).

The grid opposite (Box 2.3.1) provides an overview of some forms of family based abuse. The columns specify particular forms of abuse and the rows specify the family relationship between the victim and the perpetrator.

It would not be difficult to quote cases which illustrate each of the 16 boxes in the above figure. Box 10, for example, would include marital rape, and Box 16 would include cases in which the needs of elderly people are neglected by other family members.

In this chapter we will consider three types of physical abuse (the physical abuse of children, marital violence and elder abuse, Boxes 1, 9 and 13) and child sexual abuse (Boxes 2 and 6) will also be considered.

Violence within the Family

The family is the setting for a substantial proportion of the violence that occurs within society. Most estimates agree that in any average week at least two children in the UK die as a result of a violent attack by a parent or caregiver; many more women are seriously injured as a result of marital battering than as a result of road accidents and street violence; and violence is a significant cause of bruising and more severe injuries among old people living with relatives. Estimates of the prevalence of the various forms of family violence depend to a great extent on the definitions used, and on diagnostic criteria, but it is clear from all of the available evidence that many forms of family violence are all too common.

Box 2.3.1 Family based abuse

	Physical abuse	Sexual abuse	Emotional abuse	Neglect
Parent to child	1	2	3	4
Sibling	5	6	7	8
Marital	9	10	11	12
Elderly victims	13	14	15	16

Explanations of Family Violence

The issue of how family violence is best explained is somewhat controversial. Some authorities consider violence in families to be a 'natural' effect of the kind of society in which we live, and a reflection of the attitudes that adults generally have towards children and that men generally have towards women. Others, while not denying the relevance of the cultural climate, suggest that acts of domestic violence are 'deviant' behaviours that are explained as aggressive responses to interpersonal conflict. Such 'interactional' explanations account for physical abuse by focusing on the relationships and interactions between the assailant and the victim, particularly in conflict between the assailant and the victim, particularly in conflict and disciplinary situations, and attribute the violence to the assailant's high level of anger and low level of inhibition regarding the aggressive assault.

In trying to understand particular incidents of family violence it is useful to bear in mind the distinction between hostile and instrumental violence. Hostile violence is driven by anger and the principal motive for the action is that of hurting the victim. Instrumental violence is driven principally by a desire for certain 'gains', with aggression being used merely as a means to this end. Thus the 'mugger' is aggressive not because he wishes to hurt his victim but because he believes that his attack will enable him to steal money.

Some incidents of family violence are best explained as examples of instrumental aggression. A husband may be violent towards his wife, for example, because he believes that violence will enable him to 'get his own way' or that violence will help to maintain 'a reign of terror' which will give him the power to dominate his wife and the freedom to do as he wishes. Instrumental violence may also be used strategically to 'teach' the wife that a beating will follow if she criticizes, makes claims on resources, or refuses any demand.

On the other hand, most incidents of marital violence, physical child abuse and elder abuse are probably best understood as examples of hostile aggression. Typically, one member of the family does something which makes another member very angry, and in the absence of sufficient inhibitions the angry person then assaults the victim. This simple model suggests that in order to understand the nature of family violence we need to understand anger triggers, the way in which individuals appraise other people's behaviour, the dynamics of anger, and inhibitions against physical violence. The model also suggests that effective interventions might involve strategies for reducing anger, for increasing inhibitions, and for maintaining self-control (Frude, 1991).

The interactional model will form the basis for much of the analysis provided in this chapter, and the discussion will focus, for the most part, on hostile rather than on instrumental violence. Three types of family violence will be examined – physical child abuse, marital violence and elder abuse. But first the general issue of why violent assaults occur so frequently in so many families will be considered.

Why Is There So Much Violence Within The Family?

One reason why family violence may be considerably more common than street violence, or violence towards neighbours, friends and work colleagues, is that contact between family members is prolonged and is often intense. People who live together, eat together, sleep together and play together will be in close proximity for so much of the time that strong emotions, including anger, are likely to be generated at least occasionally. In addition, family members are locked into the family situation. It is possible to avoid or to walk away from an annoying stranger, but a demanding child or a crying baby cannot be avoided or ignored.

Irritating behaviours such as constant 'complaints' or 'nags' by one partner about the other, a child's persistent attention seeking, or a baby's continual 'grizzling', are likely to lead to extreme annoyance. Family members are interdependent, and the behaviour of one of them can affect everyone else. A person who invests a lot of time and energy in helping or caring for others is likely to feel aggrieved if there is no appreciation of the effort involved. Babies, children and the elderly infirm, especially, demand a great deal of attention and their care involves considerable costs in time, effort and money. It is understandable that a carer might become angry in response to an apparent lack of gratitude or when additional demands are made (for example, if an infant soils a nappy immediately following a change, or if a child refuses to eat food that has taken a long time to prepare).

Anger may also result when there is a conflict over the allocation of space, money or other resources, and such disputes may be especially bitter if the relevant resources are very limited (for example, if the family is poor). Thus some marital fights concern money, with one partner being accused of wasting money (for example, on drink or gambling). Other conflicts focus on the allocation of duties, responsibilities and household chores. Those who feel that they are being exploited or are being 'taken for granted' are likely to object, and their complaint will often lead to conflict.

Anger is often preceded by the judgement that someone has behaved badly or has 'broken a rule', and family life is governed by so many rules. Rules and transgressions, or supposed transgressions, are bound to feature prominently in family interactions. Verbal complaints regarding rule-breaking usually include 'should' or 'ought'. Accusations that are felt by the target to be unwarranted or unfair may lead to a protestation of innocence or to a counter-accusation. Real or supposed transgressions frequently initiate an episode which ultimately results in violence. Some parents even judge that very young babies are guilty of rule-breaking and regard certain aspects of the infant's behaviour as 'naughty' and 'blameworthy'.

Family violence is not simply a reflection of the fact that family situations frequently generate anger, but also reflects the fact that people have relatively few inhibitions in the home situation. In most other contexts expressions of anger are regularly inhibited, or at least 'toned down', but people often have few reservations about expressing their disagreement with other members of the family, making complaints to them, or even threatening them. In contrast to a disagreement arising in a work situation, for example, or a dispute with a neighbour, family conflicts may involve little verbal sparring before a rapid onslaught of insults and disparagements focuses on particularly sensitive areas. Family members know about each other's vulnerabilities and therefore have the 'advantage' being able to inflict maximum hurt.

Furthermore, inhibitions against physical aggression are often particularly low in family situations, and many people feel justified in behaving aggressively towards family members within the home. Parents may believe that it is their right to physically discipline a child by smacking them, and some men feel that they have a right to physically abuse a wife who has 'misbehaved'. If pushing, pulling or slapping a relative is regarded as acceptable, and becomes habitual, physical aggression may occasionally escalate to a dangerous level to include punches, kicks and the use of weapons. In addition, many other constraints which normally inhibit violence towards strangers may be absent in the family situation. For example, a man may assume that, if he were to attack his wife, his child, or his aged mother, his actions would not come to the attention of the police. In addition, his physical size and strength may eliminate any fear of physical reprisal by his victim. If previous assaults have passed without serious repercussions then inhibitions about a further assault may be particularly low.

Thus it appears that family aggression is relatively common because a good deal of anger is generated in family situations and because there are relatively few inhibitions that prevent this anger from being expressed in the form of physical aggression.

Physical Child Abuse

Definition and Prevalence Most estimates of the prevalence of the physical abuse of children are based on extrapolations from injuries that are known to have been deliberately inflicted. Such methods, however, may lead to a serious underestimation, since only a proportion of injuries to children are ever reported, and some which are said to be accidental probably do result from a parental attack. Some people maintain that any assault on a child which leaves a bruise should count as a case of physical child abuse, while others go further and insist that any form of physical disciplining constitutes physical abuse (in which case over 90% of parents in the UK might be described as 'abusive'). Gelles (1979) pointed out that physical methods of discipline are used in the majority of homes and that the average child is subjected to literally thousands of slaps before he or she reaches adolescence. The definition of physical child abuse is therefore a matter of some controversy. Some people equate abuse with any physical disciplining method while others maintain a sharp distinction between such 'ordinary' behaviours and those which cause serious injury to a child.

Demographic Patterns Roughly equal numbers of boys and girls are victims of attacks made by a parent or caregiver, and the attacker is equally likely to be a man or a woman. Babies and young children are much more likely to be injured by their parents than older children (hence the term 'baby battering' originally used to describe physical child abuse), partly because the very young are physically more vulnerable, but also because babies are very demanding and need continuous care. They cry a lot, the reason for their crying is not always easy to judge, and it is impossible to 'reason' with them or to cajole, beg or threaten them in order to gain compliance. Factors associated with a relatively high risk of physical abuse include poor accommodation, poverty, marital instability and social isolation. At one stage it was hoped that information about such correlational factors would permit the identification of 'high-risk' families before any damage had been done to the child, but attempts at formulating a useful 'risk index' by this means have proved impractical (Browne and Saqi, 1988). The age of the child, and the quality of the everyday relationship between the parents and the child, protracted legal proceedings and a history of frequent placement changes are associated with relatively poor outcome (Lynch, 1988), while factors associated with a positive outcome include the child's retention of a basic sense of 'trust' in adults and the presence of supportive relatives (Wolfe, 1987).

An Explanation of Physical Child Abuse

According to the interactional model of physical child abuse (Frude, 1980, 1991; Kadushin and Martin, 1981) physical abuse is best understood as a form of aggression, a hostile attack made by an angry parent who has been intensely annoyed, usually by some action of the child victim. The child's behaviour instigates a high degree of parental anger so that, in the absence of effective inhibitions against attacking the child, an assault will occur. The suggestion that the victim's behaviour plays an important role in the events leading up to an attack does not mean, of course, that children are held to be responsible for the injuries that they suffer. Certain children, however, are more vulnerable to attack than others by virtue of their physical characteristics, their behavioural style, and their response to the parents' attempts at discipline (Martin, 1976). Parents who are at high risk of abusing a child include those with an aggressive personality, those who have poor childcare and disciplining skills, those whose beliefs about children are inappropriate, and those who generally lack self-control.

Briefly, the interactional model of physical child abuse suggests that a poor parent–child relationship is likely to lead to disciplinary problems, and that frequent and badly handled disciplinary encounters are likely to escalate in seriousness and may lead to habitual low-level aggression. A fuller account of this model has been provided elsewhere (Frude, 1989b, 1991).

Therapy for Abusive Families

Some parents confide to a professional that they are under considerable stress and that their child may be at risk, and many different types of treatment can be offered to such high-risk families. Parents who frequently use severe and dangerous methods of disciplining, for example, can be guided towards the use of more refined techniques that are not only more appropriate but are also much more effective. Parents may be helped to develop effective childcare skills, to manage their anger, and to formulate a range of 'escape tactics' for emergency use when they feel that they might attack the child (Kelly, 1983). Some parents have strong pro-punishment attitudes and these may need to be challenged directly by a therapist.

Child Sexual Abuse

Sexual interference with a child is a crime which sickens, angers or frightens most people, including those who deal professionally with victims and perpetrators. However, perpetrators are less likely to re-offend, and child victims are more likely to receive the protection and help they need, if the professionals who deal with them have an understanding of the problem that is based on accurate information rather than on moral outrage.

Most victims of sexual abuse are aged between 8 and 14 years. Girls are at somewhat greater risk than boys. At one time it was thought that almost all the perpetrators of sexual abuse were male, but it is now recognized that sexual abuse by females is by no means rare. Whereas physical abuse is an aggressive act carried out in anger and intended to hurt the victim, sexual abuse is essentially self-gratificatory behaviour in which there are few, if any, hostile feelings towards the victim. Sexual abuse is sometimes, but by no means always, perpetrated by a member of the victim's family (in which case it is referred to as 'intrafamilial abuse'). The victim's older brothers are the relatives most likely to be perpetrators of intrafamilial sexual abuse, but other perpetrators include the father, uncles, a grandfather and, in a small proportion of cases, a female relative.

In a minority of cases, sexual abuse involves intercourse with the victim. More common abusive actions include oral–genital contact, masturbation, fondling, exposure to pornography, and indecent exposure. The term 'incest' is best used in the legal sense (in which case it refers to intercourse between two people who have a close blood relationship – neither need be a child). Once a child has become a victim of intrafamilial sexual abuse, the victimization is likely to continue for some time; incidents may be numbered in hundreds, and the abuse may extend over several years (Frude, 1985).

Prevalence and Definition

The most frequently quoted estimate of the prevalence of sexual abuse within the UK is 10%, based on the 1984 MORI poll of over 2000 adults who reported their own childhood experiences (Baker and Duncan, 1985). This figure includes cases in which a child had been a victim of indecent exposure in a public situation. When these cases are excluded, the prevalence figure is halved, illustrating the general point that as the definition of any form of abuse becomes narrower the prevalence figures decrease. Although it is impossible to produce an accurate estimate of the number of children who are sexually abused (for example, an unknown number of undetected cases involve abuse in early infancy), it is clear that sexual abuse is much more common than was imagined until recent times. Inappropriate sexual attention leads many children to suffer greatly both during childhood and in the longer term (Haugaard and Repucci, 1988).

Explaining Abusive Behaviour

Why do adults interfere sexually with children? The idea that sexual abuse is perpetrated mainly by adults who are 'psychopathic', or 'psychotic', or 'criminal types' can now be dismissed. Evidence has shown that the vast majority of those who sexually abuse children do not engage in other forms of serious crime and are not suffering from any psychiatric condition. The term 'paedophile' is applied to men whose sexual interests exclusively concern young children. Paedophilia is a well-documented disorder and does account for a proportion of cases of sexual abuse, but the majority of those who commit sexual offences against children are not paedophiles, and this is especially true of perpetrators of intrafamilial abuse.

One model of sexual abuse portrays the behaviour as a variation of a 'normal' seduction patterning. The age of the seduction 'target', the inability to give informed consent, and the relationship between the victim and the 'seducer', make the sexual approach aberrant and unacceptable (Frude, 1982, 1989a). The model suggests that, either because they develop an inappropriate romantic passion for a particular child, or because they have unmet sexual urges, certain adults come to find a child sexually attractive. Some of these adults (the majority of whom are men) attempt to engage the child in sexual practices, usually through persuasion and the subtle exertion of power rather than through physical force. Power is a central feature of the model, since the adult is seen to misuse his power (his adult status, his 'rights' as a trusted family member, and his greater sophistication) to gain sexual access to the child. However, power is regarded as a means rather than an end, and the principal motive for sexual abuse, it is suggested, is not the acquisition of power but the pursuit of sexual excitement.

In an earlier section of this chapter we considered the issue of why the family context is the setting for so much violence. We can ask a similar question about sexual abuse, and suggest a number of reasons why sexual abuse is so often perpetrated against young family members. A child is likely to be trusting and compliant with a close relative, and some adults take advantage of their loving relationship with the child and regard the child as a legitimate target for a sexual advance. Family members generally have little suspicion that a child might be at risk from one of their number, and a potential perpetrator is therefore likely to have many opportunities to be alone with the child. Such opportunities can be used initially to implement gradual and subtle seduction initiation procedures (sometimes labelled 'grooming strategies') and later to engage in overt and repeated abuse. The child who has been initiated into abusive activities may feel obliged to continue to comply with the perpetrator's wishes, and may be especially susceptible to threats and bribes. The adult's position and power within the family may persuade him that even if the child were to disclose to other family members his denials would be believed and that, even if his protestations of innocence were not accepted, his secret would remain safely hidden within the family.

It is likely that many adults who recognize that they have sexual feelings towards a young person in the family are horrified by the implications and strive to eliminate any thought of sexual contact with the child. Such people may avoid close physical contact with the child and resist any opportunity to be alone with the child. Others eventually succumb to temptation by making excuses and attempting to rationalize their abusive behaviour, while others may weaken when under the influence of alcohol, or when they become highly sexually aroused. Some adults, of course, exhibit no such restraint. They freely indulge in their fantasies and seek out every chance to trap and take advantage of the child.

Abusive adults use a variety of strategies to overcome their own inhibitions and those of their victims. They may insist that the victim is 'old for her years' or play upon the positive and loving nature of their relationship. The sexual approach will typically be very gradual, and may begin with the perpetrator conversing on sexual topics with the child, or indulging in various kissing, touching or tickling games. A perpetrator's inhibitions are often reduced by the victim's apparent lack of rejection or distress. Some children do protest and struggle when approached sexually but the majority behave in a compliant way (Meiselman, 1978). The victim's acquiescence may allow the perpetrator to tell himself that 'she is enjoying it', 'she doesn't mind' or 'she won't be harmed'. Perpetrators generally act as 'careful seducers' rather than as 'rapists', partly because they have no desire to hurt the victim and partly because they realize that an aggressive attack would be likely to lead to disclosure.

Consequences for the Victim

Sexual abuse may lead to physical injury. Attempts at intercourse with young children (or anal intercourse with a child at any age) may lead to bruising or to more severe injuries. Some victims contract a sexually transmitted disease and older girls who are subjected to intercourse run the additional risk of pregnancy. In the majority of cases, however, the abuse takes the form of masturbation, fondling or indecent exposure and does not leave any physical damage or any forensic evidence.

In terms of psychological effects, there is no 'post-sexual abuse syndrome' and symptom patterns vary greatly in nature and degree. Immediate effects are sometimes, but not always, traumatic and may include extreme anxiety, depression, various forms of behaviour disturbance and an abnormal interest in sexual matters (Haugaard and Repucci, 1988). Some abused children continue to show symptoms into adulthood, and some victims who appear to be relatively unscathed during childhood develop symptoms much later in life.

It is unfortunate that many people believe psychological trauma to be an inevitable consequence of sexual abuse, for the relevant research has consistently shown that many children are resilient and cope relatively well following sexual abuse (Powell and Chalkley, 1981). There is a danger that professionals who believe the myth of universal trauma will communicate their expectation of psychological damage to the children in their care. Hunting for 'latent trauma' in children who present as healthy and well-adjusted is rarely helpful and may do considerable harm. The resilience which many children show following sexual interference should be appreciated and enhanced rather than disregarded or undermined. In many cases, of course, the child will be in need of specialist psychological help, and any child who has been sexually abused needs to be carefully assessed. Traumatic effects are more likely when the child is young at the time of abuse and in the relatively rare cases in which force is used. Needless to say, sexual abuse is an appalling infringement of a child's rights whenever it occurs and whether or not it leaves the child profoundly distressed.

Difficulties of the adult survivor of childhood sexual abuse include mood disturbances (feelings of guilt, low self-esteem and depression), interpersonal difficulties (isolation, insecurity, discord and inadequacy) and sexual difficulties (sexual phobias and aversion, and sexual dissatisfaction (Jehu, 1988). Early sexual abuse also appears to be a risk factor for a variety of psychiatric disorders, including eating disorders. In recent years various therapeutic strategies have been developed to help survivors, and these are offered both by professional agencies and through voluntary and self-help groups (Hall and Lloyd, 1989).

Unfortunately, the sexual abuse of children is by no means rare, and any professional who comes into regular contact with families should be vigilant for evidence of such abuse. Child protection policies and practices in this field have developed rapidly within the past decade, and agencies have been at pains to establish guidelines which direct the actions of any professional (including teachers, nurses, general practitioners and youth leaders) who has reason to suspect that a child has been subjected to this form of victimization.

Marital Violence

There is enormous variation in the estimates of the incidence of marital violence, largely as a result of the different criteria used to define 'violence'. According to national US surveys, when 'violence' is defined to include slapping, pushing and more serious forms of attack, around a sixth of all couples experience violence within any given 12 month period (Straus, *et al.*, 1980; Straus and Gelles, 1986). The rate of 'marital' abuse is significantly higher for cohabiting couples than for married couples (Ellis, 1989, Stets and Straus, 1989), perhaps because cohabiting relationships are less well defined and may generate frequent confrontations regarding the issue of commitment.

Although some women do attack their male partners, it is clear that many more women than men are injured as a result of marital violence. Aggressive behaviour by a woman against her partner will rarely lead to serious injury, and female aggression is often retaliatory (Saunders, 1986). It has been estimated that marital violence is the single most common source of serious injury to women, being responsible for more injuries than road accidents, muggings and rape combined (Stark and Flitcraft, 1988).

Two principal models are used to explain marital violence. The sociological model suggests that wife battering is a socially approved strategy that reflects patriarchy and is used to maintain women in an inferior position in society (Dobash and Dobash, 1979). The psychological interaction model regards marital abuse as a hostile aggressive attack by an assailant on the victim, usually following a conflictual encounter between the two (Frude, 1994). It is important to recognize that although the interactional model attempts to explain violent attacks as the outcome of the behaviour of both the aggressor and the victim, the blame for the violence is attributed solely to the assailant.

The Interactional Explanation

Psychological accounts of marital violence suggest that the majority of cases of wife beating arise out of marital conflict and that most violent marriages are generally difficult and quarrelsome. Most men who beat their wives have extreme and objectionable views about how a wife should behave and judge many of the woman's actions as 'out of order'. If a man judges his wife to be unsupportive, or believes that she is failing to provide him with due attention, consideration, power or privileges, the extreme hostility that he feels may lead to physical aggression. The issue of power is clearly central to this analysis, and a wide status difference between the partners is associated with a higher frequency of violence.

Intervention

The physical and psychological effects of marital abuse are often extremely severe, and once a relationship has become violent there is a high probability of recurrent attacks. The availability of shelters or refuges is a major contribution to the safety of women and children, but around half of those who enter a shelter eventually return to live with the man who attacked them. Various forms of 'treatment' have been developed, some of which focus principally on the violent husband (e.g. anger control training) and some of which focus on victim's need to develop an effective 'personal safety plan'. A number of extensive couple-based intervention programmes aim to modify the couple's conflict interactions, to teach the assaultive husband anger-control techniques, and to help the victim to promote her own safety (Brygger and Edelson, 1987). Recent developments in social policy and law enforcement practices (for example, the setting up of police domestic violence units) are likely to make important contributions to reducing the extreme danger that so many women face within their own home, although few would deny that there is still a great deal to be done (Farrington, 1986; Sherman and Berk, 1984; Parker, 1985).

Elder Abuse

The frailty, illness and deterioration of function which often come when a person reaches an advanced age demand various adaptations in the family structure and functioning. For an elderly couple, old age may mean major changes in responsibilities and the allocation of chores, for example, as one partner becomes dependent upon the other for help with feeding and toileting. In well-established, three generation households, the increasing dependency of an elderly person may require gradual changes in family organization. And in families in which an elderly relative comes to live in a younger relative's home because he or she can no longer live independently, family life will be subject to sudden and radical changes.

Although the presence of an elderly person in the household with younger relatives often proves agreeable and successful, this arrangement frequently leads to tension, and the atmosphere often becomes fraught and conflictual. In many cases the family is subjected to increasing stress as the care demands increase due to progressive illness or disability, or as the cognitive and emotional health of the older person deteriorates. Family life may be severely disrupted as the consequences of the elderly person's condition reverberate around the family, affecting the relationships between other family members. If a general atmosphere of tension and hostility develops, even minor setbacks and annoyances may generate very strong emotional responses. These often take the form of depression or anxiety, but in some cases (especially those in which the elderly person becomes highly critical and demanding), family members feel a good deal of resentment and anger. Physical attacks on elderly people by their younger relatives are almost always driven by such anger, very few assaults being 'cold-blooded' (Zdorkowski and Galbraith, 1985).

Only a minority of cases of elder abuse ever come to light, mostly because neither the perpetrators nor the victims are likely to disclose information about an attack. Perpetrators may be profoundly ashamed of the way they have treated their elderly relative and fear the possible legal consequences, and victims may be unable or reluctant to report incidents because of their isolation, their sense of shame, fear of possible reprisal, and the fact that, even if they have been seriously assaulted within the home, they may dread the thought of being admitted to a residential institution.

Family Dynamics and the Burden of Care

We know from those cases which do come to light that an attack is rarely an isolated occurrence, and that many elderly people are subjected to prolonged emotional and physical cruelty. Many victims are made to feel a burden to the family and are held responsible for all manner of family difficulties. Sometimes the needs of the older relative are totally neglected. He or she may be confined to a small part of the house or may be exploited financially. Such cruelty or neglect usually reflects a chronic breakdown of relationships, whereas the aggressive attacks made on old people by their caregivers usually reflect acute stress and annoyance. Such feelings may be a direct response to the elderly person's demands for care, or critical behaviour, but the high level of stress experienced by a younger relative may also reflect wider family factors such as marital instability or financial hardship (Steinmetz, 1984).

Several aspects of the older person's behaviour may prove especially irritating. Memory problems may lead to endless repetition, for example, and items may be constantly mislaid. Hearing difficulties may require family members to shout, and the high volume necessary for the person to enjoy radio and television programmes may be intrusive and annoying. Constant 'aimless' wandering, and prolonged periods of silent sitting, may also prove very annoying, and erratic patterns of sleep and waking may disturb normal family interaction.

Susceptibility to the cold may lead to increased heating bills, and special mobility, dietary and toileting needs may affect the family's budget. Such costs may be resented, particularly if the family is relatively poor and if some members feel deprived as a result of the expenditure on the elderly person. Family members may also resent any loss of space and privacy consequent on the arrival of the elderly relative.

Certain actions by the elderly person may be experienced as 'interfering', or as 'careless', and the person may be accused of such 'offences' as withholding finances, or of attempting to impose outdated views about such matters as child discipline, the 'manners' of adolescent children, or the preparation of meals. The neurological effects of certain disorders lead to certain personality changes, so that some elderly people become especially cantankerous, uninhibited, or 'childish'. If no allowance is made for the disorder, and if critical and disruptive behaviours are judged to be 'deliberate' attempts to undermine the family, intense resentment may be generated.

The picture presented here of family life with an elderly person is extremely unfavourable, and it needs to be emphasized that such circumstances are by no means universal, and may be far from typical. Many families care for their elderly relatives without undue hardship or stress, and in many cases such an arrangement proves highly successful and mutually gratifying. It also needs to be emphasized that however stressful the circumstances may become, there can never be any justification or excuse for the psychological or physical mistreatment of an older relative. But we do need to appreciate the stresses, costs and irritations in order to understand how people who are normally kindly and supportive can behave violently towards a vulnerable person in their charge (Pillemer and Suitor, 1988).

Escalation and Intervention

An understanding of elder abuse demands an understanding of why anger arises and why the normally powerful inhibitions against physical aggression towards an elderly person may be nullified. One factor that can help to explain such violence is the frequent misunderstanding by the assailant of the nature and causes of the victim's annoying behaviour. Those who abuse elderly people may make inaccurate judgements, for example, about whether difficult behaviour is 'symptomatic' of some disorder, is 'accidental', or is deliberately provocative. Furthermore, those who assault elderly relatives often lack skills in managing difficult situations and gaining the compliance of those they are attempting to care for. Other relatives, friends and (especially) professionals, may be able to help caregivers to understand why an older person is behaving oddly, or disruptively, or in a challenging fashion. If the caregiver comes to realize that the person's medical condition may lead to certain psychological problems (including changes of mood, difficulties of memory, confusion and disorientation) which then give rise to awkwardness or a quarrelsome attitude, the difficult behaviour may be judged more charitably. Health professionals can often advise the family on effective ways of dealing with disruptive behaviour and, through their own interaction with the elderly person, can provide a model of skilful and tolerant care.

Ideally, potential 'at-risk' families should be monitored so that advice and help can be given as needed. As with all other forms of abuse, evidence of serious mistreatment demands the immediate attention of social work agencies and the police.

CONCLUSION

There is clearly a great deal of abuse within families, and many people are victimized by members of their family. However, there is a lack of agreement about what level of hostile action constitutes 'abuse'. Opinions differ, for example, on whether smacking a child is ever appropriate and justified. For too long, the family has been regarded by many as 'private territory' within which family members are free to regulate their own affairs, but it is increasingly appreciated that society has a right and a duty to protect individuals. Professionals who come into regular contact with families will often be the first 'outsiders' to recognize abuse, and in recent years much more has been done to produce practice guidelines to be followed when abuse is suspected. A chapter which focuses on familial abuse obviously tends to provide a negative view of family life, and we need to be reminded that many homes do provide a safe and supportive haven. Although almost all families experience serious conflict from time to time, most manage to avoid the most damaging behaviours that are sometimes provoked by a high level of anger and serious conflicts of interest.

SUMMARY

- The incidence of child physical abuse, marital violence and elder abuse indicates that violence is a significant feature within many families.
- A high proportion of violent acts are committed by one family member against another.
- At least 90% of parents occasionally smack their children.
- Marital violence is the single most common source of serious injury to women. It is responsible for more injuries than road accidents, muggings and rape combined.
- Child sexual abuse is usually motivated by a sexual drive rather than an aggressive drive.
- Many abused children are profoundly traumatized as a result of their abusive experiences. However, it appears that others are resilient, and professionals should avoid disturbing the child's own attempts at coping.
- Various therapeutic programmes can be successful in reducing the incidence of family violence.

DISCUSSION QUESTIONS

- ♦ Why is there so much violence within families?

- ♦ Discuss the issue of whether any level of physical aggression (including slapping, pushing, smacking) is appropriate or tolerable in (a) the parent–child relationship; (b) the marital relationship.

- ♦ Consider the difficulties involved in the 'diagnosis' or 'detection' of child abuse. Issues you may wish to consider include the question of accidental versus non-accidental injury in young children, and children's apparent reticence about disclosing sexual abuse.

- ♦ Imagine that you begin to suspect that there is undisclosed violence or sexual abuse within a family that you are visiting regularly for an unrelated medical problem. Discuss the action you might take if you were to suspect (a) marital violence; (b) elder abuse; (c) child sexual abuse.

FURTHER READING

Browne K Davies C and Stratton P (Eds) (1988) *Early Prediction and Prevention of Child Abuse*. Chichester: Wiley.
Useful text which examines prevention aspects of the broad spectrum of child abuse, including failure to thrive. Also examines what might be done to support families under stress.

Corby B (1993) *Child Abuse: Towards a Knowledge Base*. Milton Keynes: Open University Press.
A fairly comprehensive review of research on child abuse, with some focus on practice issues.

Frude NJ (1991) *Understanding Family Problems: A Psychological Approach*. Chichester: Wiley.
Includes chapters on marital violence and child physical abuse, emphasizing how these problems can be explained in terms of interaction between victim and perpetrator.

Gelles RJ (1987) *The Violent Home: Updated Edition*. Beverly Hills, CA: Sage.
Classic volume describing a research project which aimed to help an understanding of the causes and dynamics of marital violence and child abuse.

Hall L and Lloyd S (1989) *Surviving Child Sexual Abuse: A Handbook for Helping Women Challenge their Past*. London: Falmer Press.
A practical handbook citing many ways in which adult survivors of child sexual abuse can be helped by professionals, or can help themselves. Extremely useful, especially, for those involved in organizing 'self-help' victim groups.

Howells K and Hollin C (Eds) (1989) *Clinical Approaches to Violence*. Chichester: Wiley.
Broad-ranging text with chapters on physical child abuse, violence in the workplace and a variety of other topics.

Jehu D (1988) *Beyond Sexual Abuse: Therapy with Women who were Childhood Victims*. Chichester: Wiley.
Detailed report of a study of groups of women who presented at a sexual dysfunction clinic after having been sexually abused in childhood. Includes useful information on the long-term impact of their abuse and on useful therapeutic methods.

Wolfe DA (1987) *Child Abuse: Implications for Child Development and Psychopathology*. Beverly Hills, CA: Sage.
Excellent integrated review of work in the child abuse field, emphasizing the immediate and longer-term psychological effects on the child victim.

REFERENCES

Baker AW and Duncan SP (1985) Child sexual abuse: A study of prevalence in Great Britain. *Child Abuse and Neglect* **9:** 457.

Browne K and Saqi S (1988) Approaches to screening for child abuse and neglect. In K Browne, C Davies and P Stratton (Eds) *Early Prediction and Prevention of Child Abuse*. Chichester: Wiley.

Brygger MP and Edelson JL (1987) The Domestic Abuse Project: A multisystems intervention in woman battering. *Journal of Interpersonal Violence* **2:** 324.

Dale P, Davies M, Morrison A and Waters J (1986) *Dangerous Families: Assessment and Treatment of Child Abuse*. London: Tavistock.

Dobash RE and Dobash R (1979) *Violence against Wives*. New York: Free Press.

Ellis D (1989) Male abuse of a married or cohabiting female partner: The application of sociological theory to research findings. *Violence and Victims* **4:** 235.

Farrington K (1986) The application of stress theory to the study of family violence: Principles, problems and prospects. *Journal of Family Violence* **1:** 131.

Frude NJ (1980) Child abuse as aggression. In N. Frude (Ed) *Psychological Approaches to Child Abuse*. London: Batsford.

Frude NJ (1982) The sexual nature of sexual abuse: a review of the literature. *Child Abuse and Neglect* **6:** 211.

Frude NJ (1985) The sexual abuse of children within the family. *Medicine and Law* **4:** 463.

Frude NJ (1989a) Sexual abuse: An overview. *Educational and Child Psychology,* **6:** 34.

Frude NJ (1989b) The physical abuse of children. In K. Howells and C. Hollin (Eds) *Clinical Approaches to Violence*. Chichester: Wiley.

Frude NJ (1991) *Understanding Family Problems: A Psychological Approach*. Chichester: Wiley.

Frude NJ (1994) Marital violence. In J Archer (Ed) *Male Violence*. London: Routledge.

Gelles RJ (1979) *Family Violence*. Beverly Hills, California: Sage.

Gelles RJ (1987) *The Violent Home: Updated Edition*. Beverly Hills, CA: Sage.

Goldsmith HR (1990) Men who abuse their spouses: An approach to assessing future risk. *Journal of Offender Counseling, Services and Rehabilitation* **15:** 45.

Goldstein D and Rosenbaum A (1985) An evaluation of the self-esteem of maritally violent men. *Family Relations Journal of Applied Family and Child Studies* **34:** 425.

Green AH (1983) Dimensions of psychological trauma in abused children. *Journal of the American Academy of Child Psychiatry* **22:** 231.

Hall L and Lloyd S (1989) *Surviving Child Sexual Abuse: A Handbook for Helping Women Challenge their Past*. London: Falmer Press.

Haugaard JJ and Repucci ND (1988) *The Sexual Abuse of Children*. San Francisco: Jossey-Bass.

Hornung C, McCullough B and Sugimoto T (1981) Status relationships in marriage: Risk factors in spouse abuse. *Journal of Marriage and the Family* **43:** 675.

Jehu D (1988) *Beyond Sexual Abuse: Therapy with Women who were Childhood Victims*. Chichester: Wiley.

Kadushin A and Martin JA (1981) *Child Abuse: An Interactional Event*. New York: Columbia University Press.

Kazden AE, Moser J, Colbus D and Bell R (1985) Depressive symptoms among physically abused and psychiatrically disturbed children. *Journal of Abnormal Psychology* **94:** 298.

Kelly JA (1983) *Treating Child-Abusive Families: Intervention based on Skills-Training Principles*. New York: Plenum.

Kessler DB (1985) Pediatric assessment and differential diagnosis of child abuse. In EH Newberger and R Bourne (Eds) *Unhappy Families: Clinical and Research Perspectives on Family Violence*. Littleton, MA: PSG Publishing.

Kinard EM (1980) Emotional development in physically abused children. *American Journal of Orthopsychiatry* **50**: 686.

Lynch M (1988) The consequences of child abuse. In K Browne, C Davies and P Stratton (Eds) *Early Prediction and Prevention of Child Abuse*. Chichester: Wiley.

Martin HP (1976) Which children get abused: High risk factors in the child. In: HP Martin (Ed) *The Abused Child: A Multidisciplinary Approach to Developmental Issues and Treatment*. Cambridge: Ballinger.

Mason A and Blankenship V (1987) Power and affiliation motivation, stress and abuse in intimate relationships. *Journal of Personality and Social Psychology* **52**: 203.

Meiselman K (1978) *Incest: A Psychological Study of Causes of Effects*. San Francisco: Jossey-Bass.

Pahl J (Ed) (1985) *Private Violence and Public Policy: The Needs of Battered Women and the Response of the Public Services*. London: Routledge and Kegan Paul.

Parker S (1985) The legal background. In J. Pahl (Ed) *Private Violence and Public Policy: The Needs of Battered Women and the Response of the Public Services*. London: Routledge and Kegan Paul.

Pillemer K and Suitor JJ (1988) Elder abuse. In VB Van Hasselt, RL Morrison, AS Bellack and M Hersen (Eds) *Handbook of Family Violence*. New York: Plenum.

Powell GE and Chalkley AJ (1981) The effects of paedophile attention on the child. In B Taylor (Ed) *Perspectives on Paedophilia*. London: Batsford.

Rosenbaum A and O'Leary KD (1981) Marital violence: characteristics of abusive couples. *Journal of Consulting and Clinical Psychology* **49**: 63.

Roy M (1977) *Battered Women: Psycho-sociological Study of Domestic Violence*. New York: Van Nostrand Reinhold.

Roy M (Ed) (1982) *The Abusing Partner: An Analysis of Domestic Battering*. New York: Van Nostrand Reinhold.

Saunders DG (1986) When battered women use violence: Husband abuse or self defense? *Violence and Victims* **1**: 47.

Sedlak AJ (1988) Prevention of wife abuse. In VB Van Hasselt, RL Morrison, AS Bellack and M Hersen (Eds) *Handbook of Family Violence*. New York: Plenum.

Sherman LW and Berk RA (1984) The specific deterrents of arrest for domestic assault. *American Sociological Review* **49**: 261.

Stark E and Flitcraft A (1988) Violence among intimates: An epidemiological review. In VB Van Hasselt, RL Morrison, AS Bellack and M Hersen (Eds) *Handbook of Family Violence*. New York: Plenum.

Steinmetz SK (1984) Family violence towards elders. In S Saunders, A. Anderson, C Hart and G Rubenstein (Eds) *Violent Individuals and Families: A Handbook for Practitioners*. Springfield, IL: Charles C Thomas.

Steinmetz SK (1987) Family violence: Past, present and future. In MB Sussman and SK Steinmetz (Eds) *Handbook of the Marriage and the Family*. New York: Plenum Press.

Stets JE and Straus MA (1989) The marriage license as a hitting license: A comparison of assaults in dating, cohabiting, and married couples. *Journal of Family Violence* **4**: 161.

Straus MA and Gelles RJ (1986) Societal change and family violence from 1975 to 1985 as revealed by two national surveys. *Journal of Marriage and the Family* **48**: 445.

Straus MA, Gelles RJ and Steinmetz SK (1980) *Behind Closed Doors: Violence in American Families*. New York: Doubleday.

Tarter RE, Hegedus AE, Winsten NE and Alterman AI (1984) Neuropsychological, personality and familial characteristics of physically abused delinquents. *Journal of the American Academy of Child Psychiatry* **23**: 668.

Telch CF and Lindquist CU (1984) Violent versus nonviolent couples: A comparison of patterns. *Psychotherapy* **21**: 242.

Walker JC (1985) Protective services for the elderly. In JJ Kosberg (Ed) *Abuse and Maltreatment of the Elderly: Causes and Interventions*. Littleton, MA: John Wright PSG.

Wolfe DA (1987) *Child Abuse: Implications for Child Development and Psychopathology*. Beverly Hills, CA: Sage.

Zdorkowski RT and Galbraith MW (1985) An inductive approach to the investigation of elder abuse. *Ageing and Society* **5**: 413.

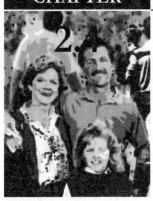

FAMILY NURSING AND COMMUNITY NURSING PRACTICE

Brian Millar

KEY ISSUES

- ■ The family, health and nursing
- ■ Nursing theory and family nursing
- ■ Exploring the components of family nursing
- ■ Analysing the potential value and benefits of a family nursing perspective

INTRODUCTION

Students who are preparing for more advanced practice in the community will have a number of opportunities to consider various theoretical perspectives concerned with the family, such as those presented in this section of the book by a sociologist and psychologist and those offered by social epidemiologists, who for example, seek to explain why families in some communities seem to be at greater risk of ill health and family breakdown, when compared with others in comparable settings. Gillis (1991), however, points to the need for developing research paradigms which move beyond those of social science to those which focus on the phenomena derived from the interaction between a nurse and the family.

In general terms, the community health nurse's ability to make a comprehensive assessment of need, together with an estimate of progress towards agreed goals, will critically influence the decision-making about the most appropriate level of intervention. Various writers in the field of family nursing (e.g. Luker and Orr (1992) and Whyte (1991) in the UK and Friedmann (1992), Gillis *et al.* (1989), and Wright and Leaghy (1987) in the USA) have drawn attention to the importance of differentiating between the family as the context within which assessment is undertaken and care is offered to an individual, and the family itself as the focus for assessment, negotiation, intervention, participation and evaluation.

This chapter will not only consider the development of family nursing theory but will also explore examples of theoretical perspectives which have particular relevance for the community health nurse. Some of the issues facing a nurse when moving from the structured and relatively predictable environment of the hospital, to the essentially unpredictable and variable environment of a family in a community setting, are also addressed.

In considering the perspective of community health nurses, questions which are likely to broaden the framework for nursing assessment in a family setting, might include: Why does the arrival of a first baby have such a significant effect on a marriage or partnership, as well as on other family relationships? In what ways can the continuing care of a chronically sick or disabled individual at home cause various kinds and levels of stress within a family? How does a pattern of family behaviour influence the recovery or rehabilitation of a family member? What kinds of coping mechanisms might be predicted in the face of specified family crises? How does the nursing framework for assessment, affect the nature of information sought and the relationship between the nurse and the family?

A nursing intervention has the potential to be beneficial in a variety of ways and in adopting a perspective which focuses on the family as a whole, it can seek to optimize the health potential of the family as a whole, as well as seeking to address individual needs where appropriate, utilizing resources and processes within the family unit itself to restore health, normal functioning and equilibrium.

The Family, Health and Nursing the Family

Whether traditional or otherwise, families have basic characteristics and structures which are uniquely expressed by each individual family. A family is perhaps most usefully seen as a unique group of individuals who engage in patterns of interaction which derive from the intimacy of their relationships. Such interactions are often characterized by reciprocity, intensity and frequency and by their potential influence on individual members of the group. The interaction itself tends to reinforce the interdependence of group members, as well as the instability/stability of the group.

From a community health nursing point of view, a family has a right and a responsibility to make choices about matters which affect its health and welfare and the interaction between family members forms the setting in which such choices (informed or otherwise) are made. The interaction between family members also provides the setting in which the nurse has opportunities to develop the capacities of individuals to participate in attitude changing and decision-making processes and to find ways to remove barriers or stumbling blocks to a family achieving its optimum health potential.

Where there is a breakdown in health, the stress or distress of one member's illness or health care problem is likely to have a powerful influence on both the level of family functioning and on individual levels of wellness, as well as on patterns of behaviour (Campbell, 1986). For example, while parents can be successfully supported in the family management of chronic conditions (Deatrick and Knafl, 1987), they can also create or exacerbate family problems by trying to live their lives through their children, gaining vicarious satisfaction from their activities and achievements (Herbert, 1988). Marriages or partnerships can also face difficult transitions which may place excessive strain on relationships; good examples include balancing the ambitions of two careers if both parents work; coming to terms with various physical and psychological limitations following a serious road traffic accident; adapting to the changes wrought by an only child leaving home to undertake further education. The particular challenge facing the community health nurse is to achieve a sufficiently productive relationship so that the interaction between the family and nurse can incorporate issues of family functioning and family development where it is deemed to be relevant for recovery or health improvement.

Health

The goal of health – its restoration, maintenance or improvement – remains a central tenet for much of community nursing practice. Exploring the various meanings that have been attached to the concept of health can usefully highlight different perspectives such as the dichotomy or continuum between health and illness; the idea that health can sometimes be conceived as a commodity with monetary currency; or health as a fluctuating dynamic state, affected by internal and external resources or stressors. In this sense, the family may be seen as 'source' of ill health or a 'resource' for enhancing health. A particular definition of health often underpins a framework for nursing practice, for example Neuman's systems model (1983). The cognitive framework which encompasses this model then becomes a paradigm for research, pulling together the combining influences of biology, social context and environment to explain relationships between nursing activity and the outcomes for an individual, family or the wider community.

Parse (1987) describes health as a 'dynamic state and process of physical, psychological, social and spiritual well-being'. Inherent in this view is the assumption that there is an optimal level of health which can be influenced by external norms and standards, as well as internal beliefs and values. Such an assumption is reflected in the results of an application for life insurance where the degree of risk to the company is based on predictive tables. Statistics for major diseases suggest, for example, that where an applicant smokes, consumes excessive amounts of alcohol, is obese and fails to take an adequate amount of exercise, there is an increased risk of having some form of circulatory disease, or of dying at an unexpectedly early age.

In a similar vein, those whose health, or health-related behaviour, deviates significantly from accepted norms, are at risk of being defined as 'sick', or of being labelled as maladaptive or dysfunctional. Within such a perspective there may be a tendency to view illness as the result of failure on the part of a person to conform to an expected level of individual responsibility for health maintenance. Ryan (1953) has suggested that such a view is akin to 'victim blaming', where the person concerned is victimized for contributing to their ill health but with little or no reference to the implications of social or environmental circumstances within which they live.

In describing health as 'the process of becoming', Parse (1987) sees the essence of family health in pattern manifestation and the focus of the health professional directed towards finding ways to improve the overall quality of life, rather than on identifying deviations from externally imposed norms. Rogers (1970) reminds us for instance, that families are characterized by growing diversity and that such diversity should not be construed as deviancy but as a creative living system, continuously developing patterns of relating, in order to meet ever changing needs and responsibilities.

Nursing

There has been considerable support in the past for the idea that individualized care equals quality care (Monitor by Goldstone and Ball (1983)). The emphasis on individualized patient care was regarded as the means to rehumanize care and to protect nursing claims to be a caring profession (Watson, 1988) but it can also create a potential dichotomy between humanism and the requirements of professionalism. Humanistic values are focused on respecting the autonomy of the patient/client but professionalism asserts expert knowledge, practice and accountability – all of which may contribute to a view of the patient/client and their family, as passive recipients of care. From this point of view, acceptance of individualized care could be interpreted as a failure to acknowledge the social or communal aspects of human care. So while individualized care may represent an achievement, we must also recognize some limitations to the concept and remember that we live in a world where people have the right to choose for themselves how they live their lives and how they manage their health. These individual rights are generally defended through our legal system and more recently have been emphasized within the NHS by such documents as the Patient's Charter (DOH, 1992).

At its simplest, interest in the family, and recognition of the need to focus on nursing the family as a whole, has developed as a result of a number of political, economic, social and professional factors. Increasing numbers of older people, re-structuring of health care, planned moves from acute institutional care to care in the community (DOH, 1991), advances in medical technology (with surgical procedures now being undertaken on an increasingly aged population), have all contributed to promoting nursing interest in alternative and creative methods of providing care.

Terms such as 'patient centred', or 'patient focused' care, have more recently been supplanted in the literature by 'family centred' or 'family focused' care (Wright and Leaghy, 1987; Gillis *et al.*, 1989; Friedman, 1992). That is not to say that interest in the family as a focus for care, is something new; nursing interest in the family dates back to the time of Nightingale (Whall, 1986a) and there have been aspects of community nursing which have always sought to address the whole family as the recipient of care (e.g. While, 1991). But assumptions about practice can sometimes lead to confusion about definitions of community health nursing and about defini-tions of family nursing (Whall, 1986a). When dealing with patients/clients in their own homes, nurses can sometimes cling to an artificial distinction between the physical and psychological well-being of the individual and that of the family.

Labels such as 'family centred' and 'family focused' are taken to imply recognition of the important needs and roles of the family regarding the health of both individuals and the community in which they live. Problems faced by families when caring or supporting those who are ill or those who have learning difficulties are seldom the result of a single cause; and a family rarely faces a problem with a single effect. So in attempting to achieve effective and equitable community health care, there is a need for increased awareness of, and attention to, the experiences, values, priorities, and expectations of the patient/client and their family, recognizing that families are a much undervalued and little understood resource for health and well-being.

In the 1980s two competing world views of the purpose and function of nursing were described by Parse *et al.* (1985) and these were labelled as the Totality Paradigm (family as context) and the Simultaneity Paradigm (family as irreducible whole). Paradigms simply refer to a particular way of looking at the world and do no more than offer a guide to the practitioner in thinking about their observations and interactions with patients/clients and their families. Gillis (1991) claimed that 'the failure to differentiate clearly between family as context and family as client, has caused considerable confusion to the further development of the field of family nursing'.

The role of the community health nurse cannot be seen, however, in isolation from the changes affecting the organization and structure of the NHS, particularly with regard to *community care* and to *primary care*, now clearly at the centre of health service provision. The community health nurse synthesizes a public health and individual perspective, providing continuing and episodic care, working with colleagues and other agencies where appropriate to achieve health-related goals and optimum quality of life. The family in this context is a critical unit for prevention and health promotion, since the health of each member is likely to affect the health of the whole family and the health status of families is likely to influence the health status of a community.

Those who are already working in the community will already be familiar with, and accustomed to, the ideas of family centred nursing, adopting family health needs assessment procedures, family problem identification and a family centred approach to resolving problems. It might seem unnecessary then to think about them again. However, familiarity with the language can sometimes mask actual confusion, as well as the potential for confusion. Taking time to explore the meaning of 'family centred' or 'family focused' care provides opportunities to reflect on the implications for practice. In summary, some of the reasons for making the family unit the focus for community health nursing include:

- Illness, traumatic injury or suffering by one individual, affects one or more other members of the family and by focusing on an individual, important information for holistic assessment may be missed.
- Since there is a strong link between family interrelationships and the health status of individual members, the family itself plays a crucial role in all aspects of health care from prevention and health promotion, through to involvement in rehabilitation.
- Community health nursing incorporates self-care education, health promotion, family support and facilitating the development of family problem solving strategies.
- The family centred nurse collaborates with a family to identify actual and potential health risks and to help in the identification of individual health needs.
- In the context of the family unit, a clearer understanding of individual functioning can be achieved.
- The family can be a vital support system in times of crisis and, when supported by community health nurses, can become an even more important health care resource for continuing care.

Theory and Family Nursing

Within the expanding family nursing literature there exist a number of theoretical frameworks for the practising nurse to explore, such as developmental, interactional, ecological, social exchange and systems theory. For a detailed explanation of these, the reader is directed to such texts as *A Science of Family Nursing* (Gilliss *et al.*, 1989) or *Family Nursing Theory and Practice* (Friedman, 1992). An outline of one particular theoretical framework – family systems theory – is described below because its particular perspective has contributed significantly to the social sciences and to the nursing literature on family nursing practice.

Family systems theory is the term applied to family nursing by Wright and Leaghy (1987). Within the literature there is general agreement that family systems nursing provides the nurse with a practical framework for understanding and working with a family. It offers the means to explore a family in terms of how it relates to others and to the outside world and how each of its members interacts with the others. It seeks to explain how individuals can affect the whole and how the whole can affect each part. According to Bradshaw (1988), for example, a positive and functioning family system is recognized by rules which are overt and negotiable, by the open seeking of adjustments to stress and the balance obtained between togetherness and individuation. The use of the systems framework has enabled health care professionals to shift their thinking from mechanistic, outcome oriented explanations of change, to more holistic process oriented explanations of change.

In the NHS of the 1990s, increased emphasis is being placed on the roles of primary care and community care for enhancing the quality of health and social service provision. This, together with the significance given to gaining participation from individuals and families, points to the need for community health nurses to look critically at their practice, analysing their activities in terms of the purpose and forms of communication used with families and to the overall aims of their assessment and intervention. Each family member may have a different perspective of a problem and this together with patterns of relating to each other, provide valuable information for the nurse and others in the primary care team. Life cycle changes, for example, place particular stress on family members, as each struggles to adapt to the entrances and exits that mark such events as marriage, birth, migration, hospitalization or death.

Beliefs and the Family Nursing Paradigm

Traditionally, nurses operating within a stated family centred framework have tended to see the role of the family as essentially passive, supplementing or reinforcing their professional expertise in the care of the patient. Such an approach raises both ethical and moral concerns and should also raise questions about why it is that some families might seem to cope very well within such a health care delivery system, while others do not.

Any nursing assessment is likely to be influenced by a paradigm or view of the world, one which usually incorporates the social model often missing from the medico-scientific paradigm. Sometimes though, the significance of the environment can be taken for granted. A nurse can see the family as external to the patient (family as context) and accept that this may be a source of positive and negative influences, as well as a potential source of stress to the patient, who reacts and adapts in ways likely to have an impact on overall health and well-being (Parse, 1985). Nursing interventions in such circumstances would focus on manipulating the environment (including the family) to maintain or restore balance to the individual patient's life. (See the discussion in Chapter 3.4 of this book, for the development of evidence based practice.)

A contrasting paradigm for nursing practice sees the individual/family/environment interaction as something which both 'evolves and changes' (Rogers, 1970). Parse claims that 'each is a co-participant in the creation of the other' and the one is instrumental in creating the other. Where a community health nurse regards the family unit as the recipient of care, there is recognition that the family as a whole, the individuals within it and the surrounding environment, are continuously evolving and this is taken into account when assessing and planning care. In the family with adolescents, for example, increasing flexibility in the setting of family boundaries will be needed to promote independence and to provide opportunities to become more competent to deal with the tasks of everyday life. A community health nurse might help in providing role play situations for the adolescent to try out ways of discussing needs with a parent in a family setting. A nursing assessment which focuses on the family's own perceptions of their quality of life has key components which include partnership, reciprocity, effective communication and shared decision-making. Listening carefully to how a family describes its experiences is regarded as critical to understanding both the meaning given to concerns about health, as well as to the options believed to exist for resolving or managing them. The use of circular questioning, a technique reported and developed by Tomm (1985) and later explored by Loos and Bell (1990) is one way of achieving both a reliable assessment and an acceptable intervention. For both the nurse and the family, the intended outcome is not to reach a closing diagnosis but to explore possibilities through continuous reciprocal dialogue, generating and validating (or not) possible hypotheses.

The application of a family system framework encourages the community health nurse to 'travel with' the family as an assessment of family functioning is made. While a position of neutrality must be retained in order to validate the approach, where there is obvious conflict, for example, it is likely that exploration of the problem will be more effective if undertaken sooner rather than later. However, where there are long-standing maladaptive patterns of behaviour, intervening at the highest point of disequilibrium or crisis is more likely to be successful than any other attempts to achieve change (Whyte, 1991).

The nurse aims to identify causal determinants of health or functional deficits, as well as resources within the family on which to draw. No intervention can be prescribed and no intervention can be decided without reference to priorities identified by the family. The family's ability to participate in the development of an acceptable programme of care, will be critical for estimating its subsequent success. In this estimation, the nurse is not only concerned with the needs of individuals and the uniqueness of their health and illness experiences, but also with the family as a self-regulating and autonomous system, which may be more or less influenced by its internal and external environment. Efran and Lukens (1985) argue that responses to change in the internal or external environment may result in an acceptable fit between individual or family resources and stressors but a point of crisis or collapse can occur at any time when there is an absence of fit between the two.

From a community health nursing point of view, the disruption to family functioning caused by the stress of acute or continuing episodes of illness may be ameliorated by a nursing strategy designed to explore the beliefs and attitudes of the family to the particular crisis. However, once the crisis is over, the energy within the family unit may have become drained and a nurse who mechanistically responds to an episode of illness may unconsciously contribute to iatrogenic complications by a precipitate withdrawal. It is the co-participation of the nurse and family which can create an environment for growth and renewal during a crisis, helping to restore the self determination of the family.

The Elements of Family Nursing

Within family nursing three levels of practice exist. Which particular level of family nursing is practised is most readily determined by the way in which the family is conceptualized and how the community health nurse works with it. Another important variable is the philosophy of the system (or trust) within which the community health nurse is operating. Work environments (health centres, GP practices, community units) are major determinants of a nurse's behaviour. Each of the three levels (Gillis, 1991; Friedman, 1992) of family nursing mentioned below, are components of family nursing.

Level 1: Family Centred Care

Family centred care views the family as the context and the patient as the primary source of need (Bozett, 1987). An example of this approach is encapsulated in the definition of family centred care supported by the paediatric associations. They define family centred care as a philosophy of paediatric health care which treats the child in the context of the family and recognizes the family as the primary and continuing provider of care. A criticism of this approach is that health care professionals who are practising family centred care tend to view the family as important only in fulfilling their (the professionals') needs. Family are used by the professionals as an additional source of care as and when the professional feels it is appropriate.

Level 2: Family Focused Care

In this type of family nursing practice, families are seen as comprising the sum of a number of parts or individuals members. Nurses who provide care and acknowledge all of the family members in their plan are said to be family focused. This particular approach is familiar to many community health nurses especially as they are often dealing with patients who are being supported by or living with other family members in their homes. Family focused care adopts the ideals of individualized care, seeing each family member as an individual, arguing that family health equals the sum of the individual family members' health. There is always the possibility, however, that within such an approach some individual family members are more powerful, or assertive, than others; equally the social relations of the family may be ignored.

Level 3: Family as Client

In this approach to care, the family is conceptualized as the client or the primary focus of assessment and care. Wright and Leaghy (1988), for example, describe this approach as based on the view of a family as an interactional system. Nurses focus on the dynamics, and relationships, family structures and function, as well as interdependence among family members and the family interaction with their surrounding community. Relationships between health and illness, between the individuals in a family and between the family and the wider community, are assessed and included in the development of any care or treatment plan, or a strategy to promote optimum wellness, quality of life, or functioning.

Community nurses practising within this third level of family care are using a different paradigm (view of the world) as their framework for assessing and caring. Essential features of this approach include holism, circularity and systems thinking. It is the integration of nursing, family therapy and systems theory, resulting in the interaction or reciprocity between family functioning, the health/illness continuum and nursing activity, that is called a 'family systems' approach to community health nursing. Community nurses practising in this way seek to listen and learn about families' concerns and their search for meaning. Interactions with a family focus on learning about a family's perceptions of their quality of life, communication and shared decision-making. Listening to a family's experiences is seen as critical to understanding both the meaning the family attaches to their health concerns and the options which they believe exist for resolving or managing them. Through co-participating in a shared dialogue with a family, acting in part as a guide and facilitator, the nurse is in a position to explore the meaning and choices that are faced in dealing with a health concern. Through such a process, the nurse and the family both change as the reciprocal interaction occurs. For both nurse and family the intended outcome is not to reach some diagnostic closure but to expand possibilities.

How a community nurse thinks about a family, be it as the context or as the primary unit of care, will have a major influence on his/her actions and behaviours in practice. Whilst it may not always be easy to distinguish between them, it is nevertheless important that the individual nurse is aware which approach he/she is taking. Clearly there are advantages and limitations with either of the paradigms mentioned for family nursing practice. Our current health care system, for example, seems to be based on the Totality Paradigm and such views are widely accepted by nurses as well as other health care professionals – and indeed some patients and their families. For a patient/client or a family, there may be particular advantages to adopting a passive role in health care. But if this approach remains unchallenged, there is the potential that it may restrict and obstruct the development of creative and innovative family nursing practice and deny productive and beneficial opportunities for individual family members to participate in planning and decision-making.

Nurses who are new to the Simultaneity Paradigm are faced with new and at first ambiguous beliefs and since it does not provide neatly packaged lists or diagnostic categories it is unlikely that it will be enthusiastically supported within the current health care system. One major advantage is that it directs nurses and families to focus more upon quality aspects of life and less on some deficit in health and because family/nurse interactions are accepted as continuously changing, evolving, they are likely to result in creative and innovative approaches to care. Just as one theory for nursing practice seems totally unrealistic given the diverse nature of nursing and of patient groups, so to is it unlikely that a single paradigm or view of the world will fit all situations. What is needed is continued debate and further research and development, of which this chapter forms only a small part.

SUMMARY

- This chapter has attempted to draw together some of the arguments which justify a shift in focus from individual to family centred care, exploring concepts related to family, health and nursing.
- Nursing paradigms and theoretical positions are introduced as a way of differentiating levels of interaction between a community health nurse and a family.
- Some of the advantages/disadvantages of a family nursing perspective are considered in the light of current practice and the environment of the health care system.

DISCUSSION QUESTIONS

- ◆ Consider the stages of family life which might form a significant part of health assessment. What are the potential sources of strain for individual family members?

- ◆ With reference to the three levels of practice in family nursing described above, identify and consider examples from clinical practice in community or primary care settings which demonstrate each level of family nursing.

- ◆ Describe one nursing problem experienced in the practice of family nursing and consider the advantages and disadvantages (for the nurse, for the patient/client and for the family) in a passive response to health care.

FURTHER READING

Friedman M (1992) *Family Nursing: Theory and Practice*, 3rd edn Norwalk, Connecticut: Appleton and Lange.
It is the unique understanding and knowledge of family nursing theories that can direct further family nursing specific inquiry and structure activities for autonomous community nursing practice. This major text serves to focus family nursing inquiry and to expand community nurses' knowledge leading to creative and meaningful practice with individual patients and their families.

Gillis C, Highley B, Roberts B and Martinson I (1989) *Towards a Science of Family Nursing*. California: Addision-Wesley.
This textbook provides a detailed discussion of the significant developments in family theory and family nursing practice. Community nurses who are interested in developing their knowledge and understanding of the theoretical and practical aspects of family nursing will find key chapters including issues in family nursing research; factors influencing family health; transitions in the family life cycle; and promoting family health during chronic illness.

Pearson A and Vaughan B (1986) *Nursing Models for Practice*. London: Heinemann.
This book is a core text for those interested in the application of nursing models to clinical nursing practice. The authors provide clear descriptions of the theory and then give examples taken from their experiences of using the models in clinical practice. A particularly useful chapter for community nurses would be 'The Health Care Systems model' (Neuman 1972).

Walsh M (1991) *Models in Clinical Nursing*. London: Baillière Tindall.
Mike Walsh guides the reader through critical questions about how to choose a model, how to use models in practice, and then provides significant examples in the application of models of nursing in hospital, community, and mental health nursing. It is written clearly and the clinical examples support the theoretical explanations given.

Journal Papers

Dunn B (1990) Health promotion and Orem Model. *Nursing Standard* **4**(40); 34.

Faucett J, Ellis V, Underwood P, Naqvi A and Wilson D (1990) The effect of Orem's self care model on nursing care in a nursing home setting. *Journal of Advanced Nursing* **15**: 659–666.
Both these papers provide an account of the application by practitioners of the self-care model and the difficulties they encountered. A wide range of literature is available on the application of other models, specifically those of Roy, Neuman and King to the family and in particular to community nursing practice.

REFERENCES

Bradshaw J (1988) *The Family – a Revolutionary Way of Self Discovery*. Florida: Health Communication Inc.

Bozett FW (1987) Assumptions, assessment and intervention. In L Wright and M Leaghy (eds) *Families and Life Threatening Illness*. Springhouse, PA: Springhouse Corp.

Campbell T (1986) The family's impact on health: a critical review. *Family Systems Medicine* **4**(203): 135–328.

Deatrick JA and Knafl KA (1987) Conceptualizing Family Response to a Child's Chronic Illness or Disability. *Journal of Family Relations* **36**: 300–304.

Department of Health (1991) *Community Care Act*. London: HMSO.

Department of Health (1992) *Patients' Charter*. London: HMSO.

Efran J and Lukens MD (1985) The World according to Humberto Maturance. *Family Therapy Networker* **9**(3): 23–28, 72–75.

Friedman M (1992) *Family Nursing – Theory and Practice*. 3rd edn. Norwalk, CT: Appleton Century Crofts.

Gillis CL, Highley BL, Roberts BM and Martinson IM (1989) *Towards a Science of Family Nursing*. Menlo Park CA: Addison-Wesley.

Gillis CL (1991) Family Nursing Research, Theory and Practice. *Journal of Nursing Scholarship* **23**(1): 19–22.

Goldstone LA and Ball JA (1983) *Monitor: An Index of Nursing Care for Acute Medical and Surgical Wards*. Newcastle-upon-Tyne Polytechnic Products Ltd.

Herbert M (1988) *Working with Children and their Families. Psychology in Action*. London: British Psychological Society and Routledge Ltd.

Loos F and Bell J (1990) Circular Questions: A Family Interviewing Strategy. *Dimensions in Critical Care Nursing* **9**: 46–53.

Luker K and Orr J (1992) *Health Visiting – Towards Community Health Nursing*. 2nd edn. Oxford: Blackwell Scientific.

Neuman B (1983) Family Intervention using the Betty Neuman Health Care Systems Model: In W Clements and FC Roberts *Family Health: A Theoretical Approach to Nursing Care*. New York: Wiley.

Parse RR, Coyne B and Smith M (1985) *Nursing Research: Qualitative Methods*. Pittsburgh, USA: Brady Communications.

Parse R (1987) *Nursing Science: Major Paradigms, Theories, and Critiques*. Philadelphia: Saunders.

Rogers M (1970) *An Introduction to the Theoretical Basis of Nursing*. Philadelphia: F.A. Davis.

Ryan B (1953) *Blaming the Victim*. London: Penguin Books.

Tomm K (1985) Circular Interviewing: A Multifaceted Clinical Tool. In D Campbell *Applications of Systemic Therapy: The Milan Approach*. London: Grune and Stratton.

Watson J (1988) *Nursing: Human Science and Human Care: A Theory for Nursing*. New York: National League for Nursing.

Whall AL (1986) *Family Therapy Theory for Nursing. Four Approaches*. Norwalk CT: Appleton Century Crofts.

Whall AL (1986a) The Family as the Unit of Analysis in Nursing. A Historical Review. *Public Health Nursing* **3**(4): 240–249.

While A, Ed. (1991) *Caring for Children – Towards Partnership with Families*. London: Edward Arnold.

Whyte D (1991) Caring for a child with chronic illness using King's Theory of Nursing. In While A (ed) *Caring for Children – Towards Partnership with Families*. London: Edward Arnold.

Wright LM and Leahey (1984) *Nurses and Families – A Guide to Family Assessment and Intervention*. Philadelphia: F.A. Davis.

Wright LM and Leahey LM (1987) *Families and Life Threatening Illness*. Springhouse, PA: Springhouse Corp.

Wright LM and Leahey LM (1988) Family Nursing Trends in Academic and Clinical Settings. In *Proceedings of the International Family Nursing Conference*, September 1989. Calgary, Alberta.

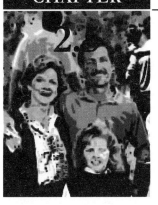

THE POLITICS OF 'LIFESTYLE': GOVERNMENT POLICIES AND THE HEALTH OF THE POOR

Tessa Davies

KEY ISSUES

■ Behaviourist strategy must be placed within an ideological context

■ The weakness of a 'lifestyle' approach to health

■ Preoccupation with risk behaviour

INTRODUCTION

The main focus of government policies towards improving the nation's health has been the emphasis placed on the need for individuals to adopt a more healthy lifestyle. The message is clear, change your behaviour, particularly with regard to smoking, alcohol, diet, exercise and sex, and this will significantly reduce your risk of ill health and premature death. All health professionals, but most directly nurses, are expected to play a key role in promoting a healthy lifestyle by education and advice. No-one could dispute the desirability of these goals, but in the absence of wider social and economic change, just how effective will this highly individualized strategy be in improving the overall health of the people?

The preoccupation with 'healthy living' has left an indelible stamp on both medical and popular culture. We are bombarded with 'lifestyle' information ranging from glossy leaflets extolling the virtues of fruit and vegetables, to earnest bi-media 'specials' urging us to lessen our risk of coronary artery disease. Though variable in degrees of evangelical zeal, there is a common 'truth' pervading almost all health promotion activity. It is that we *all* have equal opportunity to change our lifestyle, and that individual will and motivation are the main catalysts for change. But can we assume that *all* citizens have equal opportunity to 'choose' a healthy lifestyle?

Against this backdrop this chapter will concentrate on the issue of lifestyle and low income.

Ideology and Lifestyle Change

Government strategy clearly reveals that the preferred route to improving health lies with behaviour change. As the Secretary of State for Health argued in the White Paper *The Health of the Nation*:

> The reason is simple. We live in an age where many of the main courses of premature death and unnecessary disease are related to how we live our lives. (DOH, 1992: 2)

This view of health sits well with the government's broader ideological predisposition to minimize state involvement and maximize personal responsibility in all areas of social welfare. Thus the *Health of the Nation* document (England) must be placed within its ideological context. It is a free market response to a social problem.

Whether expressed in populist terms as by the redoubtable Edwina Currie (1990) that 'northerners are dying of chips' or in the more sophisticated quasi-medical language of health promotion, the message remains essentially the same. The individual is viewed as a rational actor able to choose and enact rational choices. It is a strategy that rather conveniently ensures a 'non-interventionist' role for the government, a preferred model for free market ideologues (George and Wilding, 1994). This model dictates that governments should provide information about healthy living in the form of advice, but puts all the responsibility for lifestyle on individuals, stressing the notion of personal choice. In short, responsibility for health shifts from public to private responsibility, a resonant theme in many other areas of social policy change since 1979 (Sullivan, 1994).

This highly individualized approach to health is arguably not only confined to those on the political 'right'. Coward (1993) suggests that even the supposed 'radical' or 'alternative' elements within health care can retain at their core an individualistic response to health problems. The root philosophies of many alternative or 'complementary' therapies lay great stress on the inner 'ecology' of the body. Many practices are influenced by notions of holism, and the belief that a state of positive health and well-being can be achieved by attending to and listening to one's body aided by changes in for example diet, posture, relaxation techniques etc. Controversially Coward (1993) argues that so often movements claiming themselves to be part of a 'quiet social revolution' are nothing of the sort:

> this social revolution is rarely a journey towards social rebellion, but more often an inner journey, a journey of personal transformation. (Coward, 1993: 96)

Once stripped of flowery language, there remains often a deeply moralistic philosophy, based on an individual choosing 'good' over 'bad' behaviour, not dissimilar from orthodox advice concerning healthy living. As Coward concludes:

> The quest for natural health has come to be the focus of a new morality where the individual is encouraged to exercise personal control over disease. And the principal route to this control is the route to a changed consciousness and changed *lifestyle*. (Coward, 1993: 96)

These similar conclusions drawn from two supposedly conflicting philosophies highlight the extent to which the belief that health and well-being is purely the responsibility of the individual is embedded in the national psyche. The idea that health has a moral connotation is not of course new; the equation of health with virtue has long been a deep-seated concept (Blaxter, 1990: 243; Coward, 1993: 97). The revival of political conservatism in Britain over the last 20 years has merely breathed new life into a set of values that have long been embedded in Western culture, namely that the individual is ultimately responsible for his or her actions and

> indeed that the individual is ultimately responsible for whatever happens to her in society, whether she succeeds or fails. (Coward, 1993: 97).

However, if notions of moral reprehensibility begin to dominate our view of the sick and unfortunate, this may carry grave implications for the way health care is rationed and delivered.

Lifestyle and the Rationing of Care

First, the preoccupation with risk behaviour may permeate the processes by which health care is rationed. Le Grand (1994) argues that we are already witnessing 'treatment by desert', i.e. life saving operations denied to those decreed unworthy by their personal habits. Why waste valuable resources providing, for example, coronary artery bypass grafts for those who cannot, or will not, give up smoking? It is a complex and emotive issue which this chapter does not have the scope to address. However, it is pertinent to note that the way we 'choose' to live our lives may in future years openly dictate not just the type of treatment we receive, but whether we are treated at all. This in turn has consequences for health inequalities. Given that Marsh and McKay (1994) found that smoking remained normative for the lowest income groups we may be on the way to denying health care to those already disadvantaged. What poor smokers need is not to be penalized for the ill health deriving from their 'moral reprehensibility', but an acknowledgement of the emotional and material factors that make them smoke. Although smoking rates have declined in middle and higher income groups since the 1970s, the rates amongst those on the lowest incomes have remained static at 50%, a similar picture emerges for lone parents in similar circumstances, again a static rate of 60% (Marsh and McKay, 1994). This leads Marsh and McKay (1994) to conclude that there are now entire low income communities where the health message has been understood but not heeded. The reason, they conclude, is clear:

> There is something in these people's lives that is causing them to need to smoke, expect to smoke, and not to give up. There seems only one possible candidate for this role: poverty. (Marshall and McKay, 1994: 50)

Inequalities in Health

The second charge to be levelled against the government's behavioural approach is that it masks the relationship between material conditions, socioeconomic status and health. This relationship has long been recognized from the great public health reforms of the nineteenth century, through to the Beveridge Report of 1942. In 1980 the Black Report (Black, 1980) found a great disparity in rates of morbidity and mortality between social classes. The report concluded that poverty and poor social conditions were still the main precursors to poor health and premature death. The Black Report findings were dismissed by the newly elected Thatcher government, who considered the concept of a war against poverty both ideologically and financially unpalatable. Further studies of health inequalities have confirmed many of the findings identified in the Black Report and have provided additional evidence of widening health inequalities since its publication (Whitehead, 1987; Smith *et al.*, 1990; Wilkinson, 1994; Phillimore *et al.*, 1994; Judge and Benzeval, 1993; Benzeval *et al.*, 1995).

All these studies continue to indicate that an individual's pattern of health and well-being is clearly linked to their material circumstances. The poor health record of low income groups is experienced from conception to the grave (Barker, 1992). A gap exists between the death rates of non-manual and manual workers for most causes of death in almost every age group, and it is widening. In short, those born to parents at the bottom end of the social scale are far less likely to survive the first year of life, will experience much poorer health during their life, and can, on average, expect to die 8–10 years before a contemporary born into a more affluent household. The health divide is at its most acute in the early years of life. A child born into a family where the father is an unskilled worker has twice the risk of being stillborn, or of dying in infancy compared with one born into a professional family (Whitehead, 1987). Another illustration of the health divide is the fact that 62 of the 66 major causes of death in men are more common in social classes IV and V (semi and unskilled manual workers) than in other social classes.

Of the 70 major causes of female deaths, 64 were more common in women married to men in social classes IV and V than in other social classes (Townsend *et al.*, 1988). Diseases like heart disease and lung cancer, the supposed diseases of affluence, are on closer analysis, the reverse; they are more often the diseases of poverty.

Although the evidence for a health divide is overwhelming, there is far less evidence revealing why that divide should exist. The precise reasons why some individuals may be more susceptible to disease or succumb to premature death, while others in similar circumstances survive, are largely unknown, and are likely to stem from a complex relationship between lifestyle, environment, and genetic factors (Barker, 1992; Pritchard, 1994). However, what is clear is that a very significant relationship does exist between social and economic deprivation and ill-health and premature death. The reason the government has been able to sidestep a real assault on health inequalities has rested with two main issues:

1. An 'official' view that the way health inequalities are measured is inherently flawed.
2. Even if a gap exists – the explanation lies with risk behaviour.

Inequalities in Health – the Methodological Response

It is argued (and with some justification) that evidence collected from conventional occupational class based data is inherently flawed and produces an exaggerated health divide (Illsley, 1986). Problems such as misrecording of occupation, occupational change over a lifetime, the reclassification of occupations and the changing sizes of the occupational classes themselves, could all, it is argued produce dubious results. (Carr-Hill, 1987; Illsley, 1987).

In response it could be argued that conventional class analysis (using the Registrar General breakdown of class by occupation) may actually be guilty of *underestimating* the extent of health inequalities. Social trends such as mass unemployment and the increase in economically inactive lone parents have resulted in large numbers being classified as unoccupied and thus excluded from conventional class based analysis. This exclusion of those in the main living in poverty may mean that inequalities in the health of women and children in particular are grossly *underestimated* (Roberts, 1990; Judge and Benzeval, 1993). Marsh and McKay (1994) argue that for many of those in employment income has become detached from social class, especially among families with children, and that we can no longer assume that those classified as non-manual grades are not living in poverty. It would seem then that research into inequalities in health might be better served by more explicit measures of material and social deprivation (as practised, Phillimore *et al.*, 1994) rather than reliance on conventional occupational class groupings.

Box 2.5.1. Numbers of people and children in poverty (living below 50% of average income after housing costs) in the UK (millions)
* Note the figures for people include children.
Source CPAG (1996).

	People*		Children	
	No	Proportion	No	Proportion
1979	5.0	9%	1.4	10%
1992/93	14.1	25%	4.3	33%

Poverty and Health

Further research that has examined the explicit relationship between poverty and physical and mental health has produced predictable and depressing results (Blackburn, 1991; Payne, 1991; Graham, 1993; Judge and Benzeval, 1993; Phillimore *et al.*, 1994). But let us first consider the social backdrop against which any analysis of poverty and health must take place. The most underpublicized yet damning statistic of the last 15 years has been the massive increase in the number of households calculated to be living in poverty in the United Kingdom.

The Numbers in Poverty

According to the latest figures 1 in 4 people (including children) in the UK were living in poverty in 1992/93 compared with under 1 in 10 in 1979 (Box 2.5.1). Children are even more likely to be in poverty – nearly 1 in 3 were living in poverty in 1992/93 compared to 1 in 10 in 1979 (CPAG, 1996).

There are now more children than pensioners living in poverty. In 1992/3:

*   4.3m children lived in poverty compared with 3.0m pensioners.

    This is a reversal of the situation in 1979 when:

*   1.4m children lived in poverty compared with 1.5m pensioners.

70% of the children living in poverty in 1992/3 were living in families without a full-time worker.

Who are the People in Poverty?

Different groups face different risks of falling into poverty (Box 2.5.2). Looking at family type first of all, the groups with the highest risk in 1992/93 were:

*   lone parents – 6 in 10 were in poverty

Box 2.5.2 The risk of and numbers in poverty by family type (000s)

* The risk of poverty columns show the proportion of each group in poverty, e.g. 24% of couples with children were living in poverty in 1992/3.
Source CPAG (1996).

	Risk of poverty*(%)		Numbers in poverty	
	1979	1992/3	1979	1992/3
Pensioner couples	21	26	1030	1390
Single pensioners	12	36	520	1580
Couples with children	8	24	2230	5160
Couples without children	5	12	490	1590
Single with children	19	58	470	2340
Single without children	19	58	470	2340
Single without children	7	22	540	1990
Total			5280	14 050

- single pensioners – just under 4 in 10 were in poverty.

However, it is couples with children who account for the largest group in poverty; 37% of those in poverty fell into this group in 1992/93.

Looking at economic status it is the unemployed who are at greatest risk of poverty (see Box 2.5.3). However, poverty in work has become more prevalent. In 1979 4% of those in employment were living in poverty; by 1992/3 this proportion had tripled to 12%.

Growing Divisions

Any rise in poverty must be viewed alongside the growing wealth divide in Britain. Since the late 1970s there has been a dramatic widening of the gap between rich and poor. (Joseph Rowntree Foundation, 1995). Box 2.5.4 shows that the poorest 10% (decile group) had a *fall* of 18% in their real income (after housing costs) while the average had a rise of 37% and the top 10% a rise of 61%. Between 1979 and 1993 the poorest in our society failed to benefit from the economic growth which benefited others. In short, while the rich saw their share of wealth increase enormously, the poor got even poorer.

For health professionals, the most significant issues arising from the Rowntree findings are not just concern at the human misery experienced by the poorest, but at the resultant catastrophe for health that such a wealth divide represents.

Against the backdrop of increased poverty and widening inequalities in other areas such as housing income, education and health care, it is hardly surprising that most recent studies have shown the health gap to be widening further still (Davey-Smith *et al.*, 1990; Wilkinson, 1992; Phillimore *et al.*, 1994; Benzeval *et al.*, 1995). Judge and Benzeval (1993) have shown that the health implications for the children of lone mothers on low incomes may be particularly acute. Lone mothers with dependent children who are largely reliant on social security benefits are one of the fastest growing and most disadvantaged groups in society (see Chapter 2.1). Over one million dependent children are in such families, and these children have the worst mortality record of any social group. (Judge and Benzeval, 1993).

The work of Graham (1993) and Payne (1991) has highlighted the severe strain that poverty can place on women's mental and physical health, as they try to

Box 2.5.3 The risk of and numbers in poverty by economic status

	Risk of poverty (%)		Numbers in poverty (000s)	
	1979	1992/3	1979	1992/3
Self-employed	15	25	540	1420
Single/couple, all in full-time work	1	2	100	260
One in full-time work, one in part-time work	1	4	90	300
One in full-time work, one not working	4	16	480	1270
One or more in part-time work	15	33	540	1250
Head/spouse aged 60+	20	33	1660	3340
Head/spouse unemployed	58	75	880	3090
Other	35	61	990	3120
Total			5280	14 050

* The risk of poverty columns show the proportion of each group in poverty, eg, 75% of the unemployed were living in poverty in 1992/3
Source CPAG (1996).

Box 2.5.4 Rises in real income between 1979 and 1992/93 (including the self-employed)

	Income before housing costs (%)	Income after housing costs (%)
First (bottom)	0	–18
Second	8	0
Third	12	6
Fourth	16	15
Fifth	23	23
Sixth	28	29
Seventh	32	34
Eighth	36	39
Ninth	44	47
Tenth (top)	56	61
Total population	36	37

Source CPAG (December 1995).

balance the demands of home, children and other dependants against an inadequate income. Women's pivotal role as carers and keepers of health for all family members should not be underestimated by health workers. The detrimental effect these responsibilities can have on women's own health and well-being should not be overlooked.

The issue of men's health has also recently assumed a much higher profile. The alarming rise in suicide amongst young men has fuelled the debate concerning the links between deteriorating mental health and social trends such as family break-up, poverty and unemployment. (See Chapter 1.1 for further discussion.)

The health of the poor is further jeopardized by inadequate housing. Infections, cot-deaths and accidents are the main causes of post neonatal mortality. A disproportionate number of these infant deaths occur in households in which basic amenities are lacking, people are living in overcrowded conditions or faculties are shared with other families (Fox and Goldbatt, 1982; Moore, 1990; Lowry, 1991).

Adults and children living in damp housing report more respiratory symptoms than those living in dry surroundings (Lowry, 1991). Poor living conditions are not only associated with increased *physical* ill health and mortality: research has discovered links between housing and general social and *psychological* well-being. Cramped living accommodation, lack of privacy, inadequate facilities and other housing problems can produce stress and in severe cases can be contributing factors in the onset of clinical depression (Brown and Harris, 1978; Lowry, 1991). For children the cumulative effects of socioeconomic deprivation have a devastating effect on present and future health and well-being.

Sir Douglas Black returning to the health inequalities fray in 1993 argued with some despair that the 'recurrence of monetarism over the past dozen years has again created evils that should have been relegated to history'. Referring to his committee's recommendations in 1980, he remains unrepentant as to their relevance a decade on:

Our view that poverty and its effects was the root cause of the ill-health associated with it, naturally led us to advocate a wider strategy of social measures. After all, the surest way to alleviate the effects of poverty must be to alleviate poverty itself . . . if we are serious in seeking to diminish morbidity and mortality due to social deprivation, we must return to the values of the welfare state and pursue them with greater determination. (*The Guardian*, 17 December 1993)

The Government's Response to Poverty and Health

What has been the response of the government to such evidence? They are hardly likely to heed Sir Douglas Black's call to a return to welfare state principles, when they have a clear ideological mandate to do precisely the reverse (Mishra, 1986; George and Wilding, 1994; Sullivan, 1994).

By and large the issue of poverty has been ignored (*The Health of the Nation* (DOH, 1992) did not mention the word once!). Any acknowledgement of poverty has been shrouded in the increasingly fashionable notion of an 'underclass' (Murray, 1994). Therefore the poor are judged to be an undeserving band of latter day 'brigands', characterized by illegitimacy, dependency on 'generous' welfare benefits, criminality and unwillingness to work. It is the pervasiveness of this belief of an undeserving poor that has enabled government to side-step the issue of health inequalities. Not only do this 'underclass' have dubious sexual mores and a tendency towards voluntary unemployment and crime, but they also make the health of themselves and their children unnecessarily poor by their lifestyle habits. Accordingly the inferior health of poor families can be exposed as 'just another characteristic of the underclass', the result of the ignorance, fecklessness and mismanagement of finances.

It is a simplistic, unfounded and yet seductive explanation. What is so sadly lacking in this perspective is any real acknowledgement of the way in which lifestyle choices are shaped. As Baggott (1994) illustrates it is clear that individuals do not make choices within a vacuum: eating, smoking and drinking habits, for example, are shaped by class, culture and income as well as 'personal whim' (Baggott, 1994: 249).

Whilst charges of financial mismanagement are certainly justified in individual cases, this is surely not a weakness confined to the poor. There are poor money managers at each end of the social spectrum, but it always seems to be those with least money to manage who stand accused of fecklessness. Middle class mismanagement can be hidden by credit cards, overdraughts, bankloans and other 'respectable' survival mechanisms. Mismanagement amongst the poor is more visible, carries a heavy cost (as the recent rise in 'loan shark' debt has shown), and is arguably far less prevalent than popular mythology would have us believe (Parker, 1992).

The debate surrounding the consumption and purchase of a healthy diet provides a very useful illustration of both how health choices are constrained by economic circumstance and how charges of mismanagement and ignorance are unjustified.

Food, Diet and Poverty

It is often argued that not only do those on low incomes consume a poor, 'chip-rich' diet which contributes to their burden of ill health, but also this is inexcusable given that with a modicum of sense, it is very easy to eat cheaply and healthily (Currie, 1990; Leather, 1992). But is it? Or do these views merely illustrate how easy it is to pass judgement on others from the warmth of a well equipped kitchen? Research has shown that indeed low income families do consume more high fat, high sugar foods and that higher income groups purchase more fruit, vegetables and wholemeal bread etc. (Cole-Hamilton and Lange, 1986). There is evidence that these inequalities are becoming wider (Brummer, 1987a, b; Health Education Authority, 1989; Malseed, 1990).

Often this information is interpreted as yet another example of ignorance and mismanagement by the poor. As Malseed (1990) argues 'there is a common sentiment underlying government perspectives and conventional health education that the inefficient management of domestic budgets and mis-allocation of resources are principally responsible for the poor nutritional status of low-income households'.

Thus, she argues, social inequalities in food consumption are explained away by contrasting middle class organization and responsibility with lower class disorganization and irresponsibility. The health policy implications of these attitudes are evident. 'The lower classes do not need more money to attain healthier diets only to be persuaded to manage and spend their money more wisely' (Malseed, 1990: 29).

This perspective, which dominates much healthy eating literature and many professional interventions, runs contrary to actual research findings and of course what the poor know themselves. It is *not* mismanagement or ignorance that prevents them from eating healthily, it is that the paucity of their income prevents them from doing so. As Player (1988) so aptly argues.

> The problem in poor families is not ignorance and recklessness, it is shortage of money.
> In such circumstances health education messages about how to eat wisely and homilies
> from rich ministers are worse than useless: they are a plain insult. (Player, 1988)

Given, then, that lack of income is the major barrier to a healthy diet, of most urgency to health advisers is the question of whether it is possible to purchase a *cheap* but healthy diet? Leather (1992) argues that health educators have for too long wrongly presumed that a healthy diet is 'cheaper' and therefore an option available to all irrespective of income. Under pressure from consumer groups to put this belief to the test the Ministry of Agriculture, Fisheries and Food (MAFF) published details of a cheap healthy diet which could be purchased at a cost of £10 per week per person. That is as long as poor consumers did not mind eating eight slices of bread per day, five of which were to be eaten dry and a half a fish finger. (Leather, 1992: 176). Work done by the Health Education Authority in 1989 showed that mothers in low income families have just as much concern for their children's health and knowledge of 'healthy eating' as their more affluent peers and often make sacrifices so that others may be fed. A National Children's Home survey in 1992 found that mothers on benefit frequently went without food for two or three days at a time. Charles and Kerr (1988) found that mothers frequently scrimped on food for themselves in order to maximize food for husbands and children. Far from being profligate, evidence suggests poorer families actually shop more efficiently than their more affluent peers, and employ a variety of shopping and meal planning strategies. Low income groups spend a much higher proportion of their income on food than the better off. It is usually the only flexible item in a highly constrained budget, so if cutbacks need to be made to cover unexpected emergencies such as, for example, a new pair of shoes, then food is usually the area within which budgeting taking place. All shopping is often done on the day wages or giros are received, and a 'tunnel vision' approach to shopping almost always has to be adopted. The monotony of food poverty is thus set in motion, there is no room for dalliance with 'sun dried tomatoes' and other exotica, and little risk can be taken with children's food if no replacements are available when a meal is rejected. (Health Education Authority, 1989).

Out of Town – Out of Reach?

The problem of 'food poverty' has also been exacerbated by the trend towards large out of town hypermarkets. Arguably, just at the time that we are being urged to 'choose' a more healthy lifestyle, the 'choice' for poorer groups, in terms of purchasing food, is shrinking rapidly (Henson, 1992). Ironically, it is the poorest members of society who are often paying the most for their food. Out of town developments have left many urban and rural poor with little choice but to shop in small local outlets that have a limited range of products, little in the way of fresh food, and much higher prices than the big supermarket chains.

As well as lacking cars, other resources often taken for granted such as freezers, and an adequately equipped kitchen etc., are becoming beyond the reaches of many low income groups. Many social policy changes over the last decade have indirectly exacerbated the slide into food poverty. The replacement of special needs payments with loans from the Social Fund, in 1988 has left many families bereft when replacement cookers, fridges etc., are required. Charities are reportedly swamped by the level of demand for second-hand goods. The tougher responses to non-payment of bills employed by the newly privatized utilities have left many of the poor without basics such as electricity, gas and water (D'Alessio, 1994). The crisis in housing also represents a challenge in healthy eating; it is not hard to imagine the nightmare of trying to eat healthily in bed and breakfast accommodation. The withdrawal of nutritional requirements in school meals in 1980 also dealt a blow to child nutrition, a particularly worrying area.

CONCLUSION

In the 1990s nurses are facing an unenviable task. An important function of their role is to provide information and advice in order to help promote a healthy lifestyle. This has to be undertaken at a time when it is becoming increasingly difficult for many people to incorporate healthy choices into their lives. Advice, and care, has to be offered against a backdrop of rising poverty, unemployment, racism, family breakdown and social dislocation. (See Chapter 1.2 for further discussion.)

All these factors must be of concern to nurses. This chapter has shown that there is overwhelming evidence that present and future health is adversely affected by social and economic deprivation. Yet nurses are being urged to collude with government strategies born of political expediency that ignore poverty and favour modifying individual risk behaviour. This is, as Phillimore *et al.* (1994) point out, a rather curious response given:

> if historical improvements in health throughout the population are generally attributed to rising living standards and improving material conditions, so worsening health among some groups and widening differentials must be related primarily to changes in the same factors. (Phillimore *et al.*, 1994)

In response, nurses need to make their approach to health promotion sensitive, flexible and realistic. The worried middle class may well benefit from low fat recipes and exercise videos, but the needs of the poorest may require different attention and advice. Nurses cannot 'magic' a more realistic income for such people (although this would arguably improve their health most effectively); but they can demonstrate that they recognize the many constraints on living healthily. Hence, it is essential that nurses examine how these constraints restrict choices, making it very difficult to adopt a healthy lifestyle even when familiar with 'health' advice.

This chapter has also highlighted evidence to show that living on a very low income not only affects mental and physical health, but also may provoke families into adopting unhealthy behaviour (smoking, poor diet etc.) in order to keep things together, to keep the limited budget solvent and to make sure that the children have the best of what little there is. The constant strain between 'health keeping' and 'housekeeping' places considerable strain on women's health. This can only be exacerbated by the general shift from hospital to community based care, for it is most often women who bear the brunt of such policies, and shoulder the major burden of caring (Glendinning, 1992).

As well as encouraging sensitivity in their approach to work with families, nurses also need to be able to locate health policies within a wider political and economic framework. The government's preferred strategy, to combat ill health through individual will and familial responsibility, comes at a time of increasing social dislocation when people's capacity to cope and care may well be lessening. Nevertheless research indicates that most people *have* taken on board health advice, and *are* making changes to their lifestyle, yet clear differentials remain (Blaxter, 1990: 243). The health divide *cannot* be explained away by lifestyle alone. There are obviously factors outside the control of individuals like poverty, unemployment, poor housing and environmental pollution that are affecting their health.

SUMMARY

■ Nurses need to be more critical of behavioural approaches to improving health and to recognize the ideological context within which many health promotion policies must be viewed.

■ Preoccupation with individual lifestyle has served to divert attention from the clear evidence linking poor health with material and environmental deprivation.

■ We need to recognize in practice that social and economic deprivation severely constrains lifestyle choices and exacerbates risk behaviour as health needs are often neglected in the daily struggle to survive with too little money.

■ Without attention to social, economic and environmental factors there are unlikely to be any significant improvements in the health of the poorest groups, and inequalities in health will widen.

DISCUSSION QUESTIONS

◆ Will the focus on behavioural change really deliver measurable improvements in physical and emotional health where it is most badly needed; amongst the poorest sections of the UK? (Benzeval *et al.*, 1995)

◆ Why do so few agencies involved in health promotion address the vital issue of how health behaviour might be influenced by the material conditions in which people live?

◆ Consider whether the benefit of behavioural change will be as health enhancing for the poor as it is for more affluent groups?

FURTHER READING

Benzeval M, Judge K and Whitehead M (Eds) (1995) *Tackling Inequalities in Health: An Agenda for Action*. London: King's Fund.

An excellent review of the most recent evidence for inequalities in health, and explanations as to why inequalities occur. This report not only highlights particular issues such as housing, smoking, poverty etc., but also reviews recent policy initiatives and looks at the role of the NHS and practitioners within it. A must for any nurse working in the community.

Blackburn C (1991) *Poverty and Health*. OU Press.

This is a very readable account of the relationship between poverty and health. It provides clear explanations of the problems in defining and measuring poverty and carefully chronicles how a variety of factors such as housing, diet, unemployment etc.,

influence health and the dilemmas faced by health professionals working in poor communities.

Graham H (1993) *Hardship and Health in Woman's Lives*. London: Harvester Wheatsheaf.

This book examines the domestic circumstances and responsibilities of women caring for children in 1990s Britain, and asks how women survive when responsibilities are many and resources are few. This book provides invaluable insight for health workers into the dilemmas faced by women attempting to balance 'hardship' and 'health'.

Marsh A and McKay S (1994) *Poor Smokers*. London: Policy Studies Institute.

This large scale study of who smokes and why, will provide invaluable insight and information for any health professional.

REFERENCES

Baggott R (1994) *Health and Health Care in Britain*. St Martins Press.

Barker D (1992) 'Heart attacks' determined in the womb' cited in the *Observer* 24 May 1992

Barker DJP, Meade TW and Stirling Y. (1992) Relation of foetal and infant growth to plasma fibrinogen and factor VII concentration in adult life. *British Medical Journal*, **304:** 148-152.

Benzeval M, Whitehead M and Judge K (1995) *Tackling Inequalities in Health*. London: King's Fund Institute

Beveridge W (1942) *Social Insurance and Allied Services*. London: HMSO.

Blackburn C (1991) *Poverty and Health*. Open University Press.

Black D (1980) *Report on the Working Party on Inequalities in Health*, chaired by Sir Douglas Black. London: DHSS.

Blaxter M (1990) *Health and Lifestyles*. London: Tavistock/Routledge.

Brown GW and Harris T (1978) *Social Origins of Depression: A Study of Psychiatric Disorder in Women*. London: Tavistock.

Brummer E (1987a) The heart of the matter. *London Food News*, No. 6 (Summer 1987) p 5.

Brummer E (1987b) Looking at 'Look After Your Heart'. London Food Commission Briefing Paper, London: London Food Commission.

Carr-Hill R (1987) The Inequalities in Health debate: a critical review of the issues. *Journal of Social Policy* **16**(4): 509-542.

Charles N and Kerr M (1988) *Women, Food and Families*. Manchester: Manchester University Press.

Cole-Hamilton I and Lang T (1986) *'Tightening Belts'. A Report on the Impact of Poverty on Food*. London: London Food Commission.

Coward R (1993) *The myth of alternative health*. In A Beattie, M Goff *et al.* (Eds) *Health and Wellbeing: a reader*. Macmillan (in association with The Open University Press).

Currie E (1990) *Lifelines: Politics and Health 1986-88*. London: Pan Books.

Davey Smith G, Bartley M and Blane D (1990) The Black Report on socio-economic inequalities in health 10 years on. *British Medical Journal* **301:** 373-377.

D'Alessio V (1994) The Water Poverty Trap. *Nursing Times* June 22 (1994) vol 90 no 25 p 14-15.

DOH (1992) *The Health of the Nation: A Strategy for Health in England*, Cm 1986. London: HMSO.

DSS (1994) *Households below Average Incomes, A statistical analysis 1979-1991/92*. London: HMSO.

Fox AJ and Goldblatt PO (1982) *Longitudinal Study: Socio-demographic mortality differentials, 1971-75*, series L5 (i). London: HMSO.

George V and Wilding, (1994) *Ideology and Social Welfare*. London: Harvester Wheatsheaf.

Glendinning C (1992) 'Community Care': The Financial consequences for women. In C Glendinning and J Millar (Eds) *Women and Poverty in Britain: the 1990s*. London: Harvester Wheatsheaf.

Graham H (1984) *Women, Health and the Family*. London: Tavistock.

Graham H (1987) Women's smoking and family health. *Social Science and Medicine* **25**(1): 47-56.

Graham H (1988) Women and smoking in the United Kingdom: implications for health promotion. *Health Promotion* **3**(4): 371–382.

Graham H (1993) *Hardship and Health in Women's Lives*. pp 179–183. London: Harverster Wheatsheaf.

Health Education Authority (1989) *Diet, Nutrition and 'Healthy Eating' in Low Income Groups*.

Henson S (1992) From High Street to Hypermarket, Food Retailing in the 1990s, in National Consumer Council pp 95–116.

Illsley R (1986) Occupational class, selection and the production of inequalities in health. *Quarterly Journal of Social Affairs* **2**: 151–165.

Illsley R (1987) Occupational class, selection and inequalities in health: a rejoinder to Richard Wilkinson's reply. *Quarterly Journal of Social Affairs* **3**: 213–223.

Joseph Rowntree Foundation (1995) *Inquiry into Income and Wealth in Britain*.

Judge K and Benzeval M (1993) Health Inequalities: new concerns about the children of single mothers. *British Medical Journal* **306**: 677–886.

Le Grand J (1994) Equity, Efficiency and the Rationing of Health Care. Paper for the British Association for the Advancement of Science Meetings. Loughborough, September 1994.

Leather S (1992) Less money, less choice: poverty and diet in the UK today, in National Consumer Council *Your Food Whose Choice?*, pp 72–95.

Lowry S (1991) *Housing and Health*. London: British Medical Journal Publications.

Malseed J (1990) *Bread without Dough: Understanding Food Poverty*. Horton Publishing.

Marsh A and McKay S (1994) *Poor Smokers*. London: Policy Studies Institute.

Mishra R (1986) *The Welfare State in Crisis*. Wheatsheaf Books.

Moore C (1990) Homelessness: the hidden cost. *Health Visitor* **63**(6): 196–197.

Murray C (1994) *Underclass: The Crisis Deepens*. The IEA Health and Welfare Unit. Choice in Welfare Series No 20.

National Childrens' Home (1991) *Poverty and Nutrition Survey*. London: NCH.

National Consumer Council (1992) *Your Food: Whose Choice?* London: HMSO.

Parker G (1992) Making Ends Meet: 'Women, Credit and Debt'. In C Glendinning and J Millar (Eds) *Women and Poverty in Britain: the 1990s*. London: Harvester Wheatsheaf.

Payne S (1991) *Women, Health and Poverty*. London: Harvester Wheatsheaf.

Phillimore P, Beattie A and Townsend P (1994) Widening inequality of health in Northern England, 1981–91. *British Medical Journal* **308**: 1125–1128.

Platt S (1984) Unemployment and suicidal behaviour: a review of the literature. *Social Science and Medicine* **19**: 43–52.

Player D (1988) Fair play. *Lancet* 2nd June, p. 624.

Pritchard C (1994) Connections or Coincidence? An International Comparison of Sudden Infant Death Syndrome (SIDS), Baby Homicide and Childhood Malignancies in England and Wales: A New Approach to child protection? *Social Work and Social Sciences Review* **5**(3): 186–218.

Roberts H (Ed) (1990) *Women's Health Counts*. London: Routledge.

Smith GD, Bartley M and Blane D (1990) The Black Report on Socio-Economic Inequalities in Health 10 years on. *British Medical Journal* **301**: 373–377.

Sullivan M (1994) *Modern Social Policy*. London: Harvester Wheatsheaf.

Townsend P (1979) *Poverty in the UK*. Pelican Books.

Townsend P, Davidson N and Whitehead M (1988) *Inequalities in Health: The Black Report and the Health Divide*. Harmondsworth: Penguin.

Whitehead M (1987) *The Health Divide*. London: Health Education Council.

Whitehead M, Judge K and Benzeval M (1995) *Tackling Inequalities in Health*. London: King's Fund Institute.

Wilkinson RG (1990) Income distribution and mortality: a 'natural' experiment. *Sociology of Health and Illness* **12**: 391–412.

Wilkinson RG (1992) Income distribution and life expectancy. *British Medical Journal* **304**: 165–168.

Wilkinson RG (1994) Health redistribution and growth. In D Miliband and A Glyn (Eds) *Paying for Inequality: The Economic Costs of Social Injustice*. London: Rivers Oram Press.

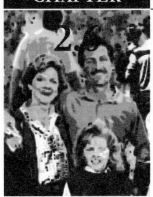

FAMILIES WITH SPECIAL NEEDS

Tony Thompson

KEY ISSUES

- The context of care
- The importance of early identification
- The design of family services
- The concept of family centred service

INTRODUCTION

The context of care identified in this chapter is one which highlights the predicament of the family and the challenge they face when a member has special needs. It reinforces the point that some families do not always see a disabled child as a single major stress. Rather, they perceive peripheral issues such as insensitive communication, arrogant professional service delivery and relationship problems as a source of distress. A disabled family member may weaken an already fragile relationship and parental confrontation with services meant to support them may occur at the most vulnerable time.

The above factors have to be balanced with the disabled member's contribution having to be viewed in ways other than in terms of disability. By taking this view the capacity for giving and receiving love, warmth and empathy should not be ignored by professionals.

The Context of Care

> The special needs of parents with a handicapped child are as specific as those of the child they love and care for. (Griffiths and Clegg, 1988)

This statement sometimes has a hollow ring for those families who provide primary care with poor input from professionals or statutory services. It is likely that in these families, input based on stereotypical notions of: (a) family, (b) special needs, and (c) learning disabilities can result in them feeling that they struggle alone with their responsibilities.

The position of the family who has a member with a learning disability is likely to reflect the dilemma of families with any other form of disability. The support networks available to the main carers in the family tend to fall into two distinct areas:

Unpaid/informal support

- Immediate family provision
- Extended family provision
- Neighbours and friends
- Ad hoc voluntary groups

Formal/paid support

- Social workers
- Health visitors
- Community learning disability nurses
- General practitioners
- Specialized therapists

It is worth observing that these structural networks tend to represent a '*client*' or '*care receiver*' focus. The significance of this is that when speaking with families they report how valuable they would find *care provider* support. Even when there is a degree of informed input of formal or informal support to the person with a disability, it is not unusual to find certain family members providing care almost 24 hours a day. This phenomenon is particularly important when the plight of young family carers is examined. In their insightful study, Jo Aldridge and Saul Becker draw attention to disturbing features of family coping by young carers. They did not find any evidence of professional support aimed expressly at young carers. Further, no professional had been involved in any discussion with young carers about their needs or their caring roles (Aldridge and Becker, 1993).

Although professional care providers often assume that some reasonable and effective support for a particular family carer would be forthcoming from the other family members, this is increasingly not the case. The above study offered evidence in relation to the duty of caring of a young family member and it is possible to draw similar conclusions in these circumstances where a family has one main significant care provider. The context is likely to be one which reflects the point that even when there are other family members in the house who could help, primary caring responsibilities tend to fall on one member. This member undertakes the major caring role either because (i) he or she cares deeply for the disabled member and consequently feels responsible for their welfare, or (ii) feels a duty to care because of a high refined sense of loyalty, or (iii) they are 'elected' to care irrespective of their feelings by other family members.

The features of the above are strongly tied to stereotyped notions of primary caring responsibilities. The notion of caring as 'women's work' is often reflected in the attitudes of potential supporting family networks.

The many historical features and myths which have surrounded people with a learning disability can add to the potential burden of a family who may be searching for appropriate help and support. At best this may result in hesitancy of community support, at worst it can result in open hostility towards the family and its individual members. Numerous explanations may account for poor support mechanisms for a family. These include:

- erosion of primary neighbourhood groupings;
- residential transience;
- political/media sentiments, e.g. no such thing as society only individuals and their families;

- uncertainty of level of commitment/support required;
- anxiety or fear of inability to cope with features of a learning disability.

Whatever the explanation offered to families, it may be that their faith in a caring 'community' can become strained at times when they most need it.

The Importance of Early Identification

Most families with a member who has special needs tend to agree about the importance of competent and accurate early identification. This is particularly true of those who have a child with profound or severe learning disabilities. A major aim of accurate identification of the phenomenon is to:

- access early inter-disciplinary assessment of the child's developmental, medical and associated problems in order to ensure that needs are met with minimum delay;
- provide appropriate counselling and support services for the family;
- initiate collaborative action between interested and responsible agencies.

It is critical for the longer-term benefit of a family that there is follow-up of any child whose preliminary examination has caused concern. This usually occurs by input from health visiting services, attendance at postnatal clinics or direct referral to the paediatrician. It is essential that a local disability/handicap team or community learning disability team, whichever is appropriate, is informed. All those concerned with the care and treatment of young children, including members of any primary care team, should know whether one or both operate in their area, and which team it is that locally concerns itself with the child with special needs. Since the 1981 Education Act (DES, 1981) there should be an established and known agreed method of local referral. Local authority social services and education departments should be informed as a matter of routine about all children with a learning disability as they are born or are identified. These agencies should contribute to the keeping of a register and should be kept fully informed of the result of any revision of assessment and or decision to which they are not party. This includes any information about additional handicaps which may affect the child's developmental progress or require particular forms of care, treatment or education during the child's lifetime (DHSS, 1984).

Detailed advice was given over a decade ago and this still remains highly pertinent to health, social services and education authorities on the specific assessment of children with special educational needs. The main aspects of this advice are contained in a joint DES/DHSS (1983) circular. It is within this guidance that the Statements of Special Educational Needs are contained.

There is evidence that when parents understand, identify with, and support, the aims of the school in relation to a child's education, they take an active interest which will make a significant impact on the life of that child (Atkin *et al.*, 1988). A good example of where these processes work well is given by Sloper and Cunningham (1991) who provide an analysis of the levels of parent/teacher links ranging from basic home–school links which is supported by written information, informal contacts, telephone calls to the more formal-professional partnership where parents are actually engaged in the educational process by contributing their own special knowledge and skills about the disabled child. Many of the lessons learned in mainstream education are likely to be equally relevant to special education.

Assessment and Intervention

Early interdisciplinary assessment should include paediatricians, nursing staff, health visiting services, professionals allied to medicine particularly physiotherapy services, speech therapy services, psychologists and social workers. The assessment process should establish the need for specialist medical screening of potentially additional handicapping or disabling conditions.

A prime focus of the assessment will be the design of a care programme aimed at meeting the needs of the child's specific health, developmental, educational, social and family needs. The family should play an active and important part in the process and it is important that their perceptions are not overlooked by overzealous professionals who may not necessarily share these perceptions and thereby run the risk of establishing inappropriate plans which are difficult for families to comprehend.

It is usual at this stage for a paediatrician to arrange comprehensive medical screening which may include:

- chromosome identification and testing;
- exclusion tests for intrauterine infection with rubella in cytomegalovirus;
- EEG for potential epilepsy;
- audiological tests;
- ophthalmological examination.

The continued monitoring of sight and hearing by the interdisciplinary team is important and in the contemporary moves to providing social care can be prone to unwitting neglect. Example of the medical or clinical emphasis includes:

- Down children being prone to palate defects and later onset development of conductive hearing deficits.
- Children with the mucopolysaccharidoses (Hurler and related syndromes) with corneal clouding, glaucoma and retinal deterioration.
- Orthopaedic handicapping conditions and locomotor abilities.
- Speech/language and hand-eye coordination problems.

The holistic assessment will consider the family circumstances and context, relationships, together with family support structures or lack of them. It is the latter which may prove vital to a disabled child's needs for stimulation and potential development.

The Design of Family Services

A major purpose of prior assessments is to facilitate appropriate services and access to these for the family. Typical questions which should be addressed include:

- What supportive options are available to the family to maintain the child with special needs at home?
- Who is likely to be the most appropriate key worker to:
  (a) the child?
  (b) the family?
- Is the child likely to benefit from early remedial intervention from personnel such as:
  (a) speech therapist?
  (b) occupational therapist?
  (c) community learning disability nurse?

(d) physiotherapists?

- would home modifications, aids or adaptations assist the child and its family?
- would playgroup, day nursery or special nursery classes be of immediate assistance?
- are there potential behavioural problems that are likely to challenge services which may benefit from earlier intervention before they become established?

For children who are very young with a learning disability, learning programmes are continually being seen as valuable by families and professionals alike. Preschool programmes such as Portage are considered to be of particular value. These highly structured and rational programmes can be used by the parent or family with guidance from a skilled and competent operator such as the community learning disability nurse or a health visitor. This scheme is used with success in increasing achievement of profoundly disabled children and those with complex needs. Such schemes are designed to meet developmental targets in short, attainable stages. The stages are graded and therefore are designed to provide positive feedback to the family and assist in maintaining their motivation.

The assessment and monitoring process continues throughout the life of the child therefore preschool, school age, young adult, adult and elderly person. Naturally the family relationships change throughout life and systematic review remains an all important part of family support mechanisms.

It is now widely accepted that even the most profoundly disabled person can continue to learn and therefore coordinated effort should be maintained to develop self-help and social/communication skills throughout a person's life. One of the most satisfying aspects of being involved in care provision is that of working closely with families. This is seen when small but important attainments are made by the disabled person and morale of both professional and family carers is lifted and another goal is set.

Families of people with disabilities sometimes find it helpful to know that if they wish, respite or short-term care may be arranged for their child. Some agencies have well established schemes which encourage the family to contact another family who will care for their child on a periodic, short-term basis enabling them to find precious space for themselves. Such schemes also include a volunteer minding scheme which can be just sufficient to allow some additional social life. Likewise, agencies provide help lines, information desks and leaflets which comprehensively describe services

Box 2.6.1. Key issues

- Informing parents of disability
- Appropriate and competent advice and counselling
- The distress of additional disabilities
- Information at appropriate stage and at level
- Taking parental perceptions seriously
- Screening
- Assessment and monitoring
- Key workers
- Sensitive suggestions of help, e.g. voluntary groups
- Keeping parents informed
- Inviting family participation
- Financial help
- Inter-agency collaboration

available together with contact addresses and telephone numbers (see 'useful addresses' at end of chapter). So far in this chapter it has been possible to reinforce the point that at all stages of life for the person with special needs or learning disabilities decisions need to be taken with the person and their families regarding the type of care and therapeutic intervention which may be needed to fulfil maximum potential.

The inputting of information and health education are important functions undertaken by health care practitioners when working with families who have a member with special needs. Early research and premises put forward by Ackerman (1958) suggested that the family is the basic unit of society and thought of the family as an organism – the basic unit of health. For many families, the health care practitioner can make the best input just by offering support and confirmation that validates that they are successfully sorting their own problems.

It is not unusual for care workers to find that families with a person with special needs can be highly creative in finding solutions to their own problems of care.

Contemporary researchers and commentators (Todd, 1993) have reflected on 'Macro' schemes intended to medically improve the life experiences and opportunities for people with a learning disability and their families. One such scheme, the All Wales Handicap Strategy (Welsh Office, 1983) went beyond an increase in service provision and promoted the improvement of the social situation, value and status of people with learning disabilities. In their research the above commentators have considered the perception of consumers regarding the meeting of ambitious aims. Amongst the most successful goals has been the provision of support services for families. Such services had typically developed from a low base provision to a higher one in a relatively short time scale. In 1990 one in three families received domiciliary support and one in four utilized short-term care. This data compared with approximately one in eight for both services in 1986 (Beyer, 1991).

For as much as they valued the support, the families expressed concern that such schemes were unstable and potentially fragile in the nature of their provision. These concerns revolve around the reality of the impact likely to be experiences when families temporarily lose such support. This is likely to be felt particularly by those families caring for a relative with high levels of dependency.

The following anecdotes are taken from the Todd *et al.* (1993) study and are used to stimulate debate and thought regarding the service user and family perspective on service strategies.

The Concept of Family Centred Service

The notion of family centred services has emerged as a philosophy for the design and provision of early information services. Families of children with disabilities clearly have unique strengths and needs that have to be understood and addressed in the process of formulating workable family – professional collaboration (Wilcox, 1993).

As Crais (1991) has indicated the professional care worker must consider children with disabilities and their parents as just one part of a network that is composed of entire families. This is important as conflict can occur within the whole family and parents with disabled children can be more sensitive to the judgements and criticism of other members of the family, simply because of the additional life stresses they carry. Further, the care worker should be mindful that although it is likely that parents will always wish that their child was not disabled, with time they often adapt their coping mechanisms and display great skills not only in child rearing but in directly assisting in therapy.

It is sometimes tempting for professionals to consider that parents only require information about the child's particular disability and direct assistance with therapeutic or behavioural management. Research contradicts this notion (Crutcher, 1991).

Parents need more than information, particularly shortly after the original diagnosis of a child's disabilities. They also require empathy, emotional support and insightful understanding as they start to cope with their personal emotions and behaviours as a reaction to the news. The quality of longer-term relationships

Box 2.6.2. Points to ponder

(extracted from Todd *et al.*, 1993)

Point   'I'd like Sharon to go into full time residential care now in a small home. But I think such places are going to those who are moving out of hospital, that's unfair.'
(On leaving home – a parent view)

Ponder.   How seriously are the families' views of future residential needs taken by services?

Point   'Moving house has been a big change. I had always lived with my mother and grandmother before. Now I've got my own independence really. Well, when I was living with my family, I couldn't go out that much.'
(On moving into his own flat)

Ponder.   How might moving from the family home heighten the experience of control over one's life and contribute to a disabled person's individual development?

Point   'Tom thought he was working in a factory before, clocking in and out. Now he's just bored. They used to do cooking and housecare, they don't do that now. The Centre used to be full of activities.'
(On missing the more traditional activities of an Adult Training Centre)

Ponder.   What might be the negative effects of services being based around a predominant ideology?

Point   'The social care worker has been a great help. We've been offered more respite care but James "don't" need it at the moment. I'd like him to have more of a social life through the social care worker. I'd like more time for him to be taken out rather than just bath him and sit with him at home.'
(On respite care offered to families)

Ponder: How could care services better offer a means valued by the family in furthering the quality of social experience of people with caring disabilities?

between the professional and the family often depends on the nature of the early intervention.

The nature of this contemporary thinking associated with family centred service highlights the need to revisit the traditional model of research into families and carers which emphasizes the stressful and difficult nature of the caring process. More recently an alternative model has been recorded which adopts a different stance. This is perceived by some as holding the potential to offer new insights into the process of family caring (Parker, 1992).

The essential nature of the type of model which is emerging, and which has particular relevance to health care professionals, is that it becomes essential to identify how carers actually cope with the variety of stresses they experience together with the features which actually help them to manage. Beresford (1994) highlights the fact that this approach redefines the issue of caring in a number of ways. Firstly, it does not pathologize caring, that is, it does not assume that caring invariably has an adverse effect on the carer. Secondly, the fact the many carers do adapt and cope with their situation is emphasized. Thirdly, carers are redefined as active agents as opposed to passive recipients of an onslaught of carer related stress. 'This shift in approach can be attributed to developments both within academic disciplines, where research on caring has taken place, and to the ways in which social and personal welfare are being reconceptualized within social policy.'

Previous research on families with a learning disabled child, in common with more generalized research in this area, tends to reinforce the commonly held view *that* perceives the situation of the family exclusively in terms of its disability and the tremendous pressures associated with facing up to the burden of care. Although the more contemporary research, which has been alluded to in previous paragraphs, aims for a more balanced view, generally speaking there is still a tendency for professionals to pathologize which is reflected in care services and therefore may, to some extent, ignore the fact that bonds and emotions exist in families with a disabled member just as any other family. Until research can look at the child as the parents do, we will never fully understand how parents manage. Parents do not look at their child and see disability; rather they look and see their child – their son or their daughter (Beresford, 1994).

The type of anecdote detailed in Box 2.6.3 can be found in many care histories. As time moves on and children like Claire may actually thrive, the parents are forced to put their trust in professional carers. In the worst scenarios, it is not unusual to find they have been subjected to the following experiences:

- being offered conflicting advice;
- lack of sensitivity during family crisis;
- lack of recognition for achieving difficult caring tasks;
- inter-professional conflicts;
- subjected to medical or scientific jargon;
- being undermined and made to feel guilty.

The lessons to be learned here revolve around sensitivity and awareness that as professionals we have the power to oppress people and add to family crisis. Quite often the problem is rooted in the professional who can only focus on the child and disabilities.

Those practitioners who have a wider focus and view the whole family are likely to be more valued by that family and more valuable to the disabled person's development.

Box 2.6.3. *Case example* : Julie, Neil and Claire

Claire arrived premature. My labour at the end wasn't so bad but in the early stages the low back pain was murder. Neil was good with me and rubbed my back until I was ready for delivery room. I was feeling 'woozy' and the doctor's voice was distant but I clearly heard him say – Sister arrange IC (intensive care). I broke into a panic! I instinctively knew that the baby was dying. I couldn't speak at first, just trembled and then I screamed and further screamed.

Whilst exhausted, the obstetrician came and tried to quieten me – he said he would explain what had happened. He told me that Claire's heart and lungs were very weak, oxygen had not been able to get to the vital organs and she could have brain damage.

He was not sure if Claire would live, but almost as an afterthought he said, 'thankfully you're ok and you will be able to try again'.

I was so furious. I didn't want other children. This was my child! and I wanted her to be made better. I was surrounded by technical machines, why couldn't they do something?

He left, Neil held me but stared blankly at the empty cot. The Sister told me I needed to stay in to get some rest as I was still emotionally unstable.

Vagg (1992) sums up the foregoing points asking 'how professionals whose objective it is to provide an appropriate effective service for families with a person with special needs can fully understand the problems encountered by their clients. The realistic answer is that they probably can't. What they can do, however, is to tread carefully and with sensitivity, assume nothing, approach each situation with an open mind uncluttered by pre-conceived, ill-informed ideas, show support without being judgemental, be realistic about the application of modern theories and parents' responses to them. Help where help is possible and stop short of making empty promises' (Vagg, 1992).

CONCLUSION

Those professionals who are able to offer skills to a disabled person should work as closely as possible with parents and families. The information and knowledge which individual professionals may have is put to maximum use if this is seen in the context of the primary carers who are usually parents. Any holes in the next of family contact will mean that important issues are likely to remain unresolved.

The chapter has indicated some important issues which are sometimes experienced by families and parents particularly. Social policy is now evolving that firmly reinforces the benefits of collaborative services. There is no more productive relationship in care than that of dignified, valued collaboration between the health care professionals and the primary carers or families.

SUMMARY

- Duty of care may fall on one family member.
- Poor support mechanisms may exist thus weakening the family unit.
- Early identification should acknowledge the child as well as the disability.
- The disabled person's mechanisms for managing their disability can reduce family pressure.

■ Holistic assessment is critical to effective interdisciplinary support to the family.

■ The nature and quality of the total family relationship directly affects how crisis and stress are coped with.

■ The competence and adequacy of professional service delivery affects the ability of the family to meet their own needs and that of a disabled member.

DISCUSSION QUESTIONS

◆ How might a practitioner identify family members who are more ready than others to learn about the person with special needs?

◆ What factors assist the practitioner assess the needs of the family?

◆ In what ways can practitioners intervene in the family?

◆ What information is likely to be of most importance to the family with a child with a learning disability:

(a) pre-school

(b) during school years

(c) during adolescence

(d) adulthood

(e) old age

FURTHER READING

Booth T and Booth W (1993) The experience of Parenthood: Research Approach. In A Craft (Ed) *Parents with Learning Disabilities*. Kidderminster: BILD.
An example of sensitive research which includes the child in the equation rather than concentrating on the sole stress of disability. Edited by one of the most respected workers in this field.

Byrne EA and Cunningham CC (1985) The effects of mentally handicapped children on families: A conceptual view *Journal of Child Psychology and Psychiatry* **26:** 847–864.
Offers a framework or construct for thinking about the impact of learning disabled children on families from a psychological perspective.

Card H (1983) What will happen when we're gone? *Community Care*, **28:** July.
A dated but poignant article highlighting parental concern regarding the enduring problems which remain when primary carers can no longer offer support.

Cork F (1992) A short break. *Nursing Times* August 12, Vol 88, No 33.
A description of the value of respite for carers from a practical perspective.

Department of Health (1993) *Services to People with Learning Disabilities and Challenging Behaviour or Mental Health Needs*: Report of the Project Group (Chairman: Professor J Mansell). London: HMSO.
A most succinct and informed account of the nature of challenging behaviour viewed from the perspective of the challenge for services and how the problems which follow are just the tip of the iceberg for families.

Grant G and McGrath M (1990) Need for Respite Care Services for Care Givers of Persons with Mental Retardation. *American Journal of Mental Retardation* **94** (6): 638–648.
A trans-Atlantic perspective which indicates the advantages of respite or short-term care as a means of furthering the chances of continued community support to families.

Haylock CL, Johnson MA and Harpin VA (1993) Parents' Views of Community Care for Children with Motor-disabilities. *Childcare, Health and Development*, **19**: 209–220.
A well researched and credible account of the specific issues associated with physical disabilities and child rearing.

Richardson A and Ritchie J (1986) Making a Break: Parents' Views About Adults with Mental Handicap Leaving the Parental Home. King Edward's Hospital Fund for London.
A balanced view of the strengths and weaknesses of parental reaction to disengagement of offspring who have up to the point of leaving home drawn on parental coping strategies.

Sherman BR (1988) Predictors of the Decision to Place Developmentally Disabled Family Members Among Family Care Providers. *American Journal of Mental Retardation*, **93**: 166–173.
A method is described which assists policy decision-makers when they wish to seek family support as the best option for care. The predictors sharply remind us that stereotypical vies can distract harmonious family care provision.

Thompson T and Mathias P (1992) *Standards and Mental Handicap – Keys to Competence*. London: Baillière Tindall.
A standard textbook which emphasizes the means of collaborative care. Specific chapters identify aspects of assessment, provision of care and the views of parents with a 'life-time of caring'.

Urey JR and Viar V (1990) Use of Mental Health and Support Services Among Families of Children with Disabilities: Discrepant views of parent and paediatricians. *Mental Handicap Research* **3**: 81–88.
A useful account which is research based and highlights the nature of ambivalence or dissonance between professionals and parents.

Wertheimer A (1989) *Self-advocacy and parents*: The impact of self-advocacy on the parents of young people with disabilities, Part of the Working Together series, Further Education Unit.
An excellent account of the effect of empowering parents and the need for inter-agency collaboration to work towards understanding valued care systems and the promotion of rights as part of advocacy.

Useful Addresses

ARC (Association of Residential Carers)
The Old Rectory
Church Lane North
Old Whittington
Chesterfield S41 9QY

Hester Adrian Research Centre
Anson House
The University
Manchester M13 9PL

APILD (Association of Practitioners in Learning Disability) formerly MHNA.
PO Box 68
Nottingham NG9 3NN

British Institute of Learning Disabilities (formerly BIMH)
Wolverhampton Road
Kidderminster
Worcestershire DY10 3PP

Disabled Living Foundation
346 Kensington High Street
London W14 8NS

Makaton Vocabulary Development Project
31 Firwood Drive
Camberley
Surrey

National Association of Mental Health
22 Harley Street
London W1N 2ED

Scope (formerly Spastics Society)
12 Park Crescent
London W1N 4EQ

King's Fund
126 Albert Street
London NW1 7NF

The Royal Society for Mental Handicapped Children and
Adults
123 Golden Lane
London EC1Y 0RT

REFERENCES

Ackerman NW (1958) *The Psychodynamics of Family Life*.
New York: Basic Books.

Aldridge J and Becker S (1993) *Children who care - inside the
world of young carers*. Department of Social Sciences,
Loughborough University in Association with
Nottinghamshire Association of Voluntary Organizations, 1
Byron Street, Mansfield, Notts.

Atkin J Bastiani J and Goode J (1988) *Listening to Parents, An
Approach to the Improvement of Home-School Relations*.
London: Croom Helm.

Beresford B (1994) *Positively Parents, Caring for a Severely
Disabled Child*. Social Policy Research Unit, HMSO.

Beyer S, Todd S and Felce D (1991) The implementation of the
All Wales Mental Handicap Strategy. *Mental Handicap
Research* **4:** 115-40.

Crais E (1991) Moving from 'parent involvement' to family
central services. *American Journal of Speech - Language
Pathology* **1:** 5-8.

Crutcher D (1991) Family support in the Home: Home Visiting
and Public Law, 99-457 a parent's perspective, *American
Psychology* **46**(2): 138-40.

DES (1981) *Effect of Provision of 1981 Education Act*. Department of Education and Science Circular 8/81.

DES/DHSS (1983) *Assessments and Statements of Special
Educational Needs*. DES Circular 1/83/HC(83)/3/
LAC(83)/2.

DHSS (1984) *Helping Mentally Handicapped People
with Special Problems*. Report of a DHSS Study Team,
DHSS.

Griffiths M and Clegg M (1988) *Cerebral Palsy: Problems and
Practice, Human Horizon Series*.

Parker G (1992) Counting care: numbers and types of informal
carers. In J Twigg (Ed) *Carers Research and Practice*.
London: HMSO.

Sloper P and Cunningham C (1978) *Helping your Handicapped Baby*. London: Souvenir Press.

Todd S, Shearn J, Beyer S and Felce D (1993) *Reflecting on
Change: Consumers' Views of the Impact of the All Wales
Strategy*. IB Mental Handicap, 13 ILD Publications
December.

Vagg J (1992) A Lifetime of Caring. In T Thompson and P
Mathias (Eds) *Standards and Mental Handicap: Keys to
Competence*. London: Baillière Tindall.

Welsh Office (1983) *The All Wales Strategy for Services for
Mentally Handicapped People*. Cardiff: Welsh Office.

Wilcox M (1993) In E Webster and L Ward (Eds) *Working with
Parents of Young Children with Disabilities*. California:
Singular Publishing Group.

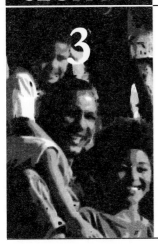

PROFESSIONAL FRAMEWORKS

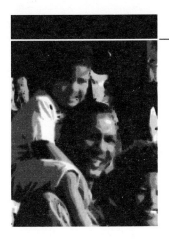

INTRODUCTION

This section considers professional issues that influence and facilitate change. The first three chapters focus on current political, ethical and legal aspects of nursing. The opening chapter is concerned with educational developments in nursing and the interface between nurse education and practice. This leads into a brief discussion of skill mix, mentorship and preceptorship and the reader is asked to consider the implications for practice of a mainly graduate workforce. The second chapter considers some current ethical issues in relation to community nursing, including a consideration of moral dilemmas, rights and responsibilities. The next chapter usefully follows with a discussion of the legal framework for ethical practice and accountability, with special reference to the duty of care and liability.

The closing chapters are concerned with issues relating to effectiveness, efficiency and resource management. The fourth chapter focuses on the importance of developing nursing services which are supported by evidence from valid and reliable research. Readers in a purchasing environment are challenged to consider justifying traditional ways of working which are not by supported research evidence. This is followed in the fifth chapter by an exploration of teamwork in a primary health care setting. In this context the advantages and possible disadvantages of teamwork are explored together with a discussion on evaluating team effectiveness. The final chapter in this section briefly introduces the reader to issues surrounding the use and impact of information systems and information technology on health care and community nursing in particular. Legal implications are discussed in relation to the *Data Protection Act* and the *Misuse of Computers Act*.

All the issues covered in this section have implications for practice in different health care settings. For some, the legal implications may be paramount, but the reader is challenged to reflect on his or her frameworks for practice in the light of topics covered in this section.

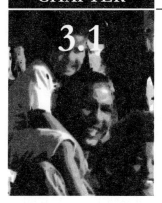

EDUCATIONAL FRAMEWORKS FOR PRACTICE

Elizabeth Porter

KEY ISSUES

■ Influences on nurse education

■ The Project 2000 nurse

■ The health care assistants

■ Community education and practice

■ Credit accumulation and transfer schemes

INTRODUCTION

This chapter will consider some of the key issues, current thinking and research influencing nurse education today. Discussion of possible educational frameworks for practice will be explored, including the preparation of graduate community health care nurses and the supporting role of health care assistants and the NVQ scheme. Whilst acknowledging the importance of the introduction of skill mix into primary health care nursing, this area will not be covered in depth in this chapter.

Influences on Education

The influences on nurse education have developed around the growing concerns about educational standards, service delivery, recruitment and retention of students, the changes in the NHS and the health needs of the population.

Purchasers, providers and other National Health Service (NHS) stake holders have a large say in how nurse education is developed to meet their needs. Yet, some seem unable to confirm the nature of their educational requirements to the Education Providers. Indeed the whole concept of self-governing NHS trusts and consortia raises anxieties as to the commitment of funding for the education of nurses. Nurses working in a community setting are finding their training needs decided by the consortia and passed to regional health authorities who place the contract and provide the funds. The risk within this system is that contracts for community nurse education can be placed with the most competitive tenderer and not with the college most suited to meet the needs of the staff (Willmott, 1990).

Wright (1994), commenting on *A Vision for the Future* (NHSME, 1993b), stated that: 'Provider units should be able to identify education that enables nurses, midwives and health visitors to develop skills associated with the overall aims of

Health of the Nation (1992), *Caring for People* (1989), the Children Act (1989) and the Patients' Charter (1991)'. This view is reinforced in *Nursing, Midwifery and Health Visitor Education*: (DOH, 1994), where the following four key points for nurse education are highlighted:

1. The need to secure adequate numbers of appropriately prepared practitioners to meet the population's health needs,
2. The need for programmes of education to be designed to satisfy the needs of the Health Commissions and meet statutory requirements as laid down by the United Kingdom Central Council (UKCC) and the National Boards for nursing, midwifery and health visiting.
3. The need for purchasers of education to forecast the nature, organization and volume of health care provision required, in order that education and training needs can be identified,
4. The need to monitor, audit and evaluate quality and outcomes of professional education and training.

The questions raised by these points revolve around the level of academic, personal and professional development required by nurses in order to deliver nursing care within a rapidly changing health service. Alongside this, the Government, as part of the Project 2000 package, set a proviso that nursing must address the issue of widening the access gate into nursing and explore the role and function of a new health care assistant/support worker (DHSS, 1988) as cited in Jowett *et al.* (1994). This development was seen as the trade off for securing Project 2000 and an inevitable consequence of the projected decline in numbers of young people available to enter nursing.

Project 2000 Nurses

Courses of preparation for Project 2000 nurses have represented a major change in nurse education. Providing an educational framework for professional practice, courses aim to produce nurses able to give a cost-effective, high quality service to the population. In the future the academic level for the Project 2000 nurse will be set at degree, but at present the preparation of the Project 2000 nurse creates a single level of practitioner able to function at diploma level in a hospital or community setting. At this level of academic ability the nurse is able to classify knowledge, make connections between fields of knowledge and begin to conceptualize and critically explore meanings in relation to professional practice. The ability to critique the contribution of research to professional practice and to raise research questions is inherent at this level.

The registered nurse (RN) is prepared for practice in either the hospital or community setting within a multidisciplinary team. The ability to work in both hospital and community settings makes maximum use of scarce resources and provides a 'knowledgeable doer' equipped: 'to make an assessment, to implement, monitor and evaluate care' (UKCC, 1986). Inherent within this role is the ability to analyse the nursing care given. However, a research study carried out by Jean Orr (1993) on behalf of the English National Board (ENB) established evidence that the Project 2000 training did not equip the nurse to work unsupervised in the community, yet managers in the research areas saw the Project 2000 nurse as the person responsible for much of the direct care given to patients and clients in the community. Despite ongoing debate about their contribution to community nursing. Project

2000 nurses are emerging from colleges of nursing with a far wider breadth of knowledge than their registered general nurse (RGN) predecessors.

Health Care Assistants (HCAs)

Nursing has always been supported by unqualified nursing staff. Voluntary workers, clerical assistants and auxiliaries are but a few examples. The introduction of HCAs to assist/support the Project 2000 nurse (UKCC, 1986) corresponded with the government scheme to rationalize vocational training whilst acknowledging that a large proportion of the nation's workforce in the United Kingdom had no recordable qualification (Rhodes, 1994).

Two types of vocational qualifications have been developed. The General National Vocational Qualification (GNVQ) and National Vocational Qualification (NVQ).

The *GNVQ* is an alternative to the General Certificate in Secondary Education (GCSE) and Advanced (A) level for students in full-time education. It is intended to lead to either higher education or directly into employment.

The *NVQ* aims to increase access to qualifications by individuals in order to encourage continuing education and learning throughout life. It also aims to recognize competence in work activities however and whenever it is required (NCVQ, 1988). The system uses five levels of vocational competence which are meant to guarantee competence to do a specific job and are designed for those who have left full-time education. As with the credit accumulation and transfer scheme (CATs) to be discussed later, the NVQ scheme also has a system of levels.

NVQ Levels

At level 1 (Basic level) the competence is seen in the performance of varied work activities most of which may be routine and predictable in prescribed settings.

At level 2 (Standard level) competence is seen in a significant range of varied work activities, performed in a variety of contexts. Some of the activities are relatively complex or non-routine and there is some individual responsibility or autonomy. Collaboration with others, perhaps through team membership, may be a requirement.

At level 3 (Advanced level) competence is in a broad range of varied work activities performed in a wide variety of contexts, most of which are complex and non-routine. There is considerable responsibility and autonomy and control or guidance of others is often required.

At level 4 (Higher level) competence is in a broad range of complex technical or professional work activities performed in a wide variety of contexts and with a substantial degree of personal responsibility and autonomy. Responsibility for the work of others and the allocation of resources is often present. It is postulated that in the future those who have attained NVQ credits at this level will be able to access Project 2000 Nurse Education programmes.

At level 5 (Professional level) competence involves the application of a significant range of fundamental principles and complex techniques across a wide and often unpredictable variety of contexts. Very substantial personal autonomy and other significant responsibility for the work of others and for the allocation of substantial resources feature strongly, as do personal accountabilities for analysis and diagnosis, design, planning, execution and evaluation (NCVQ, 1994). The present remit of the NCVQ does not extend to awarding qualifications above level 4. However, there are consultations in progress with the National Boards for Nursing, Midwifery and Health

Visiting looking at how the higher levels of professional qualification can best be articulated within the NVQ framework. As the levels of NVQ increase, 'questions are being asked both in nursing and higher education about the relationship between the two schemes' (Redfern, 1994). NVQs are now part of the world of nursing and issues such as this cannot be ignored. Indeed, underlying the NVQ qualification is the assumption that if students can show they are capable of carrying out specified tasks, they must have acquired the necessary competence. Vocational education is seen as essentially being about performance in the workplace and it is therefore logical to see NVQs in nursing fitting very well with a task/skill based approach to quality care.

It could be argued that this approach is not only a way of providing the health care assistant with a qualification, but it is also a way of maintaining and developing the skills of the registered nurse. This could be very attractive to an employer. A statement of competence is offered in the form of a number of component units which are assessed separately and certificated. Units relate to discrete groups of activity or areas of competence. This could include work experience and open learning over a given period of time where the outputs of the education/training will be clearly defined and the learning objectives derived directly from the statements of competence determined by the NCVQ. There is, however, a significant difference between knowledge to undertake a given task in a competent manner and knowledge which is capable of understanding and analyzing the results and consequences of the tasks undertaken. In the same vein it cannot be assumed that knowledge itself is associated with skills development.

Smithers (1994) as cited in Clare (1994) casts serious doubts on this approach and warns of a possible downgrading of the academic and theoretical aspects of vocational education, 'a disregard amounting to a disdain for knowledge'. Professor Smithers concludes that 'knowing how is not the same as knowing why'. Education is not simply a means to an end. Acquiring knowledge, skills and attitudes to a given area of nursing practice may not be an indication that the nurse has been educated or has gained the critical faculties necessary to decide what is good nursing practice (Jarvis, 1983). However, 'a knowledgeable practitioner who is unable to apply that knowledge is little better than a practical person who has no knowledge to apply' (Jarvis 1983).

The implications of the NVQ system for community health care nurses (CHCN) may be enormous. With the reduction in the numbers of community practice teachers (CPTs) in the early 1990s and the reduction in the numbers of community health care nurses being trained, the availability of suitably qualified assessors in the workplace could be limited. It could be that NVQ trained personnel will fill that gap. The assumption is that the knowledge and understanding which underpins the competent performance of the CHCN, and facilitates the transfer of such knowledge to the community setting, will be assessed more systematically and comprehensively by the NVQ method than in the past (NCVQ, 1988).

Both continuous assessment and assessment on demand are integral to the NVQ. Alongside this, the assessment on demand for those who acquire competence through open learning or work experience outside a formal programme of learning will put increasing pressure on those qualified to assess in the workplace. Yet, this form of assessment may provide the only practicable and cost-effective way of assessing performance. It could be that in the future the CHCN will frequently be the only person with the opportunity to observe demonstrations of performance required for assessment. This has implications for workload and skill mix.

The Community Health Care Nurse

For those registered nurses wishing to develop their knowledge and skills within the field of community nursing, The *Future of Professional Practice* document (UKCC, 1994) creates a new and unified discipline of community health care nursing (CHCN) which reflects the core skills required by all community nurse practitioners as well as the additional specialist skills required for the discrete areas of practice in district nursing, health visiting, nursing in general practice, school nursing, community mental health and community mental handicap nursing.

The preparation consists of a common core with specialist modules. The challenge for community health care nursing is in the development of programmes that provide a flexible approach, building on the best community nursing skills and developing a vision of nursing into the next century. This new model for practice is based on the nature of nursing required by communities and provides a flexible educational pathway which meets the local needs of both purchasers and practitioners whilst maintaining the standards set by the UKCC. Set at degree level, this education programme enables the Project 2000 Diplomate Nurse and others to acquire both an academic qualification at first degree level and a second professional qualification.

The evidence of educational advancement from diploma to degree status is reflected in a movement from relatively simple to more complex analysis, in increasing academic rigour and scholarship and in more specialized knowledge. This is marked by the development of a practitioner with specialist clinical expertise who has developed research skills and those specialist interpersonal skills that are necessary for professional leadership. An all graduate workforce will be expensive so purchasers of CHCNs will want assurance of the expected benefits when buying a graduate nurse. That is to say that their higher level of knowledge and clinical skills can be used to deal with clinical leadership and programme management leaving the less expensive nurse, may be the health care assistant, to develop the skills of caring using them in a variety of settings. Graduate programmes for community health care nurses must ensure that they produce a nurse able to practise in the here and now with a clear vision of the future. Working as critical thinkers, the nurse must be able to use the higher order skills required in clinical decision-making. Therefore, the programmes of preparation must deliver a nurse with an enquiring mind and the ability to be self-directed but also able to be responsive to the needs of the commissioners.

Recent and ongoing change both in the organization and delivery of primary health care means that the pace of change is so fast and the range of nursing skill required in any given situation so varied that the notion of a generic nurse who has to do anything anywhere in the community cannot be sustained. Given the current explosion in knowledge it is unlikely that a single practitioner could maintain a sufficient level of expertise to respond to all complex health needs effectively in a given area or caseload. Followed by an initial period of discipline specific preparation for practice, the foundations should be laid for ongoing professional development in response to clinical service needs. Education programmes which seek to develop the particular strengths and expertise required for practice with target groups, will go some way towards increasing the potential for effective clinical practice and collaboration. The planning and development of common core components of the degree programme should encourage course tutors to identify, teach and explore a range of transferable skills which community health care nurses can adapt to meet the health care needs in a general practice community population (e.g. diabetes, asthma, sexual health).

Reflective Practice, Mentorship and Preceptorship Programmes

Theorists (Schon, 1987; Benner, 1985) have supported the view that theory and the very essence of nursing can only be gleaned from practice. This concept will be explored in relation to reflective practice, mentorship and preceptorship.

Learning through reflection places the responsibility firmly with the undergraduate nurse. It enables the development of competencies in clinical practice through encouraging the student to reflect both on action taken by analysing and interpreting practice and reflecting on practice through knowing in practice (Fish *et al.*, 1990). Learning takes place within a practicum 'a setting designed for the task of learning' (Schon, 1987) and the student is encouraged to transfer knowledge gained from modules of learning to that of the practical situation through reflective practice. Atkins and Murphy (1993) identify the skills required to engage in reflection as self-awareness, description, critical analysis, synthesis and evaluation. The extent to which the student attains this depends, in part, on the skills of the community practice teacher (CPT) in providing suitable learning experiences for the student and demonstrating their ability to reflect both on and in practice and to facilitate this process in others. The use of a reflective chronicle is central to this process (Schon, 1987) as it enables the student to demonstrate effectively their continuing professional development through a contemporaneous record. Yet, reflective practice takes time, and for the CPT/facilitator working in a culture which puts a higher value on individual performance review and meeting identified targets of health need than on the quality of care, it may be increasingly difficult to find the time to reflect in and on practice. This is an area of concern to practitioners and educators alike.

The model of clinical skills acquisition (Benner, 1985) offers a preferred method of learning where the experienced nurse acts as a mentor to the student. My own research and that of others has found confusion with the term 'mentor' (Hagerty, 1986; Jowett *et al.*, 1994; Porter, 1994; Woodrow, 1994). In acknowledging that confusion exists, the English National Board for Nursing, Midwifery and Health Visiting (ENB) have redefined the term 'mentor' in its glossary to the regulations and guidelines pertaining to institutions and courses (ENB, 1994). This definition sees the mentor as 'an individual who has an understanding of the context of the student's learning experience and is selected by the student for the purpose of providing guidance and support'.

In this model the effectiveness of the relationship depends very heavily on the individual attributes of mentors and the individual needs of students (Woodrow, 1994). Compatibility is therefore central to this concept of mentorship where the mentor becomes a trusted adviser. Darling (1984) identified three absolute requirements for a significant relationship to work. Firstly, 'attraction' where the student is drawn to a person through admiration or desire to emulate that person in some way. Secondly 'action', where the person to be a mentor invests time and energy on the student's behalf through teaching, guiding or helping. And finally, 'affect', where the student wants the mentor to have positive feelings towards them. The ENB (1994) stipulate that the mentor is not to be an assessor to the student during the clinical placement. This is important as the success of the mentor/student relationship is built on trust and if the assessment of clinical practice is seen as part of the relationship this could present problems for both the student and the mentor. The development of mentorship could herald a move away from the one-to-one teaching, assessing and supervising role of the CPT. Against this backdrop the future scenario could see community nurse students mentored by a nurse of their choice regardless of whether or not that nurse has any particular teaching and assessing expertise and regardless of any need to undertake professional review.

This may be one way of meeting the educational needs of different student groups at a time when there is a decline in the numbers of CPTs. If mentorship is to work for the undergraduate studying for a community health care nursing qualification then the mentor must be able to act as a catalyst in developing leadership skills and motivation. The achievement and the ability to function as a leader have been identified as resulting from mentorship programmes (Smith-Hamilton, 1981). This requires of the mentor considerable experience of the job and the ability to sustain continuity of learning in their specialist area (Burnard and Chapman, 1990). Just how realistic this model is for the clinical skills training of community health care nurses remains to be seen.

In the light of skill mix reviews and moves to an all graduate profession, will there be enough suitably qualified and experienced nurses in the community from which to choose a mentor? Will educational criteria be laid down for mentorship and, if so, what form will it take? Changing staffing patterns in primary health care and the introduction of skill mix require CHCNs to have enhanced skills, particularly in organizing managing and supervising a team of nurses and support workers. According to Markham (1990) this requires 'evidence of creative thinking in the deployment of skilled staff and grades of staff to carry out nursing tasks'.

When newly registered CHCNs leave college competent to practise, they need assistance to adapt to the realities of the work environment. Preceptorship programmes are thought to reduce the 'reality shock' (Clayton, 1989) and to provide support and facilitate transmission into an environment where positive feedback and continuous learning are recommended and encouraged. This model as defined by the UKCC (1994) responds to the needs of both the employer and the employee (Porter, 1994). The recommended time for the preceptorship period is four months, with the initiation being undertaken by one key person. As the new recruit becomes more comfortable in their role and takes on greater responsibility, the preceptor's input decreases and their role becomes that of a resource person. Again, this may be difficult in practice with the growth in short-term contracts of employment.

What of the Present Community Nursing Workforce?

As the 1992/1993 professional register has less than 1000 Project 2000 nurses registered, (0.2% of the register), it will be some time before this group will make up the single source of entry into community health care nursing courses. Hence the traditionally trained existing workforce will continue to be in the majority, possibly till the end of the century (Buchan, 1994). This makes it imperative that courses leading to a specialist, community nursing qualification on the UKCC register are flexible in design to accommodate the level and variety of nurses wishing to enter community health care nursing. Whilst those with a qualification registered/recorded on the professional register have their professional integrity safeguarded, there are concerns about attaining an academic standard which equates with the newly prepared community health care nurse at degree level.

In a study of 206 health visitors working across five NHS trusts in the South West Regional Health Authority only 3.9% were found to be undertaking degree studies (Porter, 1994). Although it is increasingly possible to gain access to higher education through accreditation of prior learning (APL) or accreditation of prior experiential learning (APEL), the idea that professional experience can be quantified and compared with academic achievement is problematic. It is not clear 'to what degree professional experience can exempt a person from certain aspects of a course or whether having had professional experience facilitates the learning process' (Davis and Burnard, 1992; Howard, 1993).

The Credit Accumulation and Transfer Scheme (CATS)

The CAT scheme enables access into higher education through a more open and flexible system of learning (CNAA, 1986). This not only encourages but supports and provides the opportunities needed for continuing professional education (Selway, 1994).

Learning is accredited through the allocation of points achieved at different levels of learning as follows:

Certificate level   =   120 CATS points at level 1
Diploma level   =   120 CATS points at level 2
Degree level   =   120 CATS points at level 3
Masters level   =   120 CATS points at level M

Accreditation of prior learning (APL) is provided through a straight claim on presentation of an authentic certificate that carries institutionally accepted credit rating. The two basic functions of APL are firstly to act as an admissions function, where prior learning in the form of certificates obtained are used to admit nurses to a programme of study and secondly, to exempt nurses from certain elements of the programme that have been nominated as available for exemption by the education institution undertaking the programme.

Accreditation of prior experiential learning (APEL) is divided into three categories, specific, modified specific and general credit.

Specific APEL means the applicant can make a claim for maximum credit offered on a current validated course and provide the appropriate evidence.

Modified specific APEL means the applicant can claim for a percentage of credit offered on a current validated course by providing evidence to support a claim that the identified learning outcomes can be achieved; e.g.: if there are ten learning outcomes and the applicant can achieve five, they could claim 50% of the credit offered if the evidence is robust.

General credit APEL means the applicant can claim for a percentage of credit by providing an autobiographical account of experience in clinical practice.

APEL, general credit and autobiographical account of all other learning (e.g. study days) must be able to support learning claims with identified outcomes upon entering a formalized APL/APEL system. There are four key stages to be engaged in:

1. Reflection on experience
2. Identification of significant learning
3. Evidence to support the claim
4. Construction and submission of the evidence

These processes accumulate learning towards the acquisition of an academic qualification. In the system of credit transfer the student can learn by instalments, have breaks between studying, select from a range of courses and modes of learning at different times and gain recognition for experiential learning. Accumulation of 360 credit points, with a minimum of 120 credits at each level, normally leads to the award of an honours degree providing that an approved programme of learning has been designated and followed to attain certain learning outcomes as specified by the awarding institution.

The intention of this formal process is to evaluate the nurse's ability and highlight any shortfalls in practice. From this it is possible to identify the form and type of educational and professional development appropriate to the individual nurse. The advantage of such a system for the present workforce is that credits may be awarded and accumulated over a period of time. Short courses, open learning and experiential learning can be incorporated into the personal, professional profile of the nurse. Education is presented in modular and unitized form which incorporates packages of knowledge and training.

The CAT scheme does not allow any nurse to gain a community nursing qualification through APEL and APL. In order for a professional qualification to be recorded on the UKCC register, the nurse must have completed a (National Board validated) recognized programme of preparation including a period of taught practice and supervised practice in the specialist category of their choice. This may be district nursing, health visiting, practice nursing, school nursing, community mental health nursing, community learning disabilities nursing or occupational health nursing.

Assessment of Clinical Competence

One of the most difficult areas to overcome is that of assessment of clinical competence. The question is whether the assessor should be a skilled clinical practitioner or an experienced practitioner with teaching expertise such as the present CPT. If it is agreed that the professional development of all nurses is crucial to the advancement of clinical practice, then the assessor must be a person able to provide opportunities for reflection on clinical practice which enables the nurse to evaluate nursing interventions critically in order to solve problems. This process both enhances the individual nurse's competence and improves the culture of the workplace by providing peer reinforcement and encouragement (Spence, 1994).

Clinical Supervision

If the profession can install the right process it will have a framework in place on which to build the continuing professional, educational and training needs of community nurses. Clinical supervision may offer such a framework. In *A Vision for the Future* (NHSME, 1993b) clinical supervision is seen as a way of providing support to nurses/health visitors in the development of their practice and is a term used to describe a 'formal process of professional support and learning which enables individual practitioners to develop knowledge and competence, assume responsibility for their own practice and enhance consumer protection and safety of care in complex clinical situations'. This is seen as 'central to the process of learning and to the expansion of the scope of practice and should be seen as a means of encouraging self assessment and analytical and reflective skills' (NHSME, 1993a).

Kohner (1994) calls for such supervision to be available for all practitioners, regardless of seniority whilst Carthy (1994) reminds us that clinical supervision is only one aspect of workplace supervision and that there are a range of supervisory activities which could benefit nursing.

The nature of the supervisory relationship is difficult. Faugier and Butterworth (1994) recommend that the model nurses choose to use should address all elements of professional practice, with equal emphasis being given to educative, managerial and supportive elements of clinical supervision. The end result should be an improvement in standards and beneficial outcomes for patients/clients and their carers. In some areas of community care such as community mental health nursing and social work this form of supervision is well established and accepted. In other community nursing disciplines such a programme is in its infancy.

CONCLUSION

The remodelling of nursing can be seen as an attempt to modernize the profession (Renade, 1994). On the one level a graduate nurse is provided, working as a knowledgeable, reflective practitioner and on the other level a skills based practitioner who may be equipped with a National Vocational Qualification able to carry out nursing tasks. Nursing is facing a dilemma: 'it wants to encourage reflective practice, even to claim that it has. But, like some other professions, the structures within which community nursing operates may inhibit regular reflection in practice' (Jarvis, 1992) and constrain efforts to enhance clinical expertise.

Pushed by growing demands for a flexible, high quality community nursing service, health care providers will be forced to develop a rational approach in the allocation of resources for nurse education to meet the expanding needs of fundholding GPs and the variable health needs of local populations. Clinical effectiveness will be a priority as a consequence of being pushed into planning for the future as a provider. Employers can expect to be provided with a highly qualified, reflective practitioner and an inexpensive, task orientated nurse.

SUMMARY

- The level of academic, personal and professional development required by nurses is still under discussion by the profession.
- The implications of the NVQ system for community health care nurses may be enormous.
- Challenges for community health care nurse education are in developing programmes of learning that prepare a nurse with flexible skills and an educational pathway that meets the local needs of purchasers and practitioners whilst maintaining the standards set by the UKCC.
- The role of reflection, mentorship and preceptorship in graduate nurse education needs exploring.
- The credit accumulation and transfer scheme enables nurses to accumulate learning towards the acquisition of an academic qualification.
- Clinical supervision may provide a framework on which to build continuing professional, education and training needs of community nurses.

DISCUSSION QUESTIONS

♦ To what extent can the registered Project 2000 nurse develop their skills in relation to nursing in the community?

♦ Can you give reasons to account for Orr's findings?

♦ Do you think NVQs enhance the skills of the CHCN? If so, how, and in what way?

♦ What are the potential advantages of degree level courses for the CHCN? Do you consider this to be appropriate?

♦ What are the potential benefits (or added value) of a reflective graduate practitioner and a skills based NVQ worker from the perspective of those who:

(a) Review community nursing services?

(b) Use community nursing services?

(c) Commission/purchase community nursing services?

FURTHER READING

Atkins S and Williams A (1995) Registered nurses' experiences of mentoring undergraduate nursing students. *Journal of Advanced Nursing* **21:** 1006–1015.

This article describes a research study undertaken to explore and analyse registered nurses' experiences of mentoring undergraduate nursing students within a single Health Authority in England. The findings indicate that mentoring students is a complex and skilled activity.

Hallett C, Williams A, Orr J, Butterworth T and Collister B (1995) The implementation of Project 2000 in the community: A new perspective on the community nurses role. *Journal of Advanced Nursing* **21:** 1159–1166.

This paper considers some of the initiatives taken by community nurses in England in implementing Project 2000 programmes and identifies difficulties encountered, such as time commitment to students in a busy schedule, problems of communication between colleges of nursing and community services and the place of assessment by community nurses.

Lathlean J and Vaughan B (1994) *Unifying Nursing Practice and Theory*. Butterworth Heinemann: Oxford.

This book brings together the underlying issues that have emerged and some approaches adopted to deal with the relationship between theory and practice in nursing. Innovations in practice have been explored and the difficulties encountered in breaking down the interface between espoused and used theory.

REFERENCES

Allen D (1993) A major milestone. *Nursing Standard*, April 7, **7**(29): 21.

Atkins S and Murphy K (1993) Reflection: a review of the literature. *Journal of Advanced Nursing* **18:** 1188–1192.

Benner P (1985) *From Novice to Expert: Excellence and power in clinical practice*. Menlo Park California: Addison-Wesley.

Buchan J (1994) Licenced to practice: The nursing register. *Nursing Standard*, March 30 **8**(27): 30.

Burnard P and Chapman C (1990) *Nurse Education: The Way Forward*. London: Scutari Press.

Carthy J (1994) Band waggons roll. Viewpoint. *Nursing Standard*, June 15 **8**(38): 48–49.

Clare J (1994) Vocational courses condemned. *Daily Telegraph* Sept. 14.

Clayton M (1989) Relationship between a preceptorship experience and role socialization of graduate nurses. *Journal of Nursing Education* **28**(2): 72–75.

CNAA (Council of National and Academic Awards) (1986) *Credit Accumulation and Transfer Schemes*. London.

Darling L (1984) What do nurses want in a mentor. *Journal of Nursing Administration* October, 42–44.

Davis B and Burnard P (1992) Academic levels in nursing. *Journal of Advanced Nursing* **17:** 1395-1400.

DOH (1989a) *Caring for Patients*. London: HMSO.

DOH (1989b) *The Children Act*. London: HMSO.

DOH (1989c) *Working for Patients*, working paper 10, education and training. London: HMSO.

DOH (1991) *The Patients' Charter*. London: HMSO.

DOH (1992) *Health of the Nation*. London: HMSO.

DOH (1994) *Nursing, Midwifery and Health Visitor Education: A Statement of Strategic intent*. London: HMSO.

DHSS (1988) *Letter to the UICCC from John Moore, Secretary of State for Health and Social Security*, 20 May.

Downe S (1989) The great divide. *Nursing Times*, July 12, **85**(28): 26.

English National Board (1994) *ENB News* issue 14, Autumn.

Faugier J and Butterworth T (1994) *Clinical Supervision: A position paper*, University of Manchester, p. 51.

Fish D, Twinn S and Purr P (1990) *How to Enable Learning Through Professional Practice*, West London Institute of Higher Education.

Forester S (1994) PREP into Practice. *Health Visitor* **67**(5): 155.

Gallagher P (1989) Developing a Foundation Unit. *Nursing Standard*, Oct 25, **4**(5): 28-29.

Gott M (1990) Open learning and nursing practice. *Nursing Standard*, July 4, **4**(41): 37-40.

Hagerty B (1986) A second look at Mentors. *Nursing Outlook* **34**(1): 16-19.

Health Visitors Association (1994) *Action for Health*, Health Visitor Association, June.

Howard S (1993) Accreditation of prior learning: Androgogy in action or a cut price approach to education. *Journal of Advanced Nursing* **18:** 1817-24.

Jarvis P (1983) *Professional Education*. London: Croom Helm.

Jarvis P (1992) Reflective practice and nursing. *Nurse Education Today*, **12:** 174-181.

Jowett S, Walton I and Payne S (1994) *Challenges and Changes in Nurse Education. A study of the implementation of Project 2000*. NFER.

Kohner N (1994) *Clinical Supervision in Practice*. London: King's Fund.

Markham G (1990) Skill mix and match. *Nursing Standard* July 4, **14** (41): 46.

McManus M (1991) Credit accumulation and transfer schemes. *Nursing Standard* **6**(6): 28-30.

NCVQ National Council of Vocational Qualifications) (1988) *Developing a National System of Credit Accumulation and Transfer*. NCVQ, January.

NCVQ (National Council of Vocational Qualifications) (1994) The NVQ Framework. *The NVQ Monitor*, winter, 1993/1994, p 13.

NHSME (National Health Service Management Executive) (1993a) Framework for support and preceptorship. *NHSME EL* 93: 9.

NHSME (National Health Service Management Executive) (1993b) *A Vision for the Future*. Department of Health p 15.

O'Connell P (1978) *Health Visitor Education at University*. Edinburgh: Churchill Livingstone.

Orr J (1993) Bitter lessons in Project 2000. *Health Visitor* **66**(4): 120.

Payne D (1994) A degree of improvement. *Nursing Times* June 15, **90**(24): 18.

Porter E (1994a) Getting to know your preceptor. *Health Visitor* **67**(8): 273.

Porter E (1994b) Knowledge and Skills used in Health Visiting Practice. Unpublished MPhil thesis, University of Southampton.

Redfern E (1994) Health Care Assistants, the challenge for nursing staff. *Nursing Times* Nov 30, **90**(48): 31-32.

Renade W (1994) *A Future for the NHS*. Longman.

Rhodes L (1994) What can HCAs be asked to do? *Nursing Times* Nov 30, **90**(48): 33-35.

Schon D (1987) *Educating the Reflective Practitioner*. San Francisco: Jossey-Bass.

Selway I (1994) APL/APEL: Bringing the theory to practice. *Nursing Standard* **18**(19): 28-30.

Smith-Hamilton M (1981) Mentorhood: A key to nursing leadership. *Nursing Leadership* **4** (1): 4-13.

Spence D (1994) Curriculum revolution: Can educational reform take place without education in practice. *Journal of Advanced Nursing* **19:** 187-193.

United Kingdom Central Council (1986) *Project 2000 - a new preparation for practice*. London: UKCC.

United Kingdom Central Council (1990) *Post Registration Education and Practice*. London: UKCC.

United Kingdom Central Council (1993) Registrar's letter 1. London: UKCC.

United Kingdom Central Council (1994) *The Future of Professional Practice*. London: UKCC.

Williams K (1994) UKCC PREP proposals will cause hardship. *Nursing Standard*, July 27, **8**(44): 10.

Willmott Y (1990) Resource allocation, *Nursing Standard*, April 4, **4** (28): 46.

Woodrow P (1994) Mentorship: perceptions and pitfalls for nursing practice. *Journal of Advanced Nursing* **19:** 812-818.

Wright S (1994) A vision for the future: Targets for achievement. *Nursing Standard*, Aug 31, **8**(49): 30-34.

Wyatt J (1988) The way forward. *Quest, Nursing Times*. Nov 9, **84** (45): 75.

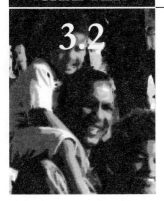

THE LEGAL BASIS FOR ETHICAL PRACTICE

David Greensmith

KEY ISSUES

- The nature of a profession
- Sources of the law affecting the ethical practice of nursing
- The Code of Professional Conduct with comments designed to assist understanding
- Professional responsibilities – powers and duties of practitioners
- Administration of medicines
- Record-keeping – how and particularly why good record-keeping is important

INTRODUCTION

The purpose of this chapter is to introduce practitioners to the concept that the law plays an important and constructive part in the achievement of ethical practice. A section describing some of the characteristics of a profession is followed by a summary of the sources of law affecting the ethical practice of nursing. There is then a detailed examination of the Code of Professional Conduct, including a word-by-word analysis of the preamble, and some comments on each numbered paragraph of the Code. There is a short examination of the professional responsibilities of community practitioners, particularly in relation to the abuse of children and elderly people, and powers under the Mental Health Act. Administration of medicines and record keeping refer the reader to the UKCC's guidance documents, draw attention to the important parts of those documents and offer some additional comments.

What is a Profession?

It is not sufficient for a member of a profession, whether a nurse, doctor, lawyer or whatever simply to do his or her job and be paid for it. Being a member of a profession demands more than this. It is therefore necessary to consider the characteristics of a profession. Some of them are set out in Box 3.2.1.

Sources of the Law Affecting the Ethical Practice of Nursing

The Nursing, Midwifery and Health Visiting professions are governed by the Nurses, Midwives and Health Visitors Act 1979 as amended by the Nurses, Midwives and

Box 3.2.1. The characteristics of a profession

- *A body of learned knowledge*
  All professions require their members to take examinations which involve academic study as well as practical knowledge. Many professions now require their members to keep up to date by continuing their education, whether by means of regular study days or residential refresher courses.

- *Which is transmitted and disseminated*
  Professions are not inward looking, nor should they keep their bodies of learned knowledge to themselves as some kind of sacred mystery. Each member of a profession should teach other members, whether newly qualified or (in relation to modern developments and new ideas) experienced. What is more, the general public, who are all actual or potential clients, should be involved so that everyone benefits from the sharing of those bodies of knowledge.

- *For the benefit of the public*
  Professions do not exist to exploit people nor primarily to be a means of acquiring wealth: each of them has a duty to serve the interests of the general public, if necessary putting the interests of that public, whether individually or collectively, ahead of their own personal interests. All professions require their members to declare financial interests, not to act in conflict with those whom they serve or by whom they are retained, and to promote the interests and well-being of their clients.

- *Subject to a code of ethics*
  All professions require their members to display the highest standards of personal conduct, and to behave in such a way as will uphold and enhance not only their personal reputations but the reputation of the profession as a whole.

- *Which is enforced ultimately by the removal of the right to practise*
  All professions have a disciplinary procedure which only applies to their members, where the ultimate sanction is the removal of a member's name from the relevant professional Register. This is not primarily a punishment, although it may feel like it, but is a protection for the public against unscrupulous, inadequate or inappropriate practitioners. The circumstances in which practitioners' names may be removed from their respective professional Registers are usually spelt out in general terms in the code of ethics mentioned above and always include situations which are neither punishable by the criminal law nor which give rise to civil liability.

- *By a Committee or Tribunal mainly composed of members of the profession elected or appointed to a governing body independent of state control*

Box 3.2.1.   *(contd.)*

All professions have governing bodies set up by Act of Parliament or Royal Charter. Members of the governing bodies are elected by members of the profession, with additional members being appointed usually by the relevant Secretary of State to bring particular expertise which members alone could not provide and to ensure some lay representation. Although subject to the provisions of the Act of Parliament or Royal Charter and although there may be close liaison with government departments, professions are substantially self-governing, particularly in matters of education, ethics and discipline.

Health Visitors Act 1992. From here on these Acts will be together referred to as 'the Act'. The Act sets out the structure of the United Kingdom Central Council for Nursing, Midwifery and Health Visiting, its functions and standing committees. There are also sections dealing with the National Boards and their relationships to the Central Council; the Professional Register; removal from and restoration to the Register; false claims of professional qualification; and midwifery practice.

Briefly, the Act provides for a United Kingdom Central Council for Nursing, Midwifery and Health Visiting consisting of 60 members, two-thirds of whom are elected and one-third of whom are appointed by the Secretary of State for Health to provide useful external expertise and fill in any gaps in areas of practice which the elections have not covered. The functions of the Council are primarily educational. They are set out in section 2 of the Act, and are mainly to do with education and training. The most important function from the point of view of professional ethics appears in section 2(v) which states: 'The powers of the Council shall include that of providing in such manner as it thinks fit, advice for Nurses, Midwives and Health Visitors on standards of professional conduct'.

Section II of the Act defines the means by which a person may be admitted to the Professional Register by reference to Rules (principally the Nurses, Midwives and Health Visitors Rules 1983 as amended) and it is important to note that admission is open only to those who both possess the requisite academic qualifications *and* who are certified to be of good conduct. The vital importance of this latter requirement is that whilst the names of nurses, midwives and health visitors may be removed from the Professional Register because they have ceased to be of good conduct, they retain their academic qualifications. This means that on restoration (subject to compliance with any requirements relating to refresher courses) it is not necessary for a person whose name has been removed for misconduct to repeat or take further examinations regarding competence.

Sections 12 and 12(A) are worth quoting from:

Proceedings about the register: procedure

12(1) The Central Council shall by Rules determine circumstances in which, and the means by which –

(a)   a person may for misconduct or otherwise, be removed from the Register or a part of it, whether or not for a specified period;

(b) a person who has been removed from the Register or part of it may be restored to it; and

(c) an entry in the Register may be removed, altered or restored.

(2) Committees of the Council shall be constituted by the Rules to deal with proceedings for a person's removal from, or restoration to, the Register or for the removal, alteration or restoration of any entry.

(3) The Committees need not be constituted exclusively from members of the Council, but the Rules shall provide, in relation to Committees constituted by them, that there shall only be a quorum if a majority of those present are members of the Council; and the Rules shall so provide that the members of a Committee constituted to adjudicate upon the conduct of any personnel selected with due regard to the professional field in which that person works.

Subsections (4) and (5) deal with procedural matters.

Cautions

12A-(1) Without prejudice to the generality of section 12, Rules under that section may make provision with respect of the giving, in the course of disciplinary proceedings, of cautions as to future conduct.

[Subsection (2) deals with keeping of records of cautions by the Council.]

(3) For the purposes of this section, "disciplinary proceedings" means proceedings for removal from the Register or a part of it for misconduct.

The Act has spawned a number of Statuory Instruments which make Rules for the practical operation of the profession. These include the Nurses, Midwives and Health Visitors (Professional Conduct) Rules 1993 Approval Order 1993 (SI 1993 No. 893) which approves in the form of a Schedule the Nurses, Midwives and Health Visitors (Professional Conduct) Rules 1993.

Much the greater part of these Rules deals with procedure, but Rule 1(2)(k) defines 'misconduct' as 'conduct unworthy of a Registered Nurse, Midwife or Health Visitor, as the case may be, and includes obtaining registration by fraud'.

This definition is of considerable importance because it places no bounds on what is or is not professional misconduct, and in effect directs the members of a Professional Conduct Committee hearing a case to use their professional experience to decide whether or not any proven allegations constitute misconduct in a professional sense.

The Code of Professional Conduct

Reference has already been made to Section 2(5) of the Act which gives UKCC power to give advice on standards of professional conduct. Such advice is contained mainly in the booklets published by UKCC, which are listed at the end of this chapter. The most important, because of its comprehensive nature, is the Code of Professional Conduct, the third edition of which was published in June 1992. It is significant to note that there have been two previous editions, because this demonstrates that ideas of professional ethics are continually developing.

Before considering some of the Code's provisions, it is important to consider what the Code is as well as what it says. In 'exercising accountability' the UK advisory document published in March 1989, the Code is said to be

- The Council's definitive advice on professional conduct to its practitioners and a clear and unequivocal statement as to what their regulatory body expects of them.
- The backcloth against which any misconduct will be judged.
- A statement of the profession's values.
- A portrait of the practitioner which the Council believes to be needed and which the Council wishes to see within the profession.
- A statement to the profession of the primacy of the interests of the patient or client.

The preamble to the Code states:

Each registered nurse, midwife and health visitor shall act, at all times, and in such a manner as to:

- Safeguard and promote the interests of individual patients and clients;
- Serve the interests of society;
- Justify public trust and confidence, and
- Uphold and enhance the good standing and reputation of the professions.

As a registered nurse, midwife or health visitor, you are personally accountable for your practice.

The words of this preamble are carefully chosen. Even the apparently less significant words repay careful study. For example:

- *Each*
  This means that the professional obligations set out in the Code cannot be delegated or assigned to others, whether by management structure, financial imperatives, or the expectation that someone else will accept responsibility (commonly called 'cover', a concept which has no place in ethical nursing practice).
- *Shall act*
  There are no options here: it is impossible to practise ethically without total acceptance of all the Code's obligations.
- *At all times*
  Professional accountability continues 24 hours a day, seven days each week, and 365 days every year. Many allegations of professional misconduct have been based on incidents which occurred whilst a practitioner was off duty, on holiday, or even asleep.
- *Safeguard and promote the interests of individual patients and clients*
  It is not sufficient merely to protect patients and clients: members of the professions should seek to improve the quality of their lives, the environment of care, and their autonomy.
- *Serve the interests of society*
  This is a command which is common to all professions
- *Justify public trust and confidence*
  It is because patients and clients trust the nurses, midwives and health visitors who attend them and advise them that the patients and clients allow them to

perform procedures which in other circumstances might be regarded as serious criminal offences.

- *Uphold and enhance the good standing and reputation of the Professions*
  It is not enough for a person to go through an exemplary professional nursing career but because of his or her inaction, leave the professions with a reputation which is no better than it was when he or she joined. It is the duty of each Nurse, Midwife and Health Visitor to work to improve the public's view of their respective professions.

The Code of Professional Conduct might well stop there and simply leave practitioners to work out for themselves how to apply the principles of ethical professional practice, but the paragraphs in the code that follow, together with all the other explanatory booklets, are designed to give specific guidelines.

In relation to each paragraph of the Code, there now follows some practical examples. They should not be regarded as exhaustive, as the situations that arise in practice are infinite in their variety.

1. *Act always in such a manner as to promote and safeguard the interests and well-being of patients and clients.*
   This looks obvious but there are examples, particularly from long stay wards where everything is a matter of routine, and primarily to do with the physical well-being and protection of the patients rather than their recovery, where bad practice leads to the interests and well-being of the staff, either individually or collectively, being those which are promoted and safeguarded. In one case a group of nurses took patients for a day out, and on the way back to the hospital left the patients in their motor coaches whilst they went to a restaurant for a meal.

2. *Ensure that no action or omission on your part, or within your sphere of responsibility, is detrimental to the interests, condition or safety of patients or clients.*
   Whilst paragraph 1 directs the practitioner to ensure that the quality of the life of patients or clients is enhanced, paragraph 2 requires practitioners to prevent harm to patients and clients, and rightly draws attention to the damage which can be caused by omission as well as commission. Many allegations of professional misconduct start with the words 'failed to'. There are many instances of practitioners failing to administer medication, leaving patients on commodes unattended, allowing them to wander away from the safety of their usual environment, and so on.

3. *Maintain and improve your professional knowledge and competence.*
   Members of all professions are under an obligation to keep up-to-date with contemporary developments so that their standards of practice may be of the highest.

4. *Acknowledge any limitations in your knowledge and competence and decline any duties or responsibilities unless able to perform them in a safe and skilled manner.*
   It is not a sin to be unable to carry out procedures in which one has not been trained, or not trained recently. It is good professional practice to decline to perform such procedures if a practitioner is not confident about his of her ability to do so safely. It must be remembered that all competencies have a 'shelf life' and that which a practitioner could perform safely several years ago may not be capable of being performed safely today.

5. *Work in an open and cooperative manner with patients, clients and their*

*families, foster their independence and recognize and ...
ment in the planning and delivery of care.*

This recognition of the valuable work done by the patients an...
selves and their family is welcome. Encouraging independence i...
ability to make informed choices about their lives and prevent the g...
'dependency culture'. Practitioners should ensure that they do not ta...
the problems of patients and clients, who are often more able to deal with ...
than has been thought.

6. *Work in a collaborative and cooperative manner with health care profession-als, and others involved in providing care, and recognize and respect their particular contributions within the care team.*

Everyone has something to contribute; domestic and portering staff, ward receptionists, paramedical staff of every kind, and nursing auxiliaries have a right to expect the support of every registered practitioner and not to be treated simply as pairs of hands.

7. *Recognize and respect the uniqueness and dignity of each patient and client, and respond to their need for care, irrespective of their ethnic origin, religious belief, personal attributes, the nature of their health problems or any other factor.*

This paragraph emphasizes the individuality of the needs of each patient and client. Who they are, where they come from, what they believe, and the condition from which they are suffering are all irrelevant to the standard of care each practitioner must deliver. The phrase 'the nature of their health problems' reflects some earlier findings of professional misconduct against practitioners who refuse to treat patients or clients who are HIV positive or suffering from full blown AIDS. Such attitudes have no place in professional practice.

8. *Report to an appropriate person or authority at the earliest possible time, any conscientious objection which may be relevant to your professional practice.*

Most practitioners know that the Abortion Act contains a 'conscience clause' which they are entitled to invoke. This is not the only conscientious issue which may arise. For example, some psychiatric nurses are opposed to the use of electro-convulsive therapy (ECT). There are conscientious arguments on both sides of the dilemma concerning the sedation or non-sedation at night of elderly confused patients. On the one side the argument is that no-one should be given medication just to enable the staff to have a quiet night, and on the other side there may be conscientious objections to preventing patients and clients from having a quiet night because of the nature of their illness or condition.

9. *Avoid any abuse of your privileged relationship with patients and clients and of the privileged access allowed to their person, property, residence or work-place.*

Close personal and intimate physical contact with patients and clients can be abused. A sexual relationship with a patient or client, borrowing their money or stealing from them, are all likely to be found to be professional misconduct. It is particularly important to community practice that practitioners realize that they are guests in the homes of their patients and clients, and that those patients and clients may behave how they choose in their own homes.

10. *Protect all confidential information concerning patients and clients obtained in the course of professional practice and make disclosures only with consent, where required by the order of a court or where you can justify disclosure in the wider public interest.*

The principles of patient confidentiality are well known, and are not difficult to understand. Patients and clients are entitled to have all matters concerning them to be kept confidential. On the other hand they would normally accept that 24 hour care cannot be provided by one person, and there needs to be a certain sharing of what would otherwise be regarded as confidential information within a team, however this is defined. So long as communication of such information is kept to a 'need to know' basis then there is no problem, but transmission of information should be limited to the team unless the patient or client consents otherwise. The phrase 'where required by the Order of a Court' must be correctly interpreted. It does not include 'where a Policeman asks a question', however important it may seem at the time. An order of a court means a witness summons in the Magistrates' Court or the County Court requiring a person to give evidence, a Subpoena in the High Court, or a verbal direction to a sworn witness to disclose information given by a Magistrate, Judge, or Chairman of a Tribunal who has power to do so. Of course a practitioner may refuse to answer a question or disclose information. If he or she does so, then a fine, or at worst imprisonment for contempt of court may follow. Justifying disclosure in the wider public interest is a matter of personal assessment as to whether the disclosure of the information will be for the ultimate benefit of a patient or client (such as a child) whilst being to the immediate detriment of perhaps another patient and client, for example the child's parent. Such disclosure should not be made lightly. A practitioner should consult with and take advice from his or her manager, trade union officer, employer or lawyer. Ultimately the decision is one for the practitioner. Full records should be made of any such disclosures, giving details of the person requesting disclosure, the person with whom there have been consultations, the advice that was given, and the reasoning behind the decision to disclose or not to disclose the information.

11. *Report to an appropriate person or authority, having regard to the physical, psychological and social effects on patients and clients, any circumstance in the environment of care which could jeopardize standards of practice.*
Note that in this and the next two paragraphs, it is not simply a matter of it being permissible for practitioners to make such reports, but an obligation on each one to do so. Obviously a clear assessment needs to be made under this paragraph of the relevant circumstances, and how the environment of care is adversely affected before such a report is made. Remember that 'an appropriate person or authority' may not be an immediate line manager, but could for example be the person with ultimate professional responsibility within the management structure, for example a Chief Administrative Nursing Officer, or event the Professional Conduct Division of UKCC if the professional conduct of some other practitioner is being called into question.

12. *Report to an appropriate person or authority any circumstances in which safe and appropriate care for patients and clients cannot be provided.*
Paragraph 11 is related to the 'environment of care' whereas paragraph 12 deals with 'any circumstances'. This could be the conduct of colleagues, inadequate resources, improper use of medication, whether prescribed by a doctor or otherwise.

13. *Report to an appropriate person or authority where it appears that the health or safety of colleagues is at risk, as such circumstances may compromise standards of practice and care.*
Nursing is a caring profession, and should not only adopt a caring attitude

towards its patients and clients, but also to those with whom nurses work. To allow a colleague to take on an excessive workload, to allow a colleague to work when unfit through some physical or mental condition, or to fail to report a colleague's drink or drug dependency is not only bad for the colleague, but creates unacceptable risk for patients and clients of which they themselves and other health care colleagues may be unaware.

14. *Assist professional colleagues, in the context of your own knowledge, experience and sphere of responsibility, to develop their professional competence, and assist others in the care team, including informal carers, to contribute safely and to agree appropriate to their roles.*

    It will be remembered that one of the characteristics of a profession is that its body of learned knowledge is disseminated. Every practitioner therefore has the duty of passing on his or her knowledge to anyone with whom they come into contact, whether or not the beneficiaries of the passing on of knowledge are formally involved in care. Any family which is encouraged by practitioners to manage the condition of one of its members takes control of the problem, enhances its own independence, and has more choice over the lives of the family members, whether they are patients and clients or not.

15. *Refuse any gift, favour or hospitality from patients or clients currently in your care which might be interpreted as seeking to exert influence to obtain professional consideration.*

    There is nothing wrong in allowing patients and clients to express their gratitude for past care by a small gift, whether of money or in kind. It is often impossible and would certainly be impolite to refuse such an expression of gratitude. To avoid the adverse interpretation which this section mentions, it is best to be open about such gifts, share those which can be shared (such as boxes of chocolates) use any money to benefit all members of the health care team involved with that patient or client, for example by contributing towards an outing or a celebration. What is absolutely not permitted is to accept a gift from a patient or client at the time when they first come into your care, as both the client and colleagues might interpret this as an inducement to show that client or patient some favour. As a footnote, if large sums of money are offered, and refusal might cause substantial embarrassment, it would be best to make a payment into an endowment fund or some charity for the relief of the condition from which the patient or client was suffering.

16. *Ensure your registration status is not used in the promotion of commercial products or services, declare any financial or other interest in relevant organizations providing such goods or services and ensure that your professional judgement is not influenced by any commercial considerations.*

    The opportunities for promoting commercial products or services may be few, but they should be resisted. Such promotion may be subtle: for example it is regarded as professionally improper to wear a uniform carrying the name or logo of a commercial company, particularly if they are involved in health care. Patients or clients might interpret this either as an endorsement of the product, or as an indication that somehow their care was being controlled by that commercial company. The 'relevant organizations' in respect of which financial or other interests would have to be declared would include nursing homes, private clinics, or pharmacies. To comply completely with this paragraph it is suggested that the financial or other interests of close relatives in such organizations should also be declared.

Professional Responsibilities

Nurses midwives and health visitors working in the community often work independently and are not subject to close management control. They can and should be regarded as prime sources of information in relation to the abuse of children and elderly people, poor housing and other social conditions, and trends in lifestyles which may be ultimately damaging to their patients and clients and their families. These responsibilities should be embraced, not shunned. If the good standing and reputation of the professions is to be enhanced, then the avoidance of responsibility in these areas must not be a feature of professional practice. Furthermore, it is not sufficient just to bring the attention of other agencies and authorities to such problems: practitioners must accept that it is their professional duty to follow up such matters and be prepared to give evidence about them in courts or tribunals. This is not a pleasant experience for anyone, but the command to serve the interests of society must be backed up by practical action, however inconvenient and uncomfortable. More information about the duties of practitioners can be found in such publications as *Working Together* (DHSS/Welsh Office, 1988).

First level psychiatric nurses have the power and duty to detain mental patients under Section 5(4) of the Mental Health Act 1983, at least for a period of six hours. Clearly it is a heavy responsibility to deprive a person of his or her freedom, but such actions should not be delayed or omitted where the safety of the patient concerned or of the general public might be put at risk. Further information on professional responsibilities can be found in *The Scope of Professional Practice* a booklet published by UKCC in June 1992, and practitioners are particularly referred to Sections 8–11, headed 'Principles for adjusting the scope of practice' and Sections 12–14 headed 'The scope and "Extended Practice" of Nursing'. Section 20 of the booklet reminds practitioners that they remain 'accountable to the Council and subject to the Council's Code of Professional Conduct, *even if their posts do not require nursing qualifications*' (emphasis supplied). The section goes on to say 'the position of such nurses is the same as that of nurses engaged in direct professional nursing practice'. This is particularly important to practitioners who are working in personal social services and the residential care sector. Sections 22 and 23 headed 'Support for professional practice' stresses that nurses, midwives and health visitors have a duty to ensure that health care assistants are and must remain the responsibility of registered practitioners, must be protected from working beyond their competence, must be members of a team, and should be encouraged to progress to professional education if they wished to do so.

Administration of Medicines

Practitioners are referred to the UKCC's booklet *Standards for the Administration of Medicines* published in October 1992. Section 5 states that 'The treatment of a patient with medicines for therapeutic, diagnostic or preventative purposes is a process which involves prescribing, dispensing, administering, receiving and recording'. Section 6 sets out the expectations that a practitioner administering a medicine may have from the prescriber and Section 7 sets out the practitioner's expectations of the dispenser. Sections 8–11 describes what the practitioner administering the medication should do, and Sections 12–16 show how the standards for administrations of medicines can be applied in a range of settings, including hospitals, domestic settings, and nursing homes. Self-administration of medicines is encouraged. Sections 28–32 set out the role of nurses, midwives and health visiting community practice in the administration of medicines, and gives valuable guidance to community psychiatric nurses, and practitioners participating in vaccination and immunization programmes. The booklet also deals with situations where the Council's standards cannot normally be applied, and discusses the administration of homeopathic herbal substances, and complementary and alternative therapies. Finally, there is guidance as to the management of errors or incidents in the administration of medicines, stressing the necessity to be honest and open about mistakes, assuring practitioners that the Council 'takes great care to distinguish between those cases where the error was the result of reckless practice and was concealed, and those which resulted from serious pressure of work and where there was immediate, honest disclosure in the patient's interests'.

Record-keeping

When added to clinical competence, and a proper understanding of the Code of Professional Conduct, good record-keeping completes the equipment which enables a nurse midwife or health visitor to practise effectively. Unfortunately it is the aspect of practice which is most disliked, and frequently skimped, if not ignored altogether. Because of the independence from immediate supervision of community practitioners, it is even more necessary for their records to be comprehensive.

Guidance on record-keeping is contained in UKCC's booklet *Standards for Records and Record Keeping* published in April 1993. Section 1 states:

Inadequate and inappropriate record keeping concerning the care of patients and clients neglects their interests through:
1.1 Impairing continuity of care:
1.2 Introducing discontinuity of communication between staff;
1.3 Creating the risk of medication or other treatment being duplicated or omitted;
1.4 Failing to focus attention on early signs of deviation from the norm, and
1.5 Failing to place on record significant observations and conclusions.

Many cases of professional misconduct arise from or are significantly affected by absent or inadequate records. One of the earliest cases concerning a health visitor which reached the Professional Conduct Committee concerned a grossly overworked practitioner who failed to complete her records contemporaneously, with the inevitable result that serious inaccuracies arose, including records of visits that had never actually been made. In another case a health visitor's diary indicated that over 1000 visits had been made over a period of several months, whilst only 100 or so were recorded.

It is important to build into programmes of work some time for record-keeping. This seemingly tedious and irritating activity must be considered as an essential part of the care of patients and clients.

Whilst the UKCC booklet mentioned above offers essential and valuable guidance on the subject of record-keeping some additional comments are appropriate.

• Each separate record should be dated, and if the record is made on a different date from the events recorded, this should be stated.

- Entries should differentiate between fact and opinion. For example, a comment regarding the cause of a minor injury to a child, like 'fell against coffee table' does not indicate whether the practitioner saw the incident or the comment was offered by the child's parent, and in the latter case whether or not the practitioner believed the explanation.
- Entries should be signed with a full signature, not simply initials.
- All records should ideally be made on the same day as the incidents recorded, and in any event within 24 hours – not after the weekend, or on return from leave. The reason for this is that in the event of a court case or similar enquiry into the events recorded, a witness would be allowed to refresh his or her memory from *contemporaneous* notes or records, but not from records made after a substantial length of time. It should be noted, however, that the records are not themselves evidence of events, but only of what was written. The witness's recollection is the primary source of evidence, assisted by the contemporaneous record.

Transmission of Records

Patients and clients move about: often community records need to be sent from one place to another. Subject to local policies, which should be taken into account but not necessarily slavishly followed if they are deficient, it is recommended that records should be sent 'recorded delivery' addressed to a named practitioner, marked 'private and confidential' and accompanied by a letter which requests an acknowledgement of receipt. If no such acknowledgement is received, a follow-up enquiry should be made after, say, two or three weeks.

SUMMARY

As a result of reading this chapter the reader should know and understand:

- The nature of professions as a whole.
- The principal Acts of Parliament and Statutory Instruments relating to the ethical practice of nursing.
- The Code of Professional Conduct and the UKCC's explanatory booklets.
- Professional responsibilities in relation to children, elderly patients and clients and those suffering from mental illness.
- The importance of administering medicines correctly
- The importance of record-keeping.

CONCLUSION

All nurses, midwives and health visitors must practise their professions not only in accordance with the law and in accordance with local procedures, but with due regard to the ethical principles governing each of them. There may be occasions when ethical duties come into conflict with managerial structures and requirements: in such cases practitioners must understand and appreciate that their ethical duties come first, and they are entitled to take such action as is necessary to ensure that their ethical duties are not compromised. They have the right to call on the assistance of United Kingdom Central Council who may bring proper pressure to bear and will support practitioners who seek to uphold and strengthen ethical principles. Good practice can only be achieved with constant effort and vigilance. It needs to be reinforced every day and the principles behind it re-emphasized, in the interests of providing the highest possible standards of patient care.

DISCUSSION QUESTIONS

♦ Do you consider the characteristics of a profession set out at the beginning of this chapter to be sufficiently comprehensive? If not, what additional characteristics do you consider to be common to all professions?

♦ What are the benefits of professions being largely self- governing?

♦ Do you consider that the professional conduct mechanism which affects nurses, midwives and health visitors to be punitive or protective? If you think it is protective, whom does it protect?

♦ Can you suggest improvements in the professional conduct process to make it more effective?

♦ How could the education of nurses, midwives and health visitors be improved to increase awareness of ethical standards?

FURTHER READING

Pyne RH (1992) *Professional Discipline in Nursing, Midwifery and Health Visiting*, Second edition. Oxford: Blackwell Scientific Publications.
This is essential reading for a proper understanding of how the nursing, midwifery and health visiting professions are regulated. The author was involved in professional conduct matters and professional ethics for many years, latterly as Assistant Registrar, Standards and Ethics, at UKCC.

DHSS/Welsh Office (1988) *Working Together*. London:
This booklet is a guide to arrangements for inter-agency cooperation for the protection of children from abuse and sets out the ways in which the various agencies concerned with the care of children should share information.

UKCC Publications

Complaints about Professional Conduct August 1993.
This advises practitioners and others about the types of cases which should be reported to the UKCC, and explains the mechanism by which complaints are handled.

Advertising
This booklet expands on what is now paragraph 16 of the Code of Professional Conduct and advises practitioners how to avoid contravening it.

Confidentiality April 1987
This booklet attempts to provide additional guidance to practitioners on problems involving confidentiality. It is (at the time of writing) slightly out of date in that the wording of paragraph 10 of the Third Edition of the code of Professional Conduct is different from the wording of the second edition, but nevertheless it is a valuable source of useful information.

Professional Conduct – Occasional Report on Selected Cases 1 April 1991 to 31 March 1992
The report summarizes 40 professional conduct cases, and sets out the information that was available to the Professional Conduct Committee and the decision that was reached.

Professional Conduct – Occasional Report on Standards of Nursing in Nursing Homes June 1994
The UKCC has been concerned at the increasing number of cases which emanate from nursing homes. the report examines the available data, sets out an agenda to improve standards, and summarizes eight cases.

REFERENCES

DHSS/Welsh Office (1988) *Working Together*. London: HMSO.

Nurses, Midwives and Health Visitors Act 1979 (c.36) London: HMSO 1979.

Nurses, Midwives and Health Visitors Act 1992 (c.16) London: HMSO 1992.

Nurses, Midwives and Health Visitors (Professional Conduct) Rules 1993 Approval Order 1993 (SI 1993 No. 893) London: HMSO 1993.

Mental Health Act 1983 (c.20) London: HMSO 1983.

UKCC Booklets (London: United Kingdom Central Council for Nursing, Midwifery and Health Visiting.)

Code of Professional Conduct, Third Edition 1992.

Exercising Accountability, March 1989.

The Scope of Professional Practice, June 1992.

Standards for the Administration of Medicines, October 1992.

Standards for Records and Record Keeping, April 1993.

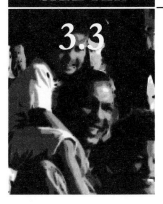

ETHICS IN PRACTICE

Pam Gastrell and Lesley Coles

KEY ISSUES

- Defining ethics: utilitarianism, egoism, formalism

- Code of Conduct and Scope of Professional Practice

- Health promotion and social control

- The internal market and consumerism

- The nurse and the health care team

- The issue of advocacy

- The concept of autonomy

INTRODUCTION

The UKCC expects that community nurses will practise ethically and legally along-side other professionals. Indeed the whole emphasis of the UKCC's code of professional practice is on personal accountability and ethical practice. In one short chapter only a few of the major areas of concern can be addressed. Hence, only some of the diverse ethical and moral issues which surround and influence community nursing practice will be considered.

In relation to community health nursing ethical dilemmas have always been with us, but as the community health care setting has changed, is changing and will continue to change, it is important that ethical concerns are identified and confronted in order that their dimensions are considered as a fundamental component of care. This view is supported by Grundstein-Amado (1993: 1710) who sees the ethical decision-making process as being 'the core element that embodies health care practice' yet at the same time acknowledges, that the emergence of new technology, scientific progress, economic constraints and higher consumer expectations, place new and complex demands upon health care providers.

Ethical considerations within nursing have frequently been concerned with the integrity of individual practitioners and of the profession collectively. In this context, ethical concerns surrounding patient/client health care have often been characterized by conflict over questions about what should be done, the amount of professional and personal autonomy involved, and the interests of differing individuals or groups (Aroska, 1987). Subsequently, the terms 'autonomy' and 'advocacy' are found extensively throughout nursing literature and are frequently framed within the context of 'empowerment' and 'partnership'. Indeed, the language of nursing has become littered with such commonplace terms, and many of these concepts are now claimed to be central tenets of the professional nurse alongside 'accountability'. These are important issues which demand closer attention and are recurring themes throughout this chapter.

Defining Ethics

Traditionally, ethics has had to do with individual decisions regarding what should be sought in life and what should be avoided; life goals, duties and obligations. With the development of new knowledge and technological advancement in health care, 'bioethics' (a discipline applying ethical thinking to the health sciences) has developed rapidly. Bioethics concerns choices and conflict around such health care issues as longevity versus freedom from pain; rights of individuals versus rights of society; and rights among individuals in the distribution of limited health care resources.

Against this backdrop, an examination of three positions in ethical reasoning will be explored: utilitarianism, egoism and formalism.

Utilitarianism

According to John Stuart Mill (1806–73) humans are pleasure seekers. 'To say that man is rational, is merely to say that he is an intelligent pleasure seeker, that he seeks pleasure and happiness with intelligence and foresight' (Kerner, 1990: 11). From this premise, the utilitarian position focuses on consequences of actions, on the greatest amount of happiness or the least amount of harm for the greatest number of individuals. This is a community orientated theory in which each person counts equally, but the consequences to future generations is taken into account. This position is in conflict with the traditional medical ethic which tends to focus on individualized patient care and may also be in conflict with some interpretations and implementation of nursing frameworks utilized by community nurses.

Egoism

The egoism position seeks the solution which is best for oneself. Hence the community nurse acting within this ethical framework would consider the solution that is most comfortable for them.

Formalism

In the formalist or deontological position, one would look neither at one's own personal position nor at the consequences of actions. Instead, one would consider the nature of the act itself and the principles or rules involved. In Kant's view for example, everything in nature happens according to laws, and humans can embark upon their actions in order to conform to those laws (Kerner, 1990). Yet all of our actions have maxims and a community nurse working within this ethical framework may therefore seek to work 'correctly', according to a moral principle, regardless of the consequences. Kant's writing on the nature of assessment of such principles highlights the possible conflict between issues which are 'technical', where all the resources of science and technology are at our disposal, and the 'pragmatic', where everything is subjective. Community nurses taking this position may be in conflict, not only within themselves, but with other professional perspectives.

Ethical theories and reasoning do not solve ethical dilemmas, but they do suggest ways of structuring and clarifying them in so far as they go beyond ethical slogans or one sentence general principles for justifying actions and decisions. For example 'Euthanasia and living wills are wrong.' According to Kerner (1990: 2), 'When you define ethics you define a problem and your definition is not to suppose, in advance, that it is solvable only in one direction'.

A search of the literature suggests that most of the current discussion of ethical issues centres upon nursing within hospital and other institutional settings with the focus upon individual care. Whilst different settings do not in themselves make a difference to the ethical concerns confronting practice, the dimensions will be different. The majority of community nurses, according to their discipline specific area of practice, will be concerned with individuals, families and communities and hence the dimension of care will be much wider.

For example, health visitors and school nurses will have a community/public health orientation for care whilst district nurses and practice nurses will often be confronted with illness needs including questions relating to the quality of life of those who are terminally ill. Community mental health nurses on the other hand will be faced with moral and ethical issues centring around the compulsory treatment and supervision of individuals with acute mental illness. (News, *Nursing Times*, 1995) Equally, community learning disability nurses may well be concerned with value systems surrounding such issues in their client group as sexual relationships, contraception including termination of pregnancies.

The whole emphasis of The United Kingdom Central Council (1992a) Code of Conduct and Scope of Professional Practice is on personal accountability. The underlying aim, Bevan (1993) argues, is to improve professionalism. Nursing, midwifery and health visiting are deemed to have come of age, and hence, practitioners are to be accountable for their own standards of practice. Each individual is charged with the task of ensuring that at all times they act within their own level of competence. If they have learning needs or gaps in their knowledge, according to the UKCC, they are now under a duty to fill them. As a consequence of this, the need for certification to carry out extended role duties has been discontinued. Thus in theory at least, practitioners have been given scope to broaden their role and to work in new ways providing they do the patient no harm.

For many community health nurses this statement may have a hollow ring as there is increasing anecdotal evidence to suggest that some of the initiatives underpinning government strategies for the organization and delivery of health care may be in conflict with some practitioners' ethical values and professional goals. This highlights the need to consider the likely/possible consequences of the community health nurse's interventions upon the autonomy of clients. It also raises questions about whose moral or ethical values are being considered or may be compromised as a result of nursing intervention. This point can be illustrated with reference to some of the targets specified in Government documents, such as England's *Health of the Nation* document (DOH, 1992b). One of the key recommendations running through-out this strategy is that targets that promote good health and prevent ill health are central planks to government policies.

Issues raised in this document and other government strategies cover many aspects of life in the United Kingdom today, including well-being and mental health. One of the key messages spelt out in all these strategies for health gain is that individuals should be encouraged to accept more responsibility for their own health and that of their children. Hence, the focus of these strategies is mainly concerned with the 'new diseases' which it is suggested are brought about by adverse lifestyles involving personal choice. Initiatives which attempt to reduce the major causes of premature death and disability, such as cessation of smoking, regular exercise, weight control and health screening, are not in themselves contentious. However, they may be difficult to evaluate in relation to mental status and emotional well-being related to environmental issues. But, if these issues give some community health nurses grounds for concern, maybe the target relating to the subject of reducing teenage pregnancies is even more contentious on ethical terms, ignoring as it does the emotional, social and economic factors which may be involved. Indeed, individual community nurses may not find it easy to carry out health policies which have been determined by central government but which may appear to have little relevance for the health and social needs of their practice population.

*Health Promotion and
Social Control*

Health education and health promotion activities cannot be seen as neutral. Indeed, Thompson *et al.* (1990) argue that health education, if used in an attempt to change individual behaviour and attitudes, raises ethical issues which should be acknowledged and explored by all nurses. Taking this argument one stage further, are community health nurses, and in particular mental health, learning disability and practice nurses, acting as agents of social control as they seek to achieve the targets set by the government? Or are they attempting to act as agents for change? Maybe some would agree with the view expressed over a decade ago in *Thinking About Health Visiting*, (RCN, 1982), that the combination of these two roles may not fit comfortably with the health visitor's role of client advocate. This is an important issue which will be explored later within this chapter.

*Professional
Boundaries and the
Internal Market*

There is evidence that in some instances, professional boundaries may serve to hinder effective collaboration. As a result there may be limited awareness of the skills of other people. This difficulty has been around for a long time, indeed, the authors of *New World: New Opportunities* (DOH, 1993b) acknowledge this, stressing that there is a continuing need for members of the primary health care team to learn from one another. However, collaboration between people needs to be matched by coordination of policies. For many community nurses the organization of the health service with its emphasis on a competing internal market with a specific contract to provide health services to health service consumers, carries its own ethical concerns in relation to equity, and there is evidence to suggest that some of the recent changes in the organization and the delivery of primary and community health care (e.g. GP fundholding) may serve to make this particular goal more difficult to achieve. At the time of writing, the rights of the patient are clearly heralded in *The Patient's Charter* (DOH, 1992a), yet, as many community nurses can testify, these issues are not clear cut; for example, the emphasis on the autonomy of the patient/client and the provision of medical and nursing care tends to ignore the fact that health care cannot be provided on the same terms as commercial industries. An example here is the promise within *The Patient's Charter* that the district nurse will visit patients by appointment within a given time span. Keeping promise is an ideal which most district nurses would agree with in principle but some may find difficult to achieve in practice because of the unpredictability of individual responses or the impact of environmental conditions.

Similarly, the allocation of scarce resources within a market economy is of current ethical concern to many community nurses. Questions about the selective or routine use of scarce resources is usually accompanied by calls for increased spending on the National Health Service, on the one hand and demands for a fairer and more equitable distribution of resources, on the other. There is little overall agreement on priorities, although there is evidence from some parts of the country that NHS trusts (Berks, *Nursing Times*) are beginning to make public the conditions they will not treat as routine NHS procedures. The publication of this information has been welcomed in some quarters as an honest attempt to make maximum use of resources for the good of the community as a whole. Others, including a group of doctors interviewed as a result of this disclosure (ITV Meridian, September 1995), insisted that doctors must have freedom to do and spend what they consider right for their patients, a view that is often shared by community nurses.

Such decisions on allocation inevitably raise questions that are as much ethical as medical and economic. Faced with daily evidence of finite resources and infinite demand it is inevitable that some form of rationing will occur. Providers of community nursing services find themselves face to face with the dilemma of whether to use nursing manpower resources to cover the identified community health needs of the population, or to ration the use of these services. For example, to limit the number of routine health visiting contacts to middle class client groups. This raises questions related to equity and moral judgements which in turn are bound up with issues relating to the achievement of actual or potential health gain versus value for money.

This throws into focus the concept that in the market for services the customer can negotiate their treatment and that health provision is planned on a basis of supply and demand. Thus the question of patients' rights and the professional duties and obligations of the nurse could be argued as being in direct conflict with the philosophy underpinning the purchaser–provider divide.

Against this backdrop, this discussion would be incomplete without reference to autonomy and empowerment, terms which crop up frequently in nursing and social work literature. These terms imply that people have the potential to achieve health for themselves, through active participation as individuals, families or community groups. Yet the paternalistic attitude so often displayed in the past by the medical and nursing professions meant that individuals were often uninformed and uninvolved in decisions affecting their care. Today, however, this attitude is changing, albeit slowly. Better press and media coverage have allowed for a more informed public. People are now questioning professional decision-making at all levels and are demanding more openness. Hence, the professional autonomy of nurses and doctors is open to public scrutiny and challenge and traditional practices will need to give way to collaborative and flexible ways of working if the concepts of patient/client autonomy and empowerment are to become a reality.

Autonomy

In relation to autonomy Gillon (1987) describes three areas of autonomy (Box 3.3.1) which together form a collective process involving thought, will and action.

This definition of autonomy encompasses the notions of individual personal liberty and freedom, which are familiar concepts to all nurses. Yet even this concept is problematic in so far as no one has the liberty and freedom to do exactly what they

Box 3.3.1. Three areas of autonomy.

- Autonomy of thought. A concept which embraces 'thinking for oneself' 'decision-making' and 'moral judgements'.
- Autonomy of will. Which embraces intentions to do something, had we the necessary strength and desire. It is acknowledged that these intentions may be diminished by disease and/or clinical agents.
- Autonomy of action. The implementation of a specific act as a direct consequence of thought and will.

like in any given situation. Nurses are constrained by their code of professional conduct and their moral judgement and responsibility. Clients and patients, with the best will in the world, are frequently powerless to influence key clinical decisions and outcomes and may not receive sufficient information on which to make a reasonable assessment of risk involved in treatment. Yet, if we are to achieve the targets specified in government strategies, community nurses will need to offer programmes of care that not only seek to facilitate and empower clients to reach their full potential, but that acknowledge people may not have the power to shape their own lives and those of their families so as to be free from disease. Hence, in the absence of policies recognizing these issues, questions of accountability are set to remain.

The Nurse and the Health Care Team

The Heathrow debate (DOH, 1994: 12) suggests that in order to supply optimal health services, there will be a need in the future, for a considerable blurring of boundaries between professions. 'In reality, there is likely to be a reallocation of tasks between nurses and others, including other professionals.' A similar point was raised in the report *New Worlds: New Opportunities* (DOH, 1993b) which stipulated that community health care would be organized around primary care and delivered by primary health care teams. Few community nurses would disagree with this conceptual framework for practice, yet others may have ethical concerns arising from the independent practitioner status of general practitioners and themselves as employees of a health authority or trust which may have different priorities for practice. However, this is not new; there has always been a possible scope for conflict in the relationship between nursing practice and medicine. This concerns the power dimension related to the medical profession's authority and status in law. Similarly, general practitioners may find themselves experiencing increasing conflict between the demands of their own professional ethics and the required business ethos that comes with their newfound role. As general practice fundholding becomes more widespread it could be that some nurse members of the primary health care team will face increasing tensions relating to interpersonal issues, interprofessional tensions and organizational changes. Commenting on this, June Huntington (1993), in a public lecture at Southampton, pointed out that practice based primary care will need to shift from a focus on individual client centred practice to an organized unit of care. Using this argument of organizational form, strategic management will be essential to accommodate these changes, Huntington argues that the overall direction and management function within the practice has to be controlled by the general practitioners who, after all, own the business. These tensions may well influence community health nurses' scope for, and accountability for, practice. Such issues are the subject of ongoing debate throughout the country and general practitioner fundholders are talking seriously about their relationship with attached nurses. (See Chapter 3.5 for further discussion on teamwork.)

The Issue of Advocacy

A further cause for concern is the threat to teamworking that acting as an advocate can throw up. Copp (1986), argues that some nurses will forgo their advocacy role in order to maintain a 'united front' with the rest of the team. This is an important consideration in relation to the nurses's role in the primary health care team, as it is often, for example, a community nurse who is aware of the social and health needs of the most vulnerable groups registered with the practice. Indeed, the notion of inequality in existing health care provision and availability of service provision has concerned health visitors for many years and one of the stated principles of health visiting is that individual practitioners should seek to influence policies affecting health (UKSC HVA, 1992). According to Fowler (1989), this model of advocacy is based on what he terms the 'Champion of Social Justice in the Provision of Health Care', a description which could usefully summarize the view of advocacy held by many community health nurses. Yet by its very nature, focusing as it does on inequalities and injustices in society and not merely or necessarily on individual needs, Fowler argues that this model of advocacy is different from those other models which deal with advocacy for individual patients.

Acknowledging the strength of this argument and the increasing governmental pressure for team working, the extent to which community health nurses can act as effective advocates for their patients/clients may be limited. This is an important observation, as the practitioner's role as an advocate for their patients/clients is implicit in the UKCC's Code of Professional Conduct (1992b) which states that, the nurse/health visitor must, in the exercise of professional accountability, 'act always in such a manner as to promote and safeguard the interests and well-being of patients and clients'.

Defining the Scope of Advocacy

Advocacy, as defined by the Audit Commission (1993), means taking a calculated risk in order to maintain our moral obligation to support and safeguard the physical, psychological and emotional well-being of patients. To do otherwise, it is argued, causes dissonance between knowing what should be done and what was actually done. Rationalizing our actions or inaction to ourselves and our peers simply reinforces the traditional ethos of nurses as 'doctors' handmaidens' and sanctions the indignity that can be suffered by patients. The degree to which individuals can carry out the function of advocacy is the subject of current debate. Writing on this, Suter (1993) even questions whether or not advocacy is a realistic goal given that many nurses have until recently lacked sufficient preparation to carry out this task. However, most community nurses have long accepted, at least in principle, that client advocacy is an important part of their role. In this context, client advocacy means informing the client/patient of their rights in a particular situation and endeavouring to ensure that they have all the necessary information required to make an informed decision. It also involves supporting them in the decision made and protecting and safeguarding their interests. The RCN working group (1982b), commenting on this in relation to health visiting, pointed out that health visitors, because of their access to other statutory and voluntary agencies, have special opportunities and responsibility for client advocacy. The group, however, argued that by accepting this responsibility health visitors may find themselves facing difficult ethical issues. Exactly the same can apply to other community nurses.

Conflict and Constraints

The advocacy role of all community nurses has been clearly heralded by the United Kingdom Central Council for Nursing, Midwifery and Health Visiting who state that all nurses are expected to act as patient advocate. Indeed the nurse's role as the patient's/client's advocate has been widely accepted. Yet, according to Tricia Reid, editor of the *Nursing Times* (1995) the whole concept of advocacy is problematic in that nurses may not be able to act independently from the constraints of their employing authority. The specific activity needed in a particular advocacy situation may create conflict between the community nurses' wish to act in their patients'/clients' interests and their ability to carry this out in practice. The community nurse who acts as an advocate on behalf of a patient, client or family may well find themselves in conflict with their employers.

Publicly pursuing the interests of individuals or groups of individuals is popularly referred to as 'whistle blowing'. This aspect of advocacy is a very real concern for some community nurses as they seek to contribute in a responsible way to public debate about the ethics of health care, resource allocation, fast track appointments for patients registered with general practitioner fundholders etc. There is a danger that in their seeking to influence policies that affect health, they will be viewed by some as trouble-makers.

It was the publicity that surrounded the case of 'charge nurse Pink' that focused attention on 'whistle blowing'. It also acted as a catalyst in the publication of *Guidance for Staff on Relations with the Public and the Media* (DOH 1993a). This report specifies that staff should express their concerns through the existing management channels and points out that staff may be punished if they ignore this advice and speak to the media.

Young, writing in the *Sunday Observer* in 1992, cited evidence to suggest that some nurses were even then too scared to express their concerns for fear of reprisals. He cited the example of a nurse who lost her job after voicing concern about the way medicines were being administered. Since then the Royal College of Nursing suggest that with the move from health authority to trust status and in some instances the renegotiating of nurse contracts this situation has worsened. Against this background some community nurses will face a dilemma between knowing the '*right*' course of action to take yet being unable or possibly unwilling to take the risk involved in adopting an advocacy role.

As a result, public pressure groups such as 'Freedom to Care' and 'Public Concern at Work' (PCAW), an independent organization funded by the Joseph Rowntree Foundation in 1993, have been established. The main aim of 'Public Concern at Work' is to ensure that when employees discover a serious fault or case of neglect at work they are not deterred from raising issues with their employers. Whilst the emergence of independent groups such as these is welcomed the fact remains that the cards are stacked against individuals who appear to be 'making waves.'

However, not everyone will agree with the view that advocacy is in itself problematic. Carpenter (1992: 1), for example, states that: 'Most of the advocacy that a nurse undertakes as part of her professional role involves no conflict.'

Client and Self-Advocacy

In the field of community nursing there may inevitably be times when advocacy has to be undertaken by the nurse, for example a nurse working with people with learning disabilities may be the most appropriate person to act as advocate on behalf of their client. Similarly a paediatric district nurse or school nurse in the absence of parents may well adopt the advocacy role when seeking to present the views of a child. In this context it may be useful to consider advocacy under the now familiar terms of client advocacy and self-advocacy.

This possible clash of perspective in relation to advocacy and accountability to employer and client is ongoing and familiar to all community nurses. Indeed, as long ago as 1982 an RCN working group raised the question as to how far the individual health visitor's accountability to the employing authority for the implementation of its policies could be seen as compatible with their accountability to clients for the advice offered. The topic of accountability is discussed in detail in an earlier chapter and will therefore not be explored here.

The Concept of Autonomy

One of the assumptions usually taken for granted is that within the limits of the law people are more or less free to act as they choose – the concept of autonomy. Within the community setting this concept is highly valued. Yet, with the best will in the world some patients, particularly the very ill and maybe people suffering from dementia, may not get the opportunity to exercise free will. In such cases decisions and actions are taken by nurses acting in the best interest of the patient. Melia (1990b), commenting on this, suggests that most nurses would regard their actions as 'doing the best they can', rather than deliberately setting out to infringe individuals' rights to autonomy.

Working in Partnership

A further consideration is that within the care of some client groups the needs of carers and/or family members must also be considered, and these may be in conflict. This raises the issue of justice. It has been argued elsewhere in this book (Chapter 5.1) that care by the community will place immense additional pressure on carers and family members who may be damaged by the experience. Against this growing pressure, community nurses will need to continue to explore new and effective ways of supporting them. One such way is to strengthen the capacity of both carers, and those they care for, to speak for themselves. This raises the understandable concern to promote advocacy and self-advocacy in an attempt to redress the balance of power. From this perspective community health nurses would hope that their visits were open and patients/clients encouraged to participate both during the core of the contact and at the planning stage.

CONCLUSION

There are many aspects of community nursing where the elements of 'right' decisions and 'best' practice are complicated by differing philosophies and value systems. Hence, the dilemmas of responsibility and ethical accountability in relation to nursing are complex and often interrelated and inherently political. Tensions and difficulties will arise where there are conflicting interests, and it will require a high level of practical application accompanied by an examination of the fundamental moral principles involved to attempt to resolve these.

SUMMARY

- Traditionally, ethics has had to do with decisions regarding what should be sought in life and what should be avoided: life goals, duties and obligations.
- With the development of new knowledge and technological advancement in health care, 'Bioethics' has developed rapidly. This concerns choices and conflict around many health care issues.
- Utilitarianism, egoism and formalization are explored in relation to ethical reasoning.
- Ethical theories and reasoning do not solve ethical dilemmas, but they do suggest ways of clarifying them.
- The emphasis of the United Kingdom Central Council's (1992) Code of Practice and Scope of Professional Practice is explored in relation to personal accountability and scope of practice.
- Health education and health promotion activities cannot be seen as neutral. If used in an attempt to change individual behaviour and attitudes

these activities raise ethical issues which should be acknowledged and explored by nurses.

■ Professional boundaries and the impact of the internal market, with its emphasis on competing internal markets with a specific contract to provide health services to health service consumers, carry ethical concerns in relation to equity, patients' rights and professional duties and obligations.

■ A team approach to care may give rise to ethical concerns centring around priorities for practice and contractual duties.

■ Advocacy, the degree to which individual nurses can carry out advocacy, is the subject of current debate and nurses engaged in this activity on behalf of their clients may find themselves facing difficult ethical decisions.

■ The dilemmas of responsibility and ethical accountability in relation to nursing are complex, often interrelated and inherently political.

DISCUSSION QUESTIONS

◆ Does the national initiative to introduce parent held and client held records raise issues of accountability and a possible clash of perspective between employers and client groups?

◆ In what ways, within the care of some client groups, may the needs of the carers and/or family members be in conflict?

◆ Demographic changes and the introduction of expensive high-technology medicine means that the health service cannot hope to meet demand, hence 'rationing' some services to some groups may be inevitable. How would you decide priorities?

FURTHER READING

Aroska MA (1980) Anatomy of an Ethical Dilemma: The theory. *American Journal of Nursing* April, 658–660.
Outlines a proposed framework for ethical decision-making. This may help to resolve the conflict between a nurse's moral values in community health nursing practice and to provide a morally accountable nursing service.

Fry ST and Spradley BW (1990) Values and ethical decision making in Community Health. Chapter 6 in *Community Health Nursing: Concepts and Practice*. London: Scott Foresran & Co.

This chapter explores values and the valuing processes which influence community health nursing practice and ethical decision-making. It discusses the meaning of values and their relationship to health and health decisions.

Grundstein-Amado R (1993) Ethical decision-making processes used by health care providers. *Journal of Advanced Nursing* **18:** 1701-1709.
This study examines and assesses how health care providers make clinical–ethical decisions in the light of a theoretical model of clinical–ethical decision-making.

REFERENCES

Aroska MA (1987) The interface of ethics and politics in nursing. Chapter 65. In BW Spradley (Ed) *Readings in*

Community Health Nursing (1991), 4th edition. Philadelphia: JB Lippincott.

Audit Commission (1993) *What Seems to be the Matter: Communication between Hospitals and Patients*. London: HMSO.

Bevan A (1993) Question of accountability: where does the buck stop? *Link 2*.

Candle S (1991) *An analysis of HV/client interaction: the influence of HV process on client participation*. King's College.

Carpenter D (1992) Advocacy. *Nursing Times* **88** (27): i–viii.

Copp LA (1986) The nurse as advocate for vulnerable persons. *Journal of Advanced Nursing* **11**: 255–6.

Department of Health (DOH) (1989) Children Act. London: HMSO.

DOH (1991) Access to Health Records Act. London: HMSO.

DOH (1992a) *The Patient's Charter*, London: HMSO.

DOH (1992b) *Health of the Nation*. London: HMSO.

DOH (1993a) *Guidance for Staff on Relations with the Public and the Media*. London: HMSO.

DOH (1993b) *New World: New Opportunities*. London: HMSO.

DOH (1994) *The Challenges for Nursing and Midwifery in the 21st Century*. London: HMSO.

Fowler DM (1989) Social Advocacy. *Heart and Lung* **1**: 18.

Gillon R (1987) *Philosophical Medical Ethics*. Chichester: John Wiley.

Grundstein-Amado R (1993) Ethical decision-making processes used by health care providers. *Journal of Advanced Nursing* **18**: 1701–1709.

Huntington J (1993) Public Lecture, University of Southampton, 19 October 1993.

Kerner GC (1990) *Three Philosophical Moralists, Mill, Kant and Satre: An Introduction to Ethics*. Oxford: Oxford University Press.

Melia KM (1983) 1. Student's views of Nursing. 2. Just passing through. *Nursing Times*. May 18: 26–27.

Montgomery-Robinson K (1987) The Social Construction of Health Visiting (Unpublished PhD). Polytechnic of the South Bank.

News (1995) Inquiry seeks compulsory treatment. *Nursing Times*, Jan 25, **91**(4): 6.

Reid T (1995) Editor's note in 'Support for Advocacy'. Jan 25, *Nursing Times* **91**(4): 28–30.

RCN (1982) *Thinking about Health Visiting*. The RCN Health Visitors Advisory Group, December.

Suter JA (1993) Can nurses be effective advocates. *Nursing Standard*, Feb 17, **7**(22): 30–32.

Thompson IE, Melia KM and Boyd KM (1990) *Nursing Ethics* 2nd edition. Edinburgh: Churchill Livingstone.

UKCC (1992) *The Code of Professional Conduct for the Nurse, Midwife and Health Visitor*, 3rd Edition. United Kingdom Central Council for Nursing, Midwifery and Health Visiting.

UKSC HVA (1992) *The Principles of Health Visiting: a re-examination*. HVA.

Young S (1992) Nurses fear to speak out as patients suffer. *Sunday Observer*, 19 April.

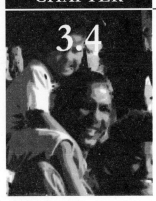

3.4

EVIDENCE BASED PRACTICE IN PRIMARY HEALTH CARE NURSING

Eileen Thomas

KEY ISSUES

- Evidence based nursing: some challenges
- Purchasing evidence based nursing
- Barriers to primary care nursing research
- Cultivating the use of evidence based practice

INTRODUCTION

National Health Service (NHS) reforms and subsequent health policy have resulted in changes in the work activity of nurses in all specialties and grades. Among the most dramatic changes have been those that have affected the work of nurses in the primary care sector, with one wave of reform rapidly following the last. Against this background of unprecedented change are emerging patterns of morbidity, a growing proportion of the elderly in the population and an increase in consumer education; all of which contribute to a predictable increase in the demand for nursing care.

Technological advances, leading to the development of new equipment, pharmaceutical products and innovative medical and surgical techniques, have also led to advances that preserve life in ways previously thought to be impossible. Where life is extended, the requirement for nursing care grows and the recent health care reforms have assured that much of this additional nursing care will be provided in the primary care sector.

Evidence Based Nursing – Some Challenges

Against the background of change surrounding nursing in primary care are demands for greater effectiveness and efficiency. Such demands mean that nurses are not only required to provide 'more' nursing but more than nursing, in terms of extending roles, with little in the way of an extended workforce. With powerful forces exerting energy in disparate directions, the decisions made by nurses in primary care are both crucial in terms of patient benefits and to the whole future of nursing.

Evidence based nursing is the process of systematically finding, critically appraising and utilizing research findings as the basis for clinical decision-making. The process fits equally as well as a basis for making effective decisions in nursing management and leadership. The use of research evidence in nursing should mean that practices based on tradition which have no proven benefit for patients are discarded and are replaced with practices for which there is evidence to support their value (Ford and Walsh, 1994).

The dictionary definition of the word evidence reads, 'facts available as proving or supporting a notion' (Allen, 1987). In terms of nursing and medicine, there are still relatively few facts available which prove or support notions beyond reasonable doubt. Where clear evidence exists in both medicine and nursing there is also widespread poor dissemination and low utilization of research findings (Haines and Jones, 1994; Mulhall, 1995).

Why should this still be the case? Medicine has long called itself a science and nursing is following closely in its research based footsteps. More than twenty years ago, The Briggs Report (DOH, 1972) underlined the importance of nursing becoming a research based profession but what are the current facts that support the use of evidence based nursing in primary care?

Nursing is currently experiencing more rigorous and stringent external reviews than at any time in its history. The major reason for such scrutiny is a desire not only to improve effectiveness but also to control the costs associated with a large nursing workforce (Skidmore, 1994). These costs are substantial and in most provider trusts, nursing is typically the largest personnel group and as a consequence is considered to have a potentially major impact on an organization's financial viability (Jelinek and Kavois, 1992). It is no wonder therefore that nursing is attracting demands for demonstrations of effectiveness. The problem with such interest is that, because much of it is focused on cost and cost reduction, it has been undertaken by organizations external to nursing rather than from within the nursing profession itself.

There are, however, special issues associated with approaches to research in primary care nursing. For example, nursing in this sector is made up of a number of different groups that are not homogeneous but have different training, qualifications and funding bodies. Approaches to research in these groups may require different methods but these issues have yet to be explored. Primary care nursing is labour intensive, consisting of around 9400 practice nurses (Atkin and Hirst, 1994), 19 800 district nurses, and 12 000 health visitors (Law, 1992), in addition to around 10 000 other nurses, in whole time equivalents (NHSE, 1993). The fact that many work on a part time basis means for example, that studies of nursing practice must involve large samples in order to allow for a wide range of variables which may result from differences in background, hours employed and geographical variations.

Nursing in the primary care sector is attracting sustained and growing interest external to the profession, by commissioners and purchasers, in addition to the growing number of general practice fundholders. This is largely due to the numbers in the workforce and the consequences of the Nurse Grading Review process. This review ensured that most primary care nurses, because of the unsupervised nature of their work, were awarded a grade, higher on the whole, than nurses in the secondary sector. Intent on obtaining maximum value for money, purchasers and commissioners increasingly asked for evidence to support the effectiveness of using highly graded nurses in primary care. In the absence of such research evidence, moves to 'dilute' the mix of staff by using lower graded and subsequently lower paid staff become commonplace in the primary care setting (Lightfoot *et al.*, 1992). To date, the only literature that demonstrates the effectiveness of using highly graded rather than lower graded staff comes from the secondary sector (Carr-Hill *et al.*, 1992).

It is against this background of emerging concern for effectiveness, and in the midst of unprecended change in health care policy and provision, that primary care nursing itself is rapidly evolving. In whatever branch nurses are employed in the primary care sector, they must more than ever, base their practice on the best available evidence, mainly in order to provide the highest standard of care possible for patients and clients but also to be able to prove their worth in terms of measurable outcomes.

There are, however, two main groups of obstacles or challenges associated with the use of evidence based practice in primary care nursing. The first is the currency of the purchaser/provider market which measures nursing on the basis of numbers of clients or patients seen. The second is the culture of nursing in this country in which research and the use of research findings on a large scale, is still relatively uncommon.

Purchasing Evidence Based Nursing

> Purchasers and providers need reliable data on the nursing contribution to health gain and patient care if such a large workforce is to be used to maximum benefit, some of the data needed can only be generated through systematic research. (Department of Health, 1993)

Providing evidence to purchasers on the effectiveness of any form of nursing is currently extremely difficult. This is mainly because work on nursing effectiveness is, in common with other health care groups, in its infancy. The only routinely collected measure of nursing is, therefore, activity. Activity as a means of assessment is widely criticized on the grounds that it is not possible to capture the multivariate, interactive nature of nursing by using simple task based counts (O'Brien-Pallas, 1992; King, 1995). Considering that nurses frequently undertake more than one 'task' at the same time it is extremely difficult to sift out bits of jobs into meaningful chunks (Hunt, 1990a).

In primary health care nursing, activity data are currently only required by community trust employed staff and not from practice nurses. Yet this group of nurses has increased at a more rapid rate than any other during the past five years (Atkin *et al.*, 1993). A major part of the primary care nursing workforce are therefore excluded from official statistics despite the fact that they work with the same patients and increasingly undertake similar work (Atkin *et al.*, 1993). The data regarding the activity of primary care nursing are incomplete and because practice nurses are currently employed by general practitioners, there are no plans to alter the collection of these statistics in the near future.

Activity measures in the form of face-to-face contacts as part of the Korner system have themselves attracted considerable criticism since their inception (Gowing, 1994), mainly on the basis that they concentrate on service utilization and not on the patients served (Hull, 1989) nor on any agreed outcome objectives. Because of this it is currently not possible to use the data to *evaluate* nursing practice. Furthermore, there are reported to be widespread errors recorded at all stages of the collection and collation process which make the resulting statistics highly unreliable (DOH Statistics Division, 1994).

Many attempts have been made to improve data collection and analysis, as a proxy for effectiveness in primary care; this has taken the form of a multitude of small-scale local projects initiated at provider or purchaser level. These initiatives have been developed with the best of intentions but without the foundation of sufficient rigour that would permit generalization. As a consequence, providers in adjoining localities frequently develop their own projects in ways that do not permit comparison (NHSE, 1994b). Even when methods have been adapted from others, the methods used are frequently misunderstood or distorted in the process of transfer (HDSS, 1983).

Overall, therefore, at the present time, the only widely available 'hard' evidence accessible to purchasers on primary care nursing is based on activity count data which are known to be incomplete and of low reliability. However, since there is no other system but activity recorded on a national scale, unreliable as they are shown to be, decisions regarding the commissioning of services will necessarily be based on this information. A system which uses activity as a means of measurement reinforces beliefs that nursing can be splintered into discrete measurable tasks, against which a standard tariff can be levied. Purchasers and commissioners of nursing services currently have little choice but to base their decisions about how much and what kind of nursing to buy on erroneous activity data.

However, there are ways in which some of these decisions could be improved. The first lies in the introduction of a new national system, which is planned for implementation by the Information Management Group. This revised Community Minimum Data Set is expected to improve radically the accuracy of information regarding nursing workload in primary care. Regrettably at the present time there are no published details which suggest that practice nurses will be required to include their work as part of these statistics. The second lies in the provision of senior nurses who are familiar with the principles of evidence based practice.

Several recent reports have urged purchasers and commissioners of health care to ensure that they have access to appropriate and experienced nursing advice (NHSE, 1994a; Benton, 1995). This has been interpreted liberally by organizations on a national level, some of whom currently obtain nursing advice in an ad hoc manner. There are, however, relatively few nurses of appropriate seniority, employed in purchasing and commissioning organizations, with relevant expertise in and knowledge of what constitutes evidence based practice, Hence, it is difficult to see how issues of nursing effectiveness and efficiency can be addressed on a strategic level, when advice is provided without the benefit of experience or overview. In terms of the provision of expert advice at purchaser and commissioner level, medical, dental and pharmaceutical opinion is obtained through the appropriate director level appointment. It is curious that the same credence is not given to the need to seek expert nursing opinion on purchasing nursing services.

The emphasis on medical effectiveness has been a growing theme in the health service since Archie Cochrane's seminal work of 1972 and by the early 1990s a sound knowledge base was considered as the foundation for successful purchasing. This means that purchasers must be able to assess the effectiveness and efficiency of medical interventions in order that resources can be used to obtain the maximum health gain for the population. That is to say, there must be an understanding of the costs and benefits of the services commissioned. The task of assessing effectiveness in medical care has widely been considered to be a matter of urgency, especially when estimates are made that only 15% of medical interventions have been of proven effectiveness (Smith, 1994).

Considerable resources have been invested in order to improve the knowledge base in the health service regarding medical effectiveness, to better inform purchasing decisions. The United Kingdom Cochrane Centre, The NHS Centre for Reviews and Dissemination, and a wide range of research and development enterprises, have been initiated in order to provide important information upon which to base medical purchasing decisions. However, given the large workforce and the costs associated with nursing, financial support for the study of nursing interventions is extremely low (Closs and Cheater, 1994). Unlike in other countries, where funding bodies have been established to support nursing research and development, there are relatively few centres of nursing research in this country and none that are focused entirely on producing systematic reviews of nursing practice.

In the absence of expert senior nursing advice in this field at the commissioner/purchaser level, and in the absence of a national movement of nursing effectiveness research, achieving a cultural change which favours research and its utilization will be a substantial accomplishment.

Barriers to Primary Care Nursing Research

The prime objective is to see that research and development becomes an integral part of health care so that clinicians, managers and other staff find it natural to rely on the results of research in their day to day decision making and longer term strategic planning. (Peckham, 1991).

The nursing literature repeatedly refers to important gaps between research evidence and its use in practice (Akinsanya, 1994; Moore, 1995; Nolan and Behi, 1995). However, the four stages of producing the scientific rigour required to be regarded as evidence are different from those likely to be part of the one-off research projects with which many nurses become involved. This process of one-off small scale study, followed by another different area of study, is said to have prevented the nursing profession from developing appropriate depth and breadth of knowledge in important areas (Hinshaw and Heinrich, 1990).

The process of finding the appropriate evidence upon which to base nursing practice has much to learn from medicine and comprises four steps which are described in Box 3.4.1.

This approach is somewhat different from classical approaches to research included in nursing texts but offers the opportunity to provide a systematic review of the available evidence by pooling all the existing available research relevant to the question. As a result of adopting and using this approach it should be possible to avoid reinventing the nursing research wheel whereby small-scale projects repeat studies already undertaken but not in such a standard manner to allow comparison or replication of results (Tierney, 1987; Freemantle, 1995).

There are important difficulties associated with the use of a systematic approach to obtaining research evidence in nursing, especially in the primary care sector. Formulating the research question is something that nurses actually do very frequently in their daily work, especially with the patient or client and frequently from

Box 3.4.1. The process of finding appropriate evidence (from Rosenberg and Donald, 1995)

- The formulation of clear clinical questions from the patients' perspective
- The search of the literature for relevant articles
- The critical appraisal of the evidence in the articles for validity and usefulness
- The implementation of appropriate findings in clinical practice

the client's point of view. The patient presents a problem and in partnership with the nurse a solution is found. Is that solution, however, based on the best available evidence, or is based on tradition that many have outlived its usefulness? A good illustration of how evidence is not informing practice was given by Cullum (1994) in a systematic review of leg ulcer treatment mainly by district nurses, who manage between 60–90% of leg ulcer patients. Compression therapy has been clearly demonstrated as the most effective approach to managing venous leg ulcers and yet there is clear evidence that this treatment is not given appropriately.

Identifying the best available evidence in any given situation requires the persistent skills of a detective but it also requires knowledge of the best way to go about it. The term 'literature search' is, in the current climate of computerization, a misnomer, since the first stage in the examination of the appropriate literature lies in accessing it in the first place. On-line computer search facilities are now commonplace in universities, colleges and libraries but access to these for nurses in primary care, working in remote geographical locations, and/or having high caseloads, means that finding the necessary amount of time to spend in the search activity is likely to be problematic. In addition, it is reported that nurses may not have the appropriate knowledge or skills required to interrogate an on-line search facility (Hunt, 1990).

The third stage in the systematic search for evidence upon which to base nursing practice is critical appraisal of the literature. This means that the relevant articles, once identified, have to be evaluated, in order to define their validity and usefulness, or otherwise (Milne and Chambers, 1993). There are currently courses available to help clinicians and purchasers learn critical appraisal skills in the form of CASP (Critical Appraisal Skills for Purchasers) workshops conducted, by many regional research and development directorates (Dunning *et al.*, 1994). These and similar programmes offer nurses and other clinicians the opportunity to learn skills which will help them to judge the quality and usefulness of research, skills which Church and Lyne (1994) say are currently lacking.

The fourth step towards basing nursing practice on evidence lies in the implementation stage. There is much written on the difficulty of utilizing research in order to develop practice (Champion and Leach, 1989; Armitage, 1990; Lacey, 1994), but there is also a considerable amount written suggesting that overall, nursing is still poorly developed in research terms (Akinsanya, 1994; Hicks, 1995; Smith, 1994). Most of the published literature relating to the standard and frequency of nursing research is based on nursing in education, either concerning teachers or students, or has taken place in this country in the secondary sector. However, given that primary care nursing faces unprecedented demands in terms of the work it is required to undertake, it is essential that a body of in-depth knowledge is established as a matter of priority. Although the systematic review process offers nursing the opportunity to pool evidence and make decisions in a more informed way, it is not the only approach that offers the chance to improve the knowledge base of primary care nursing.

Research into aspects of primary care nursing is particularly important because of the rapid changes which continue to take place, the majority of which have never been subject to sufficient evaluation. This means that many new patterns of care delivery are being implemented without prior knowledge that they will result in benefits for patients and clients. Furthermore, the lack of relevant baseline data means that measuring the consequences of these changes will in the future be extremely difficult, since if you do not know where you came from it is impossible to measure the distance you have travelled and whether the direction is helpful or otherwise.

Nursing is responding rapidly to the whirlwind of change affecting the National Health Service; this is particularly true in the primary care sector. In doing so nurses are placing themselves at risk of doing more things faster, rather than defining and choosing to do the right things.

In doing more of the present work at a faster pace, time to stop and reflect diminishes. The reflective practitioner approach (Schon, 1983), which advocates taking time to think about what worked well in the presence of a peer group and then adjusting behaviour accordingly, is also the foundation of effective research. Opportunities for reflecting on work in the community are complicated by the fact that practitioners often work on their own, usually for long periods, and sharing experiences can be hampered by extensive distances between practitioners. Increasingly large caseloads mean that many nurses feel overwhelmed by the work to be done and subsequently find little time to develop the reflective practitioner approach. The reflective approach in nursing is very similar to research, in that by finding an answer to a research question, learning from it and integrating the findings into practice, nursing effectiveness increases. The difference between the two is time, in that research has a longer time span between identification of the research question and utilization of the findings.

Time as a reason for not undertaking research is commonly given by nurses in both the primary and secondary sectors. Yet research in the area of nursing research activity shows that this may not be the case. Hicks (1995), in a national sample of 230 nurses, demonstrated that of these, 161, or 70%, had taken part in research activity. Most revealing, however, was that of this 161 who had carried out research only 16 had submitted their work for publication. Reasons for not writing up research were given as uncertainly about research methodology (66%), lack of time for writing up (45%) and general lack of confidence (5%). It is clear that aspects of self-confidence are important barriers to the submission for publication of nursing research but not, it seems, of research activity in the first place.

Confidence in any activity is obtained through practice and experience, it is also contingent in the early stages upon having good support and encouragement. Nurses in primary care may find it especially difficult to identify sufficiently experienced mentors who can help them through the critical early stages of research. Most academic nursing posts are attached to colleges or universities, the great majority of which find themselves located close to, or within, large district general hospitals.

Teachers of primary care nursing have a tradition of the rolling student intake which means that one course completes immediately prior to the next one starting. This means that like other groups of nurse teachers, there is little time available for research activity in this group (Mulhall, 1995). Primary care nursing research questions are different from those which might be asked in the secondary sector, where patients are relatively captive, at least in terms of being in the same geographical location and broadly experiencing similar problems within clinical specialties. The Project 2000 programme should result in increased opportunities for a greater body of research expertise to be built up in the primary care sector but even so the effect will not be immediate. In all fields of work there is a time lag between knowledge and practice, which is considered to be directly proportional to the distance between the creation of the theory and the position of the practitioner (McGuire, 1990). This means that if there is a perceived gap between the groups that created the knowledge and the practitioners who are expected to utilize the findings, the results of important research may take several years to implement.

For primary care nursing, special problems are presented in terms of the distance between the creation of knowledge and its use. There are, for example, problems of transferability since most nursing research has been undertaken in the secondary sector. Such knowledge does not transfer easily into the patient's or client's home and much of it has focused on nurses themselves rather than on the results of nursing work. The demography of nurses in primary care is quite different from that of secondary sector nurses; for example, a large proportion are part time and age, length of service, qualifications and experiences are different.

Cultivating the Use of Evidence Based Practice in Primary Care Nursing

> The direct, deliberate and systematic use of research findings is so rare as to be negligible. The indirect, unsystematic and opportunistic use of research findings to support policy decisions already taken on ideological or other political grounds is much more common. (Hunter and Pollitt, 1992)

Research in any field of health care requires confidence, time and expertise, especially since it is much easier and much more common for research to attract criticism rather than praise. Nursing research in this country is frequently regarded as a special interest or an extra to be added on to 'proper' work as a kind of hobby. The result of such a culture is that undertaking research or using the results is extremely difficult. According to Close and Cheater (1994), this culture has developed in part as a consequence of nursing history which makes change difficult but also because the health service as a whole still seems to undervalue research. Developments in education, such as Project 2000, are expected to have a positive influence on attitudes towards research, which will in time change the culture of nursing from within.

In the short term, the emergence of special posts which have a dual practice-research role will help to integrate research into nursing practice. In primary care terms this strongly suggests research posts in all of the nursing groups: school nursing, practice nursing, district nursing, health visiting and others. It also suggests a need for collaborative posts which examine more closely the total nursing work to be undertaken in primary care, in addition to the capacity to audit the outcomes of any innovation that is introduced as a result of research activity.

Collaboration is an important theme in primary care nursing terms, not only in respect of groups of nurses in the same geographical area working together but also by working together in multicentre trials. This would resolve criticisms of small sample sizes and convenience samples. There may be obstacles to this approach, particularly since the creation of trusts has engendered competition between areas. But in the interest of developing and clearly demonstrating good practice, ways need to be found to overcome these difficulties. Multidisciplinary research is obviously another example of collaborative working but not only in the usual manner of nurse-medical practitioner, or nurse-therapist but also nurse-leadership. In terms of clinical advice and supervision there is still much to be learned.

It is said that 'without a gardener there is no garden' and in order to cultivate a positive research culture in nursing, there is evidence that nursing leadership, which is committed to a positive research culture, is essential to the development and continuation of that culture (Champion and Leach, 1989). This implies more than the ubiquitous 'support' but action in terms of positively adopting a systematic approach to change, so that nursing strategies are based on the best available evidence regarding what constitutes effective nursing. It also strongly indicates that primary care nurse leaders must be able to tell poor research from good research, disregarding the poor for the best available.

CONCLUSION

Leadership of nursing in primary care is currently at a crossroads. New models of primary care nursing may not have access to the same clinical leadership and clear advice pathways as in the past. However, it is the development of strong, research fluent nurses in primary care that will act as guides through the many changes that are destined to influence care delivery as one century ends and another commences. Primary care delivery will probably change beyond recognition during the next decade, as it has during the previous one. The pace of that change is quickening and with it the range and type of nursing care. It is up to all nurses but, in particular, nursing leaders to ensure that the care that is offered to patients is based on the best available evidence.

SUMMARY

■ Evidence based nursing is the process of systematically finding, critically appraising and utilizing research findings as the basis for clinical decision-making.

■ The use of research evidence in nursing should mean that practices based on tradition which have no proven benefit for patients are discarded and replaced with practices for which there is evidence.

■ Purchasers and commissioners, intent on obtaining value for money, are increasingly asking for evidence to support the effectiveness of using highly graded primary health care nurses.

■ Providing evidence to purchasers on the effectiveness of nursing is a necessary but complex task.

■ Given the rate of change in the delivery and organization of primary care/community nursing, it is essential that a body of knowledge, rooted in research, be developed.

■ The development of strong research nurses in primary/community care will be essential to lead nursing through the next decade and on into the next century.

DISCUSSION QUESTIONS

♦ In what ways are the characteristics of nurses in primary care settings likely to be predictably different from those working in the acute sector? How would you account for this?

♦ What criteria has been used for assessing health care effectiveness? (See 'Effectiveness Bulletins') from York and Leeds Universities.

♦ Identify two nursing strategies with measurable outcomes based on nursing research.

FURTHER READING

Chalmers I and Altman D (1995) *Systematic Reviews*. London: BMJ Publishing Group.
A guide to critically appraising research.

Davey B, Gray A and Scale C (1995) *Health and Disease: A Reader*. Milton Keynes: Open University Press.
A collection of 62 articles on aspects of health from a variety of prespectives.

Ford P and Walsh M (1994) *New Rituals for Old: Nursing through the Looking Glass*. Oxford: Butterworth-Heinemann.
An exploration of nursing rituals still in common use and their lack of benefits to patients.

REFERENCES

Allen RE (1987) *The Oxford Dictionary of Current English*. Oxford: Oxford University Press.

Akinsanya J (1994) Making research useful to the practising nurse. *Journal of Advanced Nursing* **19**: 174–179.

Armitage S (1990) Research utilization in practice. *Nurse Education Today*. 10–15.

Atkin K and Hirst M (1994) *Costing Practice Nurses: Implications for Primary Health Care*. York: Social Policy Research Unit, University of York.

Atkin K, Lunt N, Park G and Hirst M (1994) *Nurses Count: A National Census of Practice Nurses*. York: Social Policy Research Unit, University of York.

Benton D (1995) Opportunity or threat. *Nursing Standard* 22–23.

Carr-Hill R, Dixon P, Gibbs I, Griffiths M, Higgins M, McCaughan D and Wright K (1992) *Skill mix and the effectiveness of nursing care*. York: Centre for Health Economics.

Champion VL and Leach A (1989) Variables related to research utilisation in nursing. *Journal of Advanced Nursing* **14**: 705–710.

Church S and Lyne P (1994) Research based practice: some problems illustrated by the discussion of evidence concerning the use of pressure reducing devices in nursing and midwifery. *Journal of Advanced Nursing*, **19**(3): 513–18.

Closs SJ and Cheater FM (1994) Utilization of nursing research: culture, interest and support. *Journal of Advanced Nursing* **19**: 762–773.

Cochrane A (1972) *Effectiveness and Efficiency: Random reflections on health services*. London: Nuffield Provincial Hospitals Trust.

Cullum M (1994) Leg ulcer treatments: a critical review parts I and II. *Nursing Standard* **9**: 60–63.

DOH (Department of Health) (1972) *Report of the Committee on Nursing* (The Briggs Report). London: HMSO.

Department of Health Statistics Division 2B (1994) *Patient care in the community in district nursing*. Summary Information Form KC56 London: HMSO.

Department of Health (1993) *Report on the Taskforce on the Strategy for Research in Nursing, Midwifery and Health Visiting*. London: HMSO.

Dunning M, McQuay H and Milne R (1994) Getting a grip: Getting research into practice. *Health Service Journal* **104**: 24–26.

Effectiveness Bulletins. York: Nuffield Institute/Centre for Health Economics and the NHS Centre for Review.

Ford P and Walsh M (1994) *New Rituals for Old: Nursing through the Looking Glass*. Oxford: Butterworth-Heinemann.

Freemantle N (1995) Paper given at the Nursing and Therapy Profession's contribution to Health Services Research and Development, 1994. London: HMSO.

Gowing W (1994) Operating systems. In J Keen (Ed) *Information Management in Health Services*. Buckingham: Open University Press.

Haines A and Jones R (1994) Implementing findings of research. *British Medical Journal* **308**: 1488–1492.

HDSS Operational Research Service (1983) Nurse Manpower – planning approaches and techniques. London: HMSO.

Hicks C (1995) The shortfall in published research: a study of nurses' research and publication activities. *Journal of Advanced Nursing* **21**: 594–604.

Hinshaw AS and Heinrich J (1990) New initiatives in nursing research: a national perspective In R Bergman (Ed), *Nursing Research for Nursing Practice. An Individual Perspective*. London: Chapman and Hall.

Hull W (1989) Measuring the effectiveness of health visiting. *Health Visitor Journal* **62**(4): 113–115.

Hunt J (1990a) Towards research based practice. *Nursing Standard* **5**: 48–49.

Hunt J (1990b) The activity balance. *Nursing Standard* **4**: 47.

Hunter D and Pollitt C (1992) *Rationing dilemmas in healthcare*. Birmingham: NAHAT.

Jelinek RC and Kavois JS (1992) Nurse staffing and scheduling: past solutions and future directions. *Social Health Systems* **68**: 14–15.

King (1995) Counting what counts. *Health Visitor* **69**: 1, 15–16.

Lacey EA (1994) Research utilization in nursing practice. *Journal of Advanced Nursing*, **19**: 987–995.

Law S (1992) *Community Nursing Workforce Study*. London: HMSO.

Lightfoot J, Baldwin S and Wright K (1992) *Nursing by Numbers*. York: Social Policy Research Unit.

McGuire G (1990) Putting nursing research findings into practice, research utilization as management of change. *Journal of Advanced Nursing* **15:** 614-620.

Milne R and Chambers L (1993) Assessing the scientific quality of review articles. *Journal of Epidemiology and Community Health* **47:** 169-70.

Moore PA (1995) The utilization of research in practice. *Professional Nurse* **10**(8): 536-537.

Mulhall A (1995) Nursing research: what difference does it make? *Journal of Advanced Nursing* **21:** 576-586.

NHSE (National Health Service Executive) (1993) *New World New Opportunities: Nursing in Primary Health Care*. London: HMSO.

National Health Service Executive (1994a) *Building a Stronger Team: The Nursing Contribution to Purchasing*. Leeds: NHSE.

National Health Service Executive (1994b) *Nursing in the 21st Century: The Heathrow Debate*. Leeds: NHSE.

Nolan M and Behi R (1995) Research in nursing: developing a conceptual approach. *British Journal of Nursing* **41:** 45-49

O'Brien-Pallas L (1992) Overview of nursing research in healthcare within the current economic climate. *Canadian Journal of Nurse Administration* **5:** 20-4.

Peckham M (1991) *Research for Health: A Research and Development Strategy for the NHS*. London: HMSO.

Rosenberg W and Donald A (1995) Evidence based medicine: an approach to clinical problem solving. *British Medical Journal* **310:** 1122-1126.

Skidmore D (1994) Can nursing survive: A view through the keyhole. *Nursing Ethics* **1**(4): 193-9.

Smith L (1994) An analysis and reflections on the quality of nursing research in 1992. *Journal of Advanced Nursing* **19:** 385-93.

Tierney AJ (1987) Research issues: putting research to good use. *Senior Nurse* **6**(3): 10.

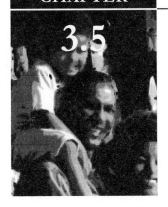

TEAM BUILDING IN PRIMARY HEALTH CARE TEAMS

Judy Gillow

KEY ISSUES

- How teamwork in primary care has evolved
- Teamwork in relation to the National Health Service agenda
- Definition of 'team'
- Membership of primary health care teams
- Advantages of teamwork
- Barriers to effective teamwork
- Evaluation of team effectiveness

INTRODUCTION

'Few things are more satisfying in life than belonging to a good team' (Adair, 1987). Some of us will have worked in good teams, others in not so good teams but what are the key influencing factors that relate to this?

Teamwork is a very complex process that often is taken for granted and it is interesting that suddenly over the last three years teamwork in primary care has become an essential ingredient to improve the quality of patient care. There has been a dearth of objective evidence for the effectiveness of teamwork but interestingly the present and future focus of care appears to work around it. This chapter will explore in depth the whole concept of team working in primary care and review recent research that is attempting to identify the key factors which relate to building positive functioning teams.

Background

The National Health Service agenda currently views primary care as the focus of health activity in the mid 1990s and into the twenty-first century. The publication of the three White Papers, *Promoting Better Health* (DOH, 1987), *Caring for People* (DOH, 1989a) and *Working For Patients* (DOH, 1989b), underlined the importance of primary care within the National Health Service. It has also been clearly identified that an important aspect in enabling primary care to move forward is the development of primary health care teams.

New World, New Opportunities (DOH, 1993) emphasized the importance of teamwork and the whole philosophy of care in the community is all about working effectively in multidisciplinary teams. However, teamwork, ideally enshrined in the concept of the primary health care team is more easily talked about and aspired to than achieved. In 1992 the Audit Commission's report *Homeward Bound* high-lighted that while many groups of professionals in primary health care teams produced a high standard of care, others were disabled by low levels of teamworking. Interestingly, a further study in Northumberland, Morpeth (Primary Care Forum, 1991) developed this theme further by finding that there were often low levels of collaboration between GPs and community nurses.

The conclusion was drawn that while many GPs, nurses and administrative staff work under the same roof it does not follow they will be working as a team.

Government reforms have forced GPs to take on a range of new tasks making it essential to build and develop a thriving primary health care team. Noakes (1992) stressed that in the future the GP will not just be producing personal doctoring to patients but will also have the responsibility for the primary care needs of a defined population. Fulfilling those needs is going to require a coordinated approach from a multidisciplinary team of professionals. This places a greater emphasis than there has ever been before on the whole culture and development of effective teamworking.

What is a Team?

All our lives, even though we may not have realized it, we have worked in teams. Some will have been formal others not so formal. Most people will remember the school sports team, the college debating team and more recently the ward nursing team. The Concise Oxford Dictionary quotes that a team is 'oxen which are harnessed together to pull a cart'. All definitions share the same theme that a team is a group of people who work together to achieve a common purpose. Firth-Cozens (1992) summarized key characteristics of a successful team:

- having a common goal
- a diversity of skills and knowledge
- mutual support for team members
- effective management of conflict

If this is broadened out into primary care it is interesting to compare these criteria with the Harding Committee (DHSS, 1981) investigation into primary health care teams. It was stated in this report that the basic prerequisites for satisfactory integration of the team were as shown in Box 3.5.1

The word 'team' is now developing into a more complex definition than just a group of people working together. Criteria for working in a team are now emerging that require at the very least coordination, cooperation, commitment and trust.

Box 3.5.1.
Prerequisites for satisfactory team integration

- A common objective for the team, accepted and understood by all members
- A clear understanding by each team member of their role, function and responsibilities
- A clear understanding by each team member of the role, function, skills and responsibilities of each other team member; and mutual respect for the role and skills allied to a flexible approach.

Membership of the Primary Health Care Team

Membership of the primary health care team is a key question that is not easily answered. This issue has long been debated and the debate continues. There is a wide variation of views from those who believe that anyone who has any contact with the patient including the patients themselves must be included and conversely those who believe that teams have a clear boundary and membership which must consist of those professionals who regularly work together.

One of the most commonly quoted definitions on the make-up of a primary health care team adopted by the Harding Committee (DHSS, 1981) is:

> An independent group of General Medical Practitioners, Secretaries, Receptionists, Health Visitors, District Nurses and Midwives.

Some will say that this definition is now outdated and too narrow. The practice nurse and practice manager, who have emerged as key team members over the last few years, are not mentioned and the definition does not include a wider range of multidisciplinary team members such as community psychiatric nurses, social workers and counsellors. Recent studies have also highlighted that the professionals themselves were not always sure of the make-up of their team.

The Southampton Primary Care Development Team undertook a study in 1993 exploring *Multi-disciplinary Audit by Primary Care Teams* and they found that some primary care team members were confused about the composition of their team, and commonly did not include community attached staff such as district nurses and health visitors. There was also a confusion on what was the 'core' team and how other potential members jointed the team such as social workers. This was backed up by further research undertaken by Poulton and West (1993) who reported that there were wide variations in team members' assessments of the size of their team. In their study it also became apparent that some practice managers classed the primary health care team as practice employed staff and of those who included attached nursing staff, many were unsure of the precise numbers of district nurses and health visitors attached to the practice. It is obvious that there was, and probably still is, confusion. Some will say does it matter, whilst others will counter that unless membership is known how can development of the team commence.

A possible model to consider for discussion is shown in Box 3.5.2:

The core team consists of professionals who concentrate on that defined practice population and are either based in the surgery or close by.

Box 3.5.2. A possible model for the primary care team

Extended team	Core team	Extended team
Physiotherapist	GP	
Chiropodist	Practice manager	
Audiologist	Practice nurse	Social worker
Speech therapist	Receptionist/ administrative staff	Voluntary and self help groups
Occupational therapist	Counsellor	
School nurse	Health visitor	
Community psychiatric nurse	District nurse	
	Midwife	
Dietician		

The extended team consists of professionals and groups who may work on a geographical or locality basis and provide a service to several practices or to the practice population.

With the development of GP fundholding and the transition of care from secondary to primary care, new core and extended team members will be identified. The challenge is how to enable these different members to work as an effective integrated team in an ever changing environment. Some would even question if it is possible. The Southampton Primary Care Development Team (1993) found that the practices they studied wanted to concentrate on team building for the core team. The extended team seemed too large and unmanageable. It is clear that further work needs to be done in this area particularly since development of locality multidisciplinary health care is high on the National Health Service agenda.

There is also emerging evidence that the make-up of the team needs to vary in different areas tailoring it to the needs of the practice population. The challenge is not only to increase the number of services that all practices provide, but to ensure that the different elements within the team work effectively.

With the encouragement of developing local services for local people, there is an emergence of locality teams which should complement and work alongside practice teams. Some professionals may be members of both which further increase the complexity of building effective teams.

Advantages of Team Work in Primary Care

There do appear to be many advantages to teamwork. Some of the key areas identified are:

- Team members offer breadth of different skills.
- The patient/client has access to a wider range of skills/specialist knowledge.
- Team members can delegate work ensuring the most appropriate person can deal with the problem.
- Team members can educate each other and pool ideas and knowledge.
- The quality of patient care can only be improved.

However, recent work undertaken by West (1993) challenges the commonly held beliefs on teamwork.

He argues that groups take longer than individuals in coming to correct solutions and do not always produce a greater quality and quantity of ideas than individuals working alone.

The Southampton Primary Care Team (1993) found in their study of primary care teams that team members felt awareness and communication had been improved since they had undertaken team building activities and it helped them improve the quality of care offered by the practice. This, however, was from the individual team members' perspective. Methods to measure this need to be more fully developed.

Barriers to Effective Teamwork

While many GPs, nurses and administrative staff work together under the same roof, it does not automatically follow that they are working as a team. There are many factors affecting teamwork, both external and internal. Often the largest barriers appear to be within the practice itself with entrenched attitudes perhaps being the most pernicious difficulty. Members of the team misunderstand or misinterpret each other's roles, expertise, objectives and professional goals. Sometimes poor teamwork results in jobs getting done twice or not at all because no clear understanding of roles within and between teams exist.

The Audit Commission's report *Homeward Bound* (1992) succinctly summarizes some of the difficulties that result in a lack of teamwork. These include separate lines of control, different payment system, professional barriers and perceived inequalities in status.

In addition it is noted that rigidity can occur in teams with members following narrow definitions of their roles which in turn can affect team morale. Poulton and West (1993) noted in their research that there was evidence of differing priorities from team members. Administrative staff focused more on practice efficiency, the practice nurses focused on health promotion targets and doctors in many cases referred to the maximization of practice income.

There can also be the attitude which teams and individual members have to the possibility of external help. The ineffective team will either reject offers of help because it fears the consequences of others finding out what the team is really like or it will seize all offers of help because there is a lack of any coherent view and is content to hand the problem over to someone else. It also appears that where effective teamwork does not exist people tend to work in isolation and neither offer nor receive help from their colleagues.

As long ago as 1981 The Harding Committee highlighted difficulties in primary health care teams of coordinated working and even then intimated that teams do not just happen, they need to be developed, supported and sustained. To be most effective team building needs to be part of the everyday culture of the primary health care team.

An increasing barrier to teamwork, which is usually identified by GPs themselves, relates to the different management structures within primary care teams.

The community attached staff such as district nurses and health visitors are generally managed by, and accountable to, GPs. There is a concern that this leads to difficulty in developing joint team objectives and reduces the flexibility of roles. With the increasing development of GP fundholding and the setting up of pilot projects to explore total GP managed teams, it will be interesting to review the outcomes of this.

Putting Theory into Practice

The Southampton Primary Care Development Team Project (1993) worked with five primary care teams and one of their key aims was to support the development of teamwork in each multidisciplinary group. Each member of the primary health care team was interviewed to elicit their views of teamwork and the results were used to help the team develop positively by using team building strategies which helped tackle the identified problems. Several common themes seen to inhibit teamwork emerged from this work. These included identification of the following by the team members:

- Shortage of time and increased workload
- Increased stress and symptoms of 'burn out'.
- Lack of time out
- Lack of appreciation of time out

- Communication – it was always felt this could be improved
- No regular team meetings
- Poor understanding of roles in teams
- Duplication of roles

The above aspects identified that the teams had no clear direction, no joint aims and objectives and no clear support systems and it further confirmed that effective teamwork does not just happen when a group of professionals are put together, everybody needs to put effort and commitment into working together.

This project, however, also identified benefits from improving teamwork and these included:

- Improved morale
- Improved communication
- Development of trust and respect which makes it easier to work together
- Learning from each other
- Peer group support
- Better understanding of roles and responsibilities
- Consistent approach to patient care
- Sharing of workload
- Reduction of duplication of roles
- Recognized benefits of taking protected 'time out'

On reviewing other research available, on teamwork, these appeared to be common issues in teams.

Peter Prichard (1994) added several other components which complement the findings of the Southampton Primary Care Development Team including:

- Shared decisions by the team reduce the pain of failure
- Sharing of knowledge to broaden everyone's horizon
- Members of effective teams are committed to the mutual tasks and to each other
- Teamwork depends on equality of status

Pritchard (1994) also agreed with the conclusions of the Southampton Primary Care Development Team such as:

- Time must be set aside for meetings.
- The meetings should have a focus and be run efficiently.
- Teamwork needs to be part of the everyday culture of the primary care team.
- Team members need to feel they can be honest about problems.
- Mistakes should provide an opportunity to learn and grow.

In addition the Southampton Project emphasized the need for practices to have 'protected' time out together on a regular basis to enable the team to reflect on the 'current state', review progress, celebrate successes and decide the next steps.

When primary health care teams have identified the pressures they are working under and the frantic pace of change, it can seem difficult to appreciate that effective time out will enhance working practice and the overall emotional status of the team. External facilitation can sometimes reduce some of the pressure by taking the primary health care team through the process of problem-solving and introducing team building strategies which remove threat and empower the team to make positive decisions about their future working.

Good Teamwork in Action

Looking at all the issues relating to teamwork it can be helpful to identify real examples which highlight the positive benefits to the patient and the team and show how minor changes can lead to major improvements.

The following examples were drawn from the work undertaken by the Southampton Primary Care Development Team (1993).

The three examples shown in Box 3.5.3 clearly document different ways a team can work together to enhance the care they give and improve the way they work together.

Team Leadership

Does a team need a leader? Particularly in relation to primary health care teams most professionals would say yes, as it is probable that without clear leadership, coordination and the wide diversity of team member's roles, little progress will be made. Baker (1993) states that the most effective teams he has encountered have been the

Box 3.5.3. Examples of teamwork

Example 1

One GP practice identified that there were unacceptable waiting times for patients to see the practice nurse. It was found that patients attending for cervical smears were booked in for a single, rather than a double, appointment. This resulted in long waiting times. This problem was highlighted during a team building exercise.

All the team members discussed the issue and agreed the following:

- The receptionist would place a notice in the waiting room asking patients to book a double appointment.
- The practice nurse would liaise with the receptionist about making appointments.
- The GP would take every opportunity to educate the patients.
- The invitation sent out to the patients would be reworded. The practice manager would coordinate this.

Example 2

Three GP practices identified problems with hospital discharge. Once highlighted it became apparent that several team members were experiencing problems (GP, district nurse, community psychiatric nurse and practice manager). The team worked together to decide what they wanted to happen and drew up a plan of action. The joint approach gave them more power to institute change and improve patient care.

Example 3

One GP practice felt that one of the biggest handicaps when working together was a lack of understanding of each other's roles and skills. They drew up a plan whereby at each regular team meeting each member undertook to do a five minute presentation to explain the key areas of their role. This stimulated much discussion and in a non-threatening way started to tackle the overlap of roles within the team.

ones with clear leaders who have been able to balance the requirements of of meeting the needs of the team and of the individuals within it. There is also the general assumption that the GP is the automatic leader but other members such as health visitors or practice managers have the skills to lead the team. It is also interesting that many GPs have not been trained in leadership skills. Pritchard and Pritchard (1992) emphasize that leadership must be learned and earned, it cannot be taken for granted. A team without a leader could be compared to a boat without a rudder, no clear direction, out of control and uncoordinated. The leadership style is also crucial to how the team functions alongside the enthusiasm and commitment demonstrated by the leader.

Evaluating Team Effectiveness

How is team effectiveness evaluated? Is it from the team members perspective, is it from the patient/client perspective or is it measured by improved outcomes in patient care? Probably it should be a mix of all these but gaining the right information to analyse is not always possible.

In the psychological literature Sundstrom *et al.* (1990) depicts team effectiveness as consisting of performance and viability. Performance relates to achievement of agreed targets and acceptability of service to consumers, whereas team viability refers to satisfaction of team members, clarity of roles and objectives and team processes such as communication and decision-making. If team viability enhances team performance and these factors contribute to team effectiveness, methods of improving viability such as communication, cohesion and shared objectives need to be reviewed. The degree to which people work, help and use each other is another indicator, for where effective teamwork does not exist people tend to work in isolation. Pritchard and Pritchard (1992) comment that evaluation of team effectiveness is a neglected subject but very essential. Poulton and West (1993) argue that there are two distinct groups of stakeholders to consider in the evaluation:

- Patients and their carers
- Health commissions (FHSA and DHAs) and fundholding GP practices

They identify that these two major groups of stakeholders may have conflicting criteria for effectiveness and suggest these could be:

1. Patient and carers to receive high quality care which in some cases may be costly.
2. Service providers to contain this care within allocated resources.

Most studies which explore the evaluation of team effectiveness use the focus of the team themselves although it is recognized that improved outcomes in patient care is also becoming an integral part of the evaluation such as concentrating on achievement of 'Health of the Nation' targets. Over the last two to three years primary health care teams have been encouraged to attend team building workshops to promote their effectiveness. Research suggests, however, that whilst these activities have a positive impact on the team members themselves, there is no proven reliable impact on team performance or task effectiveness.

The Southampton Primary Care Development Team (1993) found that in relation to benefits to team members these assumptions appeared correct. There is the view, however, that if the team feel good about themselves, have clear direction of where they are going and understand each other's roles and responsibilities, it must have a positive effect on patient care. It is, though, clearly identified that more work needs to be undertaken in this area.

CONCLUSION

The benefits of working in teams cannot be underestimated. However, this needs to be balanced against the coordination, effort and ongoing commitment it requires by all team members for the focus of care to remain in the primary setting. A multidisciplinary approach to achieve this is essential. This may involve community staff working in several teams, being adaptable, flexible and sensitive to the needs of the team. They will need to be open minded and prepared to share differences, acknowledge mistakes but most importantly celebrate successes.

For any team the patient/client must be the focus and team members must constantly review their professional practice, their communication with the patient and team colleagues and their role and responsibilities within the team. Health professionals should not be working in isolation or confine themselves to their professional group any more.

The success of providing high quality local care to local people will be dependent on strong effective multidisciplinary teams within general practice and through inter-agency team work within the geographical area. Innovative ways of enabling teams to function and the continuation of research into evaluating team work needs to continue. We need to make the recent statement in the report *New World, New Opportunities* (DOH, 1993) a reality.

Primary Healthcare in the future will be organised increasingly around General Practice and multidisciplinary teamwork will be essential for the achievement of team objectives.

SUMMARY

The following list identifies the key factors relating to teamwork in primary health care teams:

- Teams do not just happen, they need to be developed, supported and sustained.
- Teamwork is a dynamic process that needs to be constantly reviewed.
- Effective teamwork should be part of the daily culture of primary health care teams.
- There needs to be clarification of team membership with recognition that the make-up of a team will vary according to identified population health needs.
- Setting of joint objectives and having a clearly defined vision is crucial to effective teamworking.
- Good understanding of each other's roles and responsibilities within the team.
- Regular team meetings which involve all team members and include processes by which decisions can be made and conflicts resolved.
- The need for the team to generate a culture of honesty, trust and respect.
- Teams need to take 'protected time out' on a regular basis to review the current state and decide how to go forward.
- The need for effective support systems to enable the team to manage change effectively.

DISCUSSION
QUESTIONS

1. Think of teams you have worked in.
   What was good about working in the team?
   What was difficult about working in the team?
   What changes would have enabled the team to function better?

2. How can effective teamwork demonstrate positive outcomes in patient care?

3. Identify the communication networks in a team you have recently worked in:
   What were the problems?
   How could they have been improved?

REFERENCES

Adair J (1987) *Effective Teambuilding*, Second edition. London: Pan Books.

Audit Commission (1992) *Homeward Bound. A New Course for Community Health*. An Audit Commission Report. London: HMSO.

Baker R (1993) *Teamwork and Quality. Audit for Teams in Primary Care. Proceedings of a Conference (July 1993)*. Eli Lilly National Clinical Audit Centre. Department of General Practice, University of Leicester.

DOH (1987) *Promoting Better Health* Secretaries of State for Health. The Government's Programme for Improving Primary Health Care (Cm 249).

DOH (1989a) *Caring for People*. Secretaries of State for Health. London: HMSO. (Cmnd 849).

DOH (1989b) *Working for Patients* Secretaries of State for Social Services, Wales, Northern Ireland and Scotland. London: HMSO. (Cmd 555).

DOH (1993) *New World, New Opportunities. Nursing in Primary Health Care*. Secretaries of State for Health. London: HMSO.

Department of Health and Social Security (DHSS) (1981) *The Primary Health Care Team Report of a Joint Working Group of the Standing Medical Advisory Committee and the Standing Nursing and Midwifery Advisory Committee* (The Harding Report). London: HMSO.

Firth-Cozens J (1992) Building teams for effective audit. *Quality in Health Care* **1:** 252–255.

Noakes J (1992) Team spirit. *Health Service Journal*.

Poulton B and West M (1993) *Measuring the Effect of Teamworking in Primary Care. Audit for Teams in Primary Care – Proceedings of a Conference (July 1993)*. Eli Lilly. National Clinical Audit Centre, Department of General Practice, University of Leicester.

Primary Care Forum (1991). *A Journey into the Unknown*. A workbook on the formation of Primary Health Care Teams. Morpeth. Northumberland Family Health Services Authority (FHSA).

Pritchard P (1994). Effective teamwork – co-operation, competence and learning. *Primary Care Management* **4** (5).

Pritchard P and Pritchard J (1992) *Developing Teamwork in Primary Health Care. A Practical Workbook*. Oxford: Oxford University Press.

Southampton Primary Care Development Team (1993) *Multidisciplinary Audit by Primary Care Teams Project* (Funded by DOH) Southampton Community Health Services Trust.

Sundstrom E, DeMeuse KP and Futrell D (1990) Work teams, applications and effectiveness. *American Psychology*, February.

West M (1993) *The Reality of Teamwork in Primary Health Care. Audit for Teams in Primary Care*. Proceedings of a Conference, (July 1993). Eli Lilly National Clinical Audit Centre, Department of General Practice, University of Leicester.

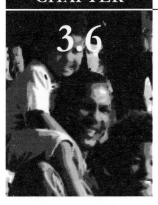

3.6

INFORMATION SYSTEMS AND INFORMATION TECHNOLOGY

Jeff Dauvin

KEY ISSUES

- An overview of information technology
- How information technology may be utilized in the primary health care setting
- Issues which may arise for the practitioner

INTRODUCTION

Information technology, its design, application and implementation, is not value free. It may be useful, liberating, enabling, restrictive or have a large number of other meanings depending on one's value system or level of knowledge. This chapter is a chance to start exploring some of the issues. The term practitioner is used of any professional member of the primary health care team but particularly a nurse, midwife or health visitor.

What are Information Systems?

Information systems are not the hardware and software of information technology. They consist of the total process by which data and information is collected, stored, processed and disseminated. It is not intended to go further than this here as it is a specialized area of study known as *informatics* which has sectors for nursing, health and medicine.

Standardization is used to bridge the gap between technology and its effective utilization. In relation to this the National Health Service Network is planned to be implemented in the near future which at an everyday level will affect patient record keeping of all sorts, such as a Standard Patient Number format. Much information is kept in code form rather than normal language which reduces the risks of ambiguity and enhances efficient analysis and processing. The NHS uses various coding systems depending on the purpose for which the data are collected. The commonly encountered codes are the International Classification of Disease, version 10 (ICD 10), the Read, Version 3, OPCS (e.g. Office of Population Censuses and Surveys, 1990) and Körner codes and are often referred to as data sets. The basic principles behind these systems is that working information is turned into coded data by data input staff. The data can then be used for various purposes by health authorities and the Department of Health for, among other things, epidemiological and population studies, planning, costing and accounting. Some of the results can be seen in publications such as *Social Trends* (HMSO) which is published annually.

The production of coded and analysed data for the Department of Health in the United Kingdom is a requirement of all bodies involved in health care provision. The source of this information is generated at all levels of the service. Traditionally it has been the role of data input and coding staff to convert much of the information on discharge summaries. For example, there are codes for diagnoses, treatments, mode of discharge, lengths of stays and much more. This conversion process is a point at which errors can take place, making the data less useful and potentially unsafe. The practitioner's role is to ensure that accurate and legible information is supplied but may not be perceived as a task which relates directly to quality client/patient care. *Data validation* is the process of sampling and measuring the accuracy. All data used for operational services must be subject to this process so that inappropriate data can be rejected. From this data the Department of Health plans much of the general strategy of health care. At the present time it is also looked at in terms of performance. Epidemiological data is contained within this large body of information. There is now a drive to generate at least some of the data from practice based, functional systems.

The Information Management Group (IMGE) of the National Health Service Executive (NHSE) is responsible for the overall coordination of Information Management and Technology (IM & T) development within the UK health service. In a Strategic Statement accompanying NHSME, CNO Professional Letter (94)3 the basis of consultation with the nursing related professions was laid down.

> SAGNIS (Strategic Advisory Group on Nurse Information Systems) is an Advisory Group of senior professional nurses, midwives and health visitors and information specialists, chaired by Mrs Yvonne Moores, Chief Nursing Officer. Its key objective is: To advise the National Health Service Management Executive on the pace and direction of information Systems and the overall development of information technology to support nursing, midwifery and health visiting.

This is an important development. If the professions do not take on the challenge others who may have different value systems may deliberately or by default take the initiative.

What are the Motives for the Use of Information Technology Systems in Primary Health Care

Motives are tied closely to value systems and value systems to roles. It is worth considering the roles and possible variations in motives.

Practitioners are assumed to be motivated by the best interest of individual patients and clients. Therefore a system may be looked at in one of two ways: firstly as a tool to enhance practice, such as system to produce an assessment or plan of care in such a way as to help the patient/client in some direct way or improve team communication, secondly a system may be seen as easing a necessary but indirect care function to allow more time for direct practice such as semi- or automatic calculation or collection of mileage, workload or dependency. In this way there is a direct justification for use of a system.

A *manager* may be an indirect carer but may have different motives due to their role being towards groups rather than individuals. They need to manage carers of all sorts as a resource and they need to meet performance targets not orientated to individuals but maybe to monetary ones. The manager may not be a carer at all and have quite different reasons for their actions. A career business manager may see health care simply as a profession in itself. This will cause and has caused conflict. An example of this may be seen in the collection of necessary data. The provision of a functional system, as above, may be seen as a luxury when the professional could type it in directly. The manager will want evidence that the system will not only provide the function the practitioner wants but also improve standards, efficiency and output.

The *politician* has an even wider remit than the manager and decisions made at a hierarchical level may eventually revolve solely around financial and electoral considerations. The result being conflict between the profession and the organization that is providing the care.

Commercial interests of software and hardware vendors should not be overlooked. It is important that mechanisms exist to ensure that the health services purchase appropriately. Many practitioners have been involved with very suspect or unusable systems sold as a package rather than being supplied to fulfil a specific function. Implementation of information technology systems should only take place as part of a properly financed project. This involves identification of needs, specification of requirements, costing, tendering and evaluation. The IMG have detailed project information in the form of PRINCE (PRojects IN Controlled Environments) project management program obtainable from the address below. European legislation strictly controls the purchase of systems over a certain price, about £1 million at present.

Resource management implementation has been a prime mover in the purchase of information technology in hospitals. The community services are fast catching up. Resource management is not an information technology solution to a problem. Resource management (RM) is the provision of appropriate, accurate and up-to-date information so that resources can be used most efficiently. Obviously information technology can help provide this so is closely associated with RM. *Case mix* is a natural development of RM schemes. Case mix software facilitates the drawing together of information from different functional systems to facilitate effective decision-making and planning (Box 3.6.1).

Functional Systems

Functional systems serve the user. The practitioner has a role to carry out, such as care planning. For the manager a functional system may rely on data from the practitioner. The risk is that the manager may supply the practitioner with a system which turns them into a data input operator, an expensive addition to their role. Ideally the practitioner's functional system overcomes this by generating the required data in the

Box 3.6.1. Case mix

Functional systems	Case mix	Output
Nursing		
Midwifery		Planning
Stores		Research
Pharmacy		Costing
Appliances	→	Charging
Medical		Audit
Personnel		Coding
Patient administration		Budgeting
Financial		

course of carrying out a useful task. As functional systems are implemented then one function above all others must occur, that is single input of data and uniform updating. In how many places may an address be wrongly recorded on paper records? With networks a single update must result in all records being updated.

Primary Health Care Information Systems

Below is an overview of primary health care information systems where information technology may make a specific contribution. These are functional systems. The systems are looked at in the light of their possible contribution to the application of information technology. Specific software is not referred to as it is changing so rapidly and may have only very local application.

Patient/client dependency measurement is important in setting priorities for care and is for managerial reasons associated with workload and resourcing. A straightforward manual system may consist of using assessment data to generate figures to be acted on. This could also be done with a handheld electronic organizer. The codes are entered against the patient and the result automatically calculated. Such systems are currently in use by community nurses at various locations. Bar codes and readers are often used to ensure good data integrity as a description of the code is given along with it. The bar codes eliminate errors which may occur when typing in codes manually.

A *functional midwifery or nursing system* may hold and retrieve useful clinical information in a way which enhances the information handling by the practitioner. The use of such a system should be an advance over a manual record. If it were now possible to link the dependency and workload to the components of the planned care it is possible to eliminate the need for secondary conversion of information to data and separate entry. Imagine the handheld organizer being plugged into a network at the end of a shift. The days data would be downloaded (transferred to the primary system) for analysis and other purposes by the manager who would then upload (transfer information to the practitioner's secondary system) information for the practitioner's next shift.

Add to this a patient/client biographical data system, diary and e-mail and there would be no need for the calculation of workload, mileage and time sheets. These could all be downloaded and calculated on demand. At the same time as increasing accuracy as the computer will do the working out and printing.

Skill mix analysis could be developed from the systems above.

Developments and Progress

There are, now, only organizational bars to electronic payment of practitioners by transferring the data electronically to the appropriate departments. The foundation of charging is also here.

The mouse and barcode readers already facilitate reduced keyboard input. Developments are occurring in relation to voice recognition. The user would speak into the system which would then convert the sound waves to text. This may produce useful results in the near future.

The *care assessment, planning and recording system* as described above has other implications with regard to the continuing development of multidisciplinary team approaches to care. Collaborative care planning is likely to become a standard mode of practice, rather than the interdisciplinary modes now common, with each professional having a separate but integrated contribution to the patient/client's care. The information technology systems based around networks could facilitate this much more easily than at present when a huge effort may be involved in getting together the team for a case conference. It is already possible to radio network via a cellular telephone. The possibilities of computer conferencing exist. The situation of the patient/client in this case must be carefully considered if a holistic philosophy of care is to be pursued.

Nursing and midwifery audit is a well developed technique (Wheeler, 1993) and the medium of the computer is useful here as it also is in the areas of *clinical research* where data storage and analysis were one of the first functions of computers. The enhancements to *communications* is an area yet to be fully exploited in clinical practice. With appropriate adaption e-mail can reduce the problem of contacting someone on a phone as they travel across over a wide geographical area. Once certain protocols of sending and answering are established and used the time saved can be quite significant.

Access to *databases* of local information such as community profiles and target groups and the like by electronic means can increase accuracy of data (the computer will not just overlook data) and speed the access. How long would it take to identify all women in a practice between the ages of 30 and 45 having two or more children and living in a specific postal area using a manual system? 10 000 records on a microcomputer could be interrogated and produce the information in seconds or minutes.

Prescription systems are well developed. They can increase patient safety by monitoring dose prescription and frequency and producing a completely legible prescription. If an attempt is made to produce a repeat prescription at too short an interval it is possible for it to alert the user. Manual systems often fail with patients obtaining huge quantities of drugs.

Access and Confidentiality

Access is considered to be the ability to get to the information held in a system. In a manual system this could be simply trying to find files or get a key to unlock the cupboard where they are locked. The legibility of the record may be a problem. With an information technology system, access is governed by the ability to use the machinery, even at a basic level of being able to turn on the machine, the ability to use the software to find what is required. Lack of training may be an absolute bar to the successful implementation of an IT system.

Access to information technology systems is governed by security systems usually involving passwords. *Security* is the control of access and is a vital consideration to any system holding personal information and is an issue of law. Security of access and confidentiality are different but closely related issues. Secure information technology systems do not guarantee confidentiality. The access to the system may be perfectly secure but the use of it may flagrantly disregard confidentiality simply by letting someone see the screen contents, leaving printouts laying around or talking about the screen content in a situation where the participants can be overheard. It is often surprising to note that some users seem to abandon normal precautions just because a computer is being used.

Security, access and confidentiality of patient/client information should not be considered primarily as an information technology issue. The importance of the issues is demonstrated by their re-occurrence throughout this chapter. There are many reasons for loss or inappropriate dissemination of information. These range from theft, through blackmail, malice, vandalism to professional ineptitude, misconduct and commercial interest.

All information is vulnerable to misappropriation. Physical removal, reading or copying of *hardcopy* (paper) records has always been a problem. Theft of hardcopy is relatively easy for a person with shoplifting or robbery skills – leaks to the press demonstrate this. However, the amounts of information removed are limited by physical bulk or ability to copy surreptitiously. In general it is easy to detect the removal of hardcopy, the loss is likely to be detected.

The form in which information is held therefore affects its security. Electronic records by their nature may be lost, stolen or disseminated in a number of ways which may be quite undetectable. Loss may occur due to physical damage or theft of hardware. Backup and storage of data onto different media, like tape, at another site is the normal method, as fire rather than theft is the greatest threat to hardware.

Portable systems by their nature are valuable and vulnerable. This may increase the risk of car theft or physical attack that a practitioner may be subject to in the community setting.

Electronic theft is the most serious threat especially on networks. Breach of security systems may give the user no indication of the loss and the dissemination can be enormous. It must be stressed that with the breach of a security system on a wide-area network (WAN) a user from the other side of the world could be perpetrating the theft while the user is using the system.

Security

Security of IT systems must operate at two levels, physical and operational. Physically the hardware needs to be securely located and lockable. Operationally, software security systems are used. This is usually via an identity and password system such as that used with cashcard machines (automatic teller machines – ATM). The user's identity may be widely know for e-mailing but the password is totally confidential to the user. The systems do not show the password as it is typed, it has a minimum length (usually seven characters), cannot be reused and forces the user to change it at frequent intervals.

Now that networks can be operated via cellular as well as domestic telephones the chances of interception increase. The situation involving cellular telephones and the Royal Family demonstrates this well.

Professional and Legal Issues Relating to the Use of Information Technology

Professional conduct

The United Kingdom Central Council for Nursing, Midwifery and Health Visiting (UKCC) *Code of Professional Conduct* (UKCC, 1992) relates to all spheres of practice and personal behaviour (see also Chapter 3.2). The use of information technology does not affect the applicability of the Code. The preface of the Code ends with the words 'As a registered nurse, midwife or health visitor, you are personally accountable for your practice and, in the exercise of your professional accountability must . . .' This is a statement of professional imperative. The use of information technology in practice or elsewhere does not affect the applicability of the Code. Three sections of the Code are discussed as being particularly significant to the use of IT.

Section 3 'maintain and improve your professional knowledge and competence' and *Section 4* 'acknowledge any limitations in your knowledge and competence and decline any duties or responsibilities unless able to perform them in a safe and skilled manner' have similar implications. In the light of the general content of this chapter there is a need to be aware of the effects that information technology is having on the practitioner's role at any time and ensure that they are able to use it effectively or safely. This could be to do with the provision of appropriate and accurate data to the skilful use of equipment. The latter could be the skill of using an electronic thermometer correctly or the ability to teach the parents the safe use of a portable apnoea monitor.

These issues cannot be divorced from the legal implications associated with litigation involving the practitioner and employer.

Section 10 'protect all confidential information concerning patients and clients obtained in the course of professional practice and make disclosures only with consent, where required by the order of a court or where you can justify disclosure in the wider public interest'. In the community situation where appropriate information flow and communications are well developed information technology may very well enhance this. Thoughtful use will prevent inappropriate dissemination. A few examples will demonstrate this – the ability to print and distribute patient/client information easily and the wider distribution via e-mail. The practitioner needs to be aware of the address lists used. At a very simple level the fact that a VDU can be easily read at distance needs to alert the practitioner of the siting of such equipment. Organizers and the like need to be securely stored and their vulnerability in cars is a problem. For example a break-in may cause the loss of a limited number of hardcopy records but the theft of a portable computer may result in the information of a whole caseload being stolen and disseminated very widely and quickly.

Legal Issues

The Data Protection Act 1984

The Act is specifically designed to protect members of the public from the misuse of personal data held on computer and in electronic processing systems, it does not relate to written records. The Act does not mention the use of computers; the reference is to automatically processed data. The Act lays down legal requirements for organizations and individuals who hold 'personal data', a term defined in the Act. The principal requirements are that the owner or manager of a system, rather than a specific computer or program, must register that system at three yearly intervals. In the health care sector the registered data user would be a nominated manager within a health authority, trust, practice or organization. This requires the submission of documentation and payment of a fee. Contravention of the Act may result in a number of enforcement procedures and ultimately criminal prosecution of the registered data user, their agents or anyone else who gains access to the data.

Most practitioners will be acting as agents for a registered data user. All requirements of the Act will probably be seen as reasonable. All match the standards required by the UKCC Code of Professional Conduct as discussed later. At first, though, some components of the Act may not seem relevant. The issues which must be addressed follow.

The Act can generally be summed up in the 'Eight Principles' listed in Box 3.6.2. These are referenced to specific points of practice as necessary. The wording of the principles is that of 'Data Protection Act 1984, The Guidelines' (Data Protection Registrar, 1994).

Box 3.6.2. The eight principles of the *Data Protection Act* (1984)

Principle 1 'The information to be contained in personal data shall be obtained, and personal data shall be processed, fairly and lawfully.' All information sources have to be registered. Therefore when adding information to a computerized system the user must be sure that it is appropriate. An example may be that the only registered information source is from a consented, written patient/client record. To enter a verbal record would contravene the Act. Likewise to enter a different class of information from that registered would be illegal, e.g. enter a marital status if it was not a registered enquiry. Users should be aware of the limits of their system.

Principle 2 'Personal data shall be held only for one or more specified and lawful purposes.'

Principle 3 'Personal data held for any purpose or purposes shall not be used or disclosed in any manner incompatible with that purpose or those purposes.'
Principles 2 and 3 are related. It would not be reasonable to make a socioeconomic status report from a system registered for the specific and only purpose of arranging foot care, even if that data could be practically generated from the system. This would require application for re-registration for the system. In practice a complete system would not be as narrowly defined as this but it is important to bear in mind the limits of registration.

Principle 4 'Personal data held for any purpose or purposes shall be adequate, relevant and not excessive in relation to that purpose or those purposes.'

Principle 5 'Personal data shall be accurate and, where necessary, kept up to date.'
Principles 4 and 5 are related and make it clear that it is not appropriate to keep 'extra' information 'just in case'. This is reasonable as a practitioner should only be collecting the best and most accurate information. The issue is not one only relating to electronic data.

Principle 6 'Personal data held for any purpose or purposes shall not be kept for longer than is necessary for that purpose or those purposes.' This is a case where the person registering the system must take into account all of the possible uses of the system for registration purposes. It is obviously also tied up with legislation regarding medical records.

Box 3.6.2. *(contd.)*

Principle 7 'An individual shall be entitled –
(a) at reasonable intervals and without undue delay or expense –
  (i) to be informed by any data user whether he holds personal data of which that individual is the subject; and
  (ii) to access to any such data held by a data user; and
(b) Where appropriate, to have such data corrected or erased.'
The registered system manager must produce a procedure to fulfil the requirements of the Act. The practitioner's role is to be familiar with this procedure which will usually involve the filling in of an application form and payment of a fee. To simply show the patient/client the information on screen does not fulfil the requirement and may contravene Section 8 unless the registered system allows them to see their personal data on screen.

Principle 8 'Appropriate security measures shall be taken against unauthorized access to, or alteration, disclosure or destruction of, personal data and against accidental loss or destruction of personal data.' This involves security of hardware, output, disks and anything else which gives access to the system. Poor positioning of VDUs and printers is the single easiest way to breach security. Unauthorized access due to loss of a password is the responsibility of the user.

The Misuse of Computers Act 1990

Whereas the Data Protection Act is designed to protect the use and dissemination of personal data, and especially confidentiality and security, the Misuse of Computers Act has much wider remit and makes illegal some of the things that may be done *with* a computer and also *to* a computer system. The first may be demonstrated by a brief editorial report (BJHCC, 1994). A 'nurse' who procured a doctor's identity and password changed a child's prescription to a fatal drugs cocktail which was fortunately intercepted by an effective practitioner. This resulted in a three month prison sentence for the nurse. This case demonstrates well the responsibilities of all concerned. 'Never let anyone find out your password.' This means not writing it down, disclosing it or letting people see the keystrokes involved.

The second part of the Act could be the introduction of a computer virus into a system, physically or software damaging a computer system. A *computer virus* is not to be confused with the real organism. It is a maliciously written program which can destroy software and data. It can be transferred from system to system by disks. Networks are very vulnerable due to their large number of connections, of which the user will be quite unaware. Most systems have protecting software and procedures for users to protect the system. These procedures need to followed exactly if accidental infection of a system is to be avoided.

CONCLUSION

The chapter has taken a broad view of the topic considering the possibilities, the applications and professional and legal view. What is required is an ongoing discussion. The practitioner cannot hide behind ignorance nor avoid the inevitable. They must be informed and have input into the developments of systems. As can be seen from the discussion there are no instant solutions to problems in an existing manual information system by the application of information technology. What appears to happen is that practitioners who are professionally aware and proactive are likely to comprehend the possibilities and problems associated with developments and system implementations. This knowledge and skill will ensure that the systems serve the professional requirements of the practitioner in relation to patient and client care. To this end some discussion topics are given below.

SUMMARY

Two issues recur throughout this chapter:

■ The speed of changes in the development of hardware and software. This should not be surprising to the professions. The health care services and the world around is in a similar state. This is the main reason for the discussions of this topic being in terms of principles – a concrete approach would be out of date in months rather than years.

■ Security, access and confidentiality are issues of importance to both aspects of the discussion, the professional and the technical. This is only right as it is not possible to consider the use of any innovation which does not take them into account.

DISCUSSION QUESTIONS

♦ What are the direct and indirect effects of information technology on practitioner patient/client relationships?

♦ Information technology – help or hindrance? Consider the statement as a practitioner, as a manager and as various members of a multidisciplinary team.

♦ Who controls the use of information technology in the primary health care team? Who should? Who will?

♦ Does IT centralize or share control?

♦ Is IT systems implementation desirable and/or inevitable? How should the practitioner respond?

♦ Refer back to Section 2 Chapters 2,4,5 and 6 and Section 3 Chapters 2,3,4 and 6 and consider the issues there in the light of the use of IT.

♦ Who owns and controls the use of information? Does the form of the data affect ownership? Does the ownership of the system affect the ownership of the information?

♦ Will information technology unify or diversify the primary health care team?

♦ Who bears the cost? Will there be quantifiable financial, or quality of care benefits?

Useful Sources of
Information

- *The British Computer Society, Nursing Specialist Group*. 1 Stanford Street, Swindon, Wiltshire, SN1 1HJ
  An active group promoting the interests of professional nurses in the whole area of information technology in health care.
- *The Office of The Data Protection Registrar*, Springfield House, Water Lane, Wilmslow, Cheshire, SK9 5AX
  A good range of publications explaining the implications of the use of information technology and the Data Protection Act.
- *NHS Executive, Information Management Centre*, Information Management Group, 15 Frederick Road, Edgbaston, Birmingham B15 1JD
  A large number of publications are available covering all areas, technical and professional. Updated regularly. Important source of current thinking of the Department of Health.

FURTHER READING

Journals

British Journal of Health Care Computing

Health Informatics

Computers in Nursing (USA)

The Health Services Journal
  All professional journals have articles relating to the current use and application of information technology.
  Many newspapers have general information technology interest sections which often include 'medical' applications which may have a bearing on the primary health care team.

Useful Database Search Terms

Computer; Computers; Computer-Hardware; Databases; Diagnosis-Computer-Assisted; Hardware; IT; Information; Information-Systems; Information-Technology; Local-Area-Networks; Logistics; Microcomputers; Networks/working; Nursing/Health-Informatics; Nursing-Information-Systems; Software; Systems; Technology; Wide-Area Networks.

REFERENCES

BJHCC (1994) Editorial. *British Journal of Health Care Computing* **11:** 7.

Data Protection Registrar (1994) *Data Protection Act 1984 – The Guidelines, Third Series November 1994*, Office of The Data Protection Registrar, Wilmslow.

Langley D and Shain M (1985) *Macmillan Dictionary of Information Technology*, 2nd ed. London: Macmillan.

NHS Centre for Coding and Classification (1995) *The Read Codes*, Version 3. Leeds: NHS Executive.

Office for Population Censuses and Surveys (1990) *Tabular List of the Classification of Surgical Operations and Procedures*, 4th revision, consolidated version 1990. London: HMSO.

UKCC (1992) *Code of Professional Conduct*, 3rd edn. London: UKCC.

Wheeler D (1993) Auditing Care using the Nursing Quality Measurement Scale, *British Journal of Nursing* **3**(6): 230–232.

WHO (1993) *International Statistical Classification of Disease and Related Health Problems*, vol. 2, *Instruction Manual*, 10th revision. Geneva: World Health Organization.

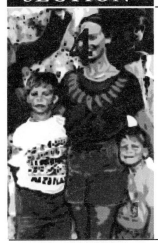

SHIFTING THE BOUNDARIES

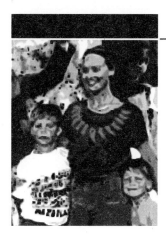

INTRODUCTION

This section explores the boundaries of practice in specific areas of community health care nursing. The linking theme throughout this section is on current practice, policy development and service delivery. The first chapter seeks to explore specific issues in relation to one specialist area of community health care nursing, and opens with a discussion on recent developments in nursing quickly moving into a consideration of 'new nursing' and 'liberation nursing'. This is followed by a discussion on developing clinical expertise. The chapter concludes with a brief exploration of clinical supervision. The theme of clinical expertise is continued in the second chapter which explores the impact of technology and its effect on nursing in the home. Indeed, throughout this chapter the reader is challenged to explore some of the major changes impacting upon society and nursing.

In the third chapter the emphasis moves to practice nursing. The development of practice nursing is reviewed against the background of change within primary health care. Policies and influences affecting the role of practice nurses are discussed together with a consideration of the potential for integrating a range of community nursing resources within primary health care settings.

The next chapter centres around the public health role of the health visitor. The chapter opens with a discussion on the meaning and purpose of 'public health', moving on to explore the developments of the new 'public health', the links between public health, health promotion and primary health care. The principles of health visiting are used as a framework to explain how public health permeates practice.

The fifth chapter discusses some of the issues surrounding the provision of paediatric community nursing services, including, a consideration of the organization and delivery of the service and the influences on current paediatric nursing practice.

The section concludes with an exploration of the factors that have influenced and are influencing the role of the nurse practitioner. Discussion centres around the development and role definition of nurse practitioners, how a nurse becomes a nurse practitioner and concludes with a brief discussion concerning future opportunities and concerns about the concept and role.

These six examples have been used to explore some of the changing frameworks for practice within community nursing settings. Other examples would be just as valid and readers may care to reflect on their own practice and consider what factors are currently shaping and influencing their framework(s) for practice.

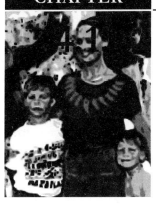

DEVELOPING CLINICAL EXPERTISE IN COMMUNITY NURSING

Kate Billingham and Maggie Boyd

KEY ISSUES

Recent developments in nursing including:

- The 'new nursing'
- Liberation nursing
- Clinical expertise and the community nurse
- Developments in community nursing
- Innovations in practice

INTRODUCTION

The purpose of this chapter is to explore the concept of the clinical expert, what it means for community nurses and the ways that expertise can be uncovered, understood and developed in practice. Drawing on the literature and the lessons we have learned from our own experience of development work in community nursing (Cope Street Project, Billingham, 1989; Strelley Nursing Development Unit and Premier Health Trust's Primary Care Development Unit), we seek to demonstrate the essential link between clinical expertise and the development of community nursing practice. In order to do this we need to look at recent changes that have taken place within nursing and have led to the development and application of the concept of the 'expert practitioner'.

If you were asked to describe what an expert community nurse was, the chances are that you would think of a particular nurse rather than a list of the characteristics that make up an expert nurse. Individuals stand out in our memory as key role models who provided us with inspiration and insight during our own personal journeys towards expertise. Describing the elements that make up an expert practitioner remains elusive and difficult to articulate. Yet without that description the expertise that makes up community nursing remains hidden, learners are left to travel in the dark and the experts are not given the recognition they deserve. Moreover, if we fail to describe 'the expert' how can we recognize the 'in-expert'?

Recent Developments in Nursing

The role of the nurse and how we describe an expert nurse reflects and is shaped by the social, cultural and historical context within which nursing takes place. The changes in nursing theory and practice that have taken place in recent years are inextricably linked to wider societal and ideological changes that have impacted on the health care system, the welfare state as a whole and the ideological thinking behind health care. Nursing is a social process, and whilst not determined solely by social structures, nursing thinking and practice has to be seen within its historically specific social context (Robinson, 1993).

Before engaging with expert practitioner theory from the USA it is helpful to develop an overview of how nursing shapes and is shaped by social forces to gain some critical insights in applying these notions to the UK.

Changes in Health Care

There can be no doubt that the 1990s is a period of enormous change in health care in the UK. There has been a reduction in the length of hospital stay, a dramatic increase in day surgery, boundaries between health and social care and hospital and community care are being redrawn (Marks, 1991), the focus is on health promotion and an internal market has been introduced into health care.

The imperatives behind these changes can be summarized as in Box 4.1.1

All of these impact on nursing and have caused us to reflect on our contribution to health and to account for our presence in the service. During the last decade nurses have responded to these changes and have struggled to have their caring therapeutic role valued and recognized by often sceptical managers and policy-makers (Hart, 1991). This climate has produced a rich theoretical debate about the nature of nursing and resulted in exciting innovations in practice.

The 'New Nursing'

The concept of 'new nursing' (Salvage, 1990; Beardshaw and Robinson, 1990) encompasses the 'unstoppable movement' (Wright, 1992) within nursing where nurses and their patients/clients are partners in care rather than givers and receivers. The nurse and the patient share their expertise and knowledge with the patient

Box 4.1.1. Factors behind changes in health care

- Demographic change – an ageing population
- Economic decline – stimulating the search for cost-effective care
- Changing patterns of disease – increase in chronic conditions and the recognition of the preventability of many diseases
- Social changes – increasing inequalities in health and social divisions in society
- Ideological changes – the patient is no longer seen as a passive recipient of care but as an active consumer with rights and choices. Individual freedom rather than collective responsibility for health has become the guiding philosophy
- Technological developments – home-based care and treatment now a possibility for many conditions and reduced need for hospitalization (Marks, 1991)
- Knowledge – the iatrogenic affects of hospitalization have been recognized and the value of hospitalization for conditions such as myocardial infarction and strokes has been questioned (Marks, 1991).

playing an active role in his/her own health care, with the nurse as an educator. In 'new nursing' the goal is empowerment and practice is patient centred and individualized to meet patient needs. The move from task orientated to patient centred care has placed the nurse/patient relationship at the centre and has challenged the biomedical ties of nursing to medicine (Butterworth, 1992; Williams, 1993). Recognizing and valuing the emotional aspects of caring has meant supplementing a biomedical approach with an holistic one, seeing the patient in their social context, acknowledging the multifactorial influences on health, illness and recovery and working with the family rather than just the individual. (See Chapter 2.4 for a more detailed discussion of family centred nursing.)

The strength of these developments in both the philosophy and process of care is that they are embedded in the practice of nursing. A feature of new nursing is that it has come not from managers, academics or educationalists but from practitioners (Wright, 1992). The development of primary nursing, nursing beds, the growth of nursing development units and the named nurse concept grew from the clinical setting and whilst it is difficult to ascertain what their impact has been on the everyday work of nurses, the principles and models have become a powerful force for change receiving legitimation in official documents (NHSME, 1993a, 1993b).

Liberation Nursing　　More recently Ford and Walsh (1994) have coined the phrase 'liberation nursing'. Incorporating the ideas of the liberation theologist Paulo Friere and feminist thinking into the 'new nursing', Ford and Walsh focus on the oppression of nursing as a gendered profession that has led to ritualistic practice on the one hand and on the other hand a tendency to adopt the latest ideas naively and uncritically. Liberation nursing seeks to challenge hierarchical and authoritarian structure in nursing and as such confronts 1980s management style.

Developments in Community Nursing

Despite sharing a common training with other nurses and a similar core function within the health service, there are salient divergences between community nursing and hospital nursing. First of all, they have different historical origins and the organization, management and education of community nurses has remained separate until recently. It was only in 1974 that district nursing, school nursing, health visiting and community midwifery came into the NHS and the primary health care team is a recent arrival in community nursing. Secondly, whilst all nurses have, until Project 2000, begun their professional lives in a hospital, the movement from hospital to community tends to be one way, with few nurses returning to hospital once they have experienced nursing in a community setting (Armitage, 1991).

However, whilst community nursing has evolved as a specialist branch of nursing it has shared the same influences outlined in the previous section. Similar developments can be seen in the philosophy of care and in changes in the practice and organization of care. The nature of community nursing and its different setting has, moreover, resulted in some aspects of new nursing being taken further than in the hospital context, for example the long established use of patient-held records in district nursing, and more recently in health visiting and school nursing. Similarly needs-based profiling and various projects involving groupwork, partnership and community empowerment demonstrate the changing face of community nursing (Dalziel, 1992; Davies, 1990; Billingham, 1989).

Current changes in the organization of health care suggest that closer integration of community and hospital nursing will take place in the future. Project 2000 training prepares nurses to work in both settings; the role of the acute hospital is coming under critical scrutiny and 'community-like' institutions, i.e. community hospitals, nursing homes, hostels and group homes, are growing in number. It is therefore likely that cross-fertilization of ideas will become more common and that the specific clinical expertise developed in the community will be seen to have application in other areas.

The Clinical Expert

It is against this background that debates on the nature of clinical expertise have taken place. The writings of Benner (1984) and Schon (1983) have provided a particularly rich source of ideas for nursing in the UK. Underpinning the notion of the clinical expert is the idea that nursing should be regarded as more of an art than a science, with the central notion of rational technical expertise being replaced by the concept of 'intuitive artistry' (Schon, 1983). Nursing often means dealing with situations of uncertainty, instability, uniqueness and value conflict which are not covered by technical rationality. In coping with these situations nurses demonstrate an intuitive artistry, a process of decision-making that cannot be readily described or explained. This 'knowing-in-action' where knowledge is revealed through the action itself is seen as the key to professional practice.

This has been described by Benner (1984) in terms of the stages that a nurse passes through on the journey from being a novice to an expert. This long and complex process results in a clinical expert who combines experience with knowledge of the clinical setting to bypass rational, structured decision-making. The nurses' perceptual acuity enables them to displace rules at an unconscious level and to become guided by principles and patterns. Intuition and 'gut feeling' are used in decision-making rather than structured, logical, directed thinking (Snyder, 1993). The nurse intuitively grasps the situation as a whole and can identify, anticipate and predict events before they happen, focusing on the problem and making a decision without attending to rules and procedures. Indeed, according to Benner (1984) such a practitioner is constrained by these regulations. This 'automaticity' (Snyder, 1993) enables practitioners to redirect energy from the clinical task being performed to attend to wider patients need, listening and looking for the unexpected – for what is different about a situation, not what is unchanged. At the same time the expert nurse reflects on the impact of her/his care, considers the options, analyses and evaluates the intervention. This level of understanding and expertise is essential to the development of nursing practice. Moreover, expertness is always to be found in the clinical setting where creativity arises from direct patient care (McGee, 1992).

Taking the work of Benner and descriptions of new nursing and liberation nursing, it is possible to identify the following key elements of clinical expertise, including educational, experiential and personal factors (McMurray, 1992):

- experience of practising in a clinical setting
- knowledge
- reflection on practice
- intuitive decision making
- critical/analytical thinking
- self-understanding and inter-personal skills (Williams, 1993)

Implicit in this description of the 'expert' practitioner is a set of values, viz:

- teamwork – collaboration rather than individualism
- empowerment of both nurses and patients/clients
- partnership/equality with patients/clients
- individualized and patient centred care

Benner's work has been contested on the grounds that the focus on experience and intuition has been at the expense of science (English, 1993; Luker and Kendrick, 1992) and this fits in with a tendency, in the nursing literature on clinical expertise, to describe different approaches in dichotomous terms as in Box 4.1.2

This can lead to 'either–or thinking [which] puts an embargo on both/sometimes-the-one, sometimes-the-other possibilities' (Oakley, 1992: X1). Perhaps then an expert nurse should be able to see these polarities as ends of a continuum, recognize their strengths and move along as appropriate in each situation.

Clinical Expertise and the Community Nurse

There is an implicit assumption in the literature that nursing equals hospital nursing and community nursing is either ignored or taken to be the same as hospital nursing but in a different setting. But can we transpose hospital based models to community nursing? How relevant are theories originating from the USA, where community nursing is notable by its absence? Community nurses often have a healthy scepticism towards some of these developments such as the nursing process, the named nurse, nursing-led care and primary nursing, either because of the practical difficulties associated with their introduction in their field or because community nurses are already working in this way, for example the named nurse and nursing-led care. At the end of the day community nursing remains under-researched and the findings from hospital settings cannot be automatically transferred into the community (Luker and Kendrick, 1992).

It is therefore important that the specialist expertise required for nursing in the community is described, researched and developed. This will entail the setting up of structures that support the development of community nursing and value existing expertise so that it is not lost under increasing medicalization and in the power struggles between health and social services.

Community nursing is different from hospital nursing for a variety of reasons and there is a need to look at these differences as they not only determine the specialist skills of community nurses, but also both hinder and facilitate the development of community nursing practice. Clinical expertise in the community is affected by the factors listed in Box 4.1.3

Lack of Predictability

Nursing in the community means coping with uncertainty and unpredictability. The infinite number of variables that impact on health and illness means that it is more difficult to assess, to predict health needs and to anticipate nursing outcomes

Box 4.1.2 Dichotomous terms

intuition	— rationality
art	— science
practice	— theory
doing	— knowing
technical expertise	— artistry
biological	— social
nursing	— medicine

Box 4.1.3. Factors which affect clinical expertise in the community

- The lack of predictability
- The nurse/client relationship
- Professional autonomy
- Public health approach
- Long-term outcomes
- Resources
- Developments in primary care

(Cowley, 1993). Community nurses are, therefore, often working with varying degrees of risk. Decision-making means assessing the complex interaction of social, environmental and psychological factors on health, therapeutic regimens and the course of illness at individual, family and community levels. Expert community nurses thus need to build up a wide range of scenarios if they are to make effective decisions and separate the abnormal from the normal.

Client/Nurse Relationship

Effective nursing care in the community is dependent on a partnership existing between the nurse, the client and the carer. The nurse spends only a small amount of time directly with the patient, so much of their work will be geared towards enabling self-care. In this context the nurse and client are co-workers. Providing information, promoting self-confidence with empowerment, is at the centre of community nursing practice. The home is the private space of the client where the nurse is a guest so an expert community nurse is one who has skills in communication, listening and negotiation to develop a productive relationship in this special setting.

Professional Autonomy

With professional autonomy comes greater responsibility. The community nurse usually works alone, often unsupervised with their work hidden from view in the private arena of people's homes. There may be little or no medical direction with the nurse being responsible for identifying need, assessing risk, determining treatments and interventions and coordinating the work of others. Expert decision-making and a wide range of knowledge, clinical skills and experience is therefore essential (Orme and Maggs, 1993).

A Public Health Approach

An expert community nurse is continually maintaining an overview, standing back from the individual and family and assessing the public health implications. This means making links between the individual client's health status and social policies, environmental influences and community factors that need addressing. This requires knowledge of public health approaches and the ability to work with local communities on health promoting strategies. A patient-centred approach also means a community-centred approach. (See Chapter 4.4 for a more detailed discussion of public health.)

Long-term Outcomes

Many community nurses have long-term relationships with their clients lasting for a number of years. The impact of their intervention may not be apparent for many years and the unpredictable nature of their work may mean that the outcomes are unexpected. This means that demonstrating their effectiveness to others may be difficult and any changes in the service not noticeable for some time to come. This is as true of innovations in practice as well as any reductions in services. Those undertaking developments in community nursing will need to apply different benchmarks and measures to those working in acute settings. (See Chapter 5.3 for further discussion of benchmarking.)

Resources

Working in people's homes means working with individuals, families and carers, taking account of their resources, tailoring information to individual circumstances and being creative and flexible with the materials available in the home. This is a very different scenario from working in a hospital where equipment and resources are at hand.

Whilst all nurses, wherever they work, share the essential elements of clinical expertise, it is factors such as those just described that mean that skills will be manifested in different ways in the community. Developing clinical expertise means continually learning, reflecting, trying out new ways of doing things and evaluating their outcomes. All of this takes place within a moral framework, with a philosophy of care which underpins both the practice and process of development.

The second half of this chapter describes the mechanisms that encourage and sustain the development of community nursing.

Developing Community Nursing: Encouraging Innovation in Practice

When considering how to encourage the development of community nursing it is worth recognizing how nursing in the community, by its very nature, has particular barriers that will need to be overcome. Many of these can be seen to represent the downside of professional autonomy.

1. Community nursing is largely private and hidden from scrutiny by colleagues and others. This can lead to professional isolation, the perpetuation of outdated practices and difficulties in understanding and describing what practice takes place, although advances in information technology will provide opportunities for sharing patient/client records.
2. Community nursing tends to be isolated from academic centres and educational institutions (Luker and Kendrick, 1991).
3. Reductions in the number of health visitors and district nurses being trained, by 20% and 33% in 1991/92, respectively (ENB, 1992), may result in a lack of new ideas with many nurses using knowledge obtained some years ago.
4. Community nursing, along with community health services in general, has been the poor relation of hospital and acute nursing. As a result community nursing has been under-researched, undervalued and misunderstood.
5. Community nursing is a divided branch of nursing. Practice nurses, health visitors, district nurses and community midwives in particular are divided by separate management structures, training and professional representation. In the past this has led to defensive practices, inter-professional rivalries and distrust (Butterworth, 1988). For community nursing to move forward an integrated team approach is essential and a common training is to be welcomed (UKCC, 1994).
6. Finally, nursing in the community has an important element of indirect patient/client care. Nurses undertake advocacy work, they act as coordinators of care and their public health work involves influencing social policies. Nursing developments are likely to be multidisciplinary and to take place in aspects of work such as liaison, profiling, record keeping, case conferences and community-based activities that may not involve direct patient care.

To facilitate the development of clinical expertise the barriers outlined above need to be removed and structures within organizations fostered to initiate and sustain development work.

Successful development is characterized by:

1. A direct improvement on patient/client care.
2. Initiation by and belonging to practitioners.
3. Arising from a clinical setting.
4. The integration of research and practice.
5. Being sustained well beyond the project phase.
6. Impacting on practice, both locally and nationally.

Achieving all of these is not an easy task. The key mechanisms that encourage sustained development in community nursing are described below.

Team Approach

Community nurses belong to both functional and multidisciplinary teams, with the latter becoming more important as the primary health care team develops as the organizational focus of community health care. Effective community nursing requires both an understanding of the specialist skills that different community nurse disciplines embody combined with multidisciplinary teamwork that offers a wider variety of skills to meet diverse population needs.

Rolls (1991) defined a team as a group of people who focus on a task in which shared goals and objectives are accomplished. An effective team will display a range of characteristics, including commitment to the task, to the team and to resolving conflict. Shared objectives, high levels of trust with communication and negotiating skills are all essential for the team to function well. Teams do not just happen, they need to be developed through team-building, shared projects, (e.g. client-held records, health profiling and wound care); common client groups and activities that help nurses to understand each other's roles. (See Chapter 3.5. for a more detailed discussion of team building.)

Team Philosophy

Establishing a philosophy of care for a team of nurses is a necessary precursor to development work. A common philosophy will underpin the models of care that evolve and will strengthen the team under a set of shared beliefs and values (Ford and Walsh, 1994).

There are two facets to developing a set of shared values as a basis for practice. One is to do with an actual philosophy of care and the other to do with a team philosophy, a set of principles for team conduct, for example involving everyone in decision-making. In Strelley Nursing Development Unit (NDU) the former was encapsulated by a commitment to address health inequalities, recognizing the structural causes of poverty.

Health Profiling

Teams need to work towards a common goal. Shared objectives should be focused on the needs of the population, rather than on the individual interests of the nurses. Assessing the needs of the population through profiling is therefore essential to community nursing development. Practice and community health profiles that involve a team approach are a valuable means for sharing health information and ensuring that community nurses set objectives for their team that are based on need, not custom and practice.

Reflective Practice

The notion of the 'reflective practitioner' has become a popular way of encouraging professionals to systematically question and challenge traditional practice. It is a method of describing, analysing and evaluating exactly what goes on in practice. This deconstructive mode necessitates a standing back and questioning of the 'taken-for-granted'. To develop as clinical experts, practitioners need to reflect on what they do in some detail.

The approach involves problematizing instances of professional performance so they are opened up as learning situations which allow personal growth and professional development (Jarvis, 1992; Darbyshire, 1993; Reid, 1993). Strelley NDU have used this approach to examine and question practice. Several methods have been used by the team to explore aspects of health visiting practice, including:

- tape-recording of HV/client interactions
- reflective diaries
- the presentation and discussion of case studies
- joint visiting

Reflecting on practice can highlight the importance of intuition, assessment, flexible care planning and responding to diverse needs. Strelley NDU has used a whole team approach to reflect on: the professional/client relationship; the management of child protection cases; being open and honest with parents and attendant difficulties; the timing of the primary visit; client perception of health visitor visits; and methods of assessing health needs. In the NDU reflective practice has allowed a shift from task-oriented care to an holistic approach involving all the family and has resulted in changes in patterns of home visiting and shared record writing with parents.

Clinical Supervision

Community nursing can be isolated and stressful and there are few formal mechanisms in place that provide support and supervision. These are well established within midwifery and psychiatric nursing, but are yet to be incorporated into other branches of community nursing apart from child protection monitoring and supervision. Clinical supervision is essential in particular where care is relationship based rather than dependent on technical proficiency (Butterworth, 1992).

Clinical supervision is a recognized way of developing expertise and ensuring improved standards of care. It also supports staff working in demanding and difficult situations and those going through periods of change. Suggested guidelines (Kohner, 1994) for clinical supervision are:

1. All staff should be involved in planning a system of clinical supervision.
2. All supervisors should receive training.
3. All supervisors should also receive supervision.
4. Ground rules should be negotiated and agreed.

5. Boundaries should be well defined and the relationship between supervisor and supervisee should be formally constituted.

Client Participation

If developments in community nursing are to be responsive to client/patient needs then methods of obtaining their views and ideas need to be in place. As mentioned earlier, patients/clients are no longer passive recipients of care and community nurses should promote the development of patient rights and choices in health care. This ideological shift has provided an opportunity for recipients of care to shape service provision. Thus developments in clinical practice are both informed by users and driven by practitioners.

Client/patient participation can take place at both an individual and collective level. An expert practitioner will ensure that clients play an active role in assessing their own health needs, planning their care and evaluating its effectiveness and quality. Commonly used tools for systematically obtaining 'consumer' views are:

- questionnaires
- focus groups
- interviews

Support Structures

In our experience clinical development is more likely to take place if certain non-clinical aspects are also attended to. These create the necessary framework and organizational culture for the promotion of creative thought and practice in community nursing.

Using a 'project framework' ensures that this takes place and that developments are legitimated and protected. A useful project format includes the following headings:

- background to/reasons for proposed changes
- summary of relevant research
- aims and objectives
- time scale
- lead person
- evaluation methods
- review/completion date
- dissemination methods

Academic Links

Dynamic nursing is dependent on rigorous research. There is a continual need to increase knowledge about what has worked and what has not worked in clinical practice. Research acts as a stimulus to good practice, education and management (NHSME, 1993a). Community nurses tend to be remote from academic centres which can lead to 'idiosyncratic practices' that are not informed by the relevant research (Luker and Kendrick, 1991). Community nurses, therefore, need guidance and support if they are to incorporate developments in theory and knowledge into their practice. In order to do this greater integration needs to take place between practitioners and academics. In an environment where confidence is built and knowledge is shared practitioners acquire research skills, knowledge and awareness and educationalists and researchers are kept in touch with practice.

In the difficult area of evaluation expert support is necessary if new methods are to be replicated elsewhere. (See Chapter 3.4 for further discussion of evidence based practice.)

Clinical Leadership

Successful teams have good leaders. The leader acts as a change agent facilitating nursing development and this is seen as crucial to success (Shaw and Bosanquet, 1993). The function of a clinical leader is to enable the team to develop by facilitation, acting as a catalyst, by providing an overview of organizational and nursing agendas, by coordinating the work of the team and by bringing knowledge and clinical expertise. To be effective the clinical leader should be in a non-hierarchical position and capable of 'leading from behind'. Successful clinical leaders do not seek power or glory, rather they enthuse, empower and enable everybody to contribute to the full. Different models of clinical leadership exist with the role being taken by a team member or a designated extra-team person who supports developments across the organization.

Management Support

In order to develop their practice community nursing teams require autonomy. In the community managers tend to be too far removed from the client/patient to make decisions about patient care. Managers who seek to control and direct the work of practitioners can constrain innovation and improvements in patient care. Self-management by community nurses, with professional support and development, will encourage care that is responsive to local needs and decision-making will take place as near to the patient as possible. Managers in this situation take on a facilitative role creating the conditions which nurture clinical expertise, enabling practitioners to try out new ways of working and freeing them from unnecessary policies and procedures and paperwork (Billingham, 1994).

CONCLUSION

In this chapter community nursing, in its broadest sense, has been described as a specialist branch of nursing with skills and expertise that need to be made explicit if practice is to move on and nurses' contribution valued. The current changes in the organization of community health services, namely greater autonomy for the primary health care team and locally run services, provide long overdue opportunities for nursing developments to become both practitioner-led and client-focused.

Practice developments do not need to take place in a development unit, indeed NDUs have been criticized for their elitism (Ford and Walsh, 1994). The mechanisms described here do not depend on formal structures and external support, rather they recognize that knowledge about community nursing can be generated by nurses working in the clinical setting. What is needed are expert, experienced nurses who can think critically, reflect on their practice, explore different ways of working and collaborate with their colleagues. It is for the wider organization to create a suitable environment for these nurses to grow and lead community nursing into the twenty-first century.

SUMMARY

- Nursing is a social process which has to be seen in its historical context.
- These changes have been accompanied by new conceptualizations of practice: new nursing, with its patient centredness, and liberation nursing, with its critique of hierarchical structures.

- Community nurses have been able to put these new ideas into practice to a greater extent than many hospital practitioners.
- Intuitive artistry and knowing-in-action is the basis of clinical expertise.
- Clinical tasks are expedited and a focus on wider patient needs is facilitated and the development of reflexivity encouraged.
- Community nursing based on valuing and practising teamwork, partnership, empowerment and patient-centredness.
- The development of community nursing expertise requires recognition of its distinctive features, viz:

  wide range of scenarios needed because of the lack of predictability;
  development of partnership with clients;
  the responsibilities contingent on professional autonomy;
  public health approach which links the individual to surroundings and work with communities to promote health;
  the long-term nature of much of the work implies different evaluation criteria to work in acute settings.
- barriers to development:

  work is largely hidden in the homes of patients;
  reduction in new entrants – lack of new ideas;
  under-researched and undervalued;
  divisions within the field;
  broad mutlidisciplinary nature of the work involving much indirect patient care.
- Overcoming barriers and sustaining development involves:

  a team approach;
  an agreed philosophy;
  health profiling;
  reflective practice;
  clinical supervision;
  client participation;
  a variety of support structures, viz: project framework, academic links, clinical leadership, supportive management and organization culture.

DISCUSSION QUESTIONS

- Is liberation from management and medicine necessary if nursing practice is to develop in its improvement of patient care through clinical expertise?

- How do beginners become experts?

- What stimulates community nurses to develop their practice?

- How should we support community nurses in developing and sustaining their clinical expertise?

FURTHER READING

Ford P and Walsh M (1994) *New Rituals for Old: Nursing through the Looking Glass*. Oxford: Butterworth and Heinemann.
Stimulates thoughts around why traditional nursing practice becomes embedded as the 'norm' and suggests some ways forward of deconstructing ritualistic practice.

Robinson J (1993) *Problems with Paradigms in a Caring Profession in Nursing*. London: Chapman & Hall.

REFERENCES

Armitage S (1991) *Continuity in Nursing Care*. London: Scutari Press.
Beardshaw B and Robinson R (1990) *New for Old? Prospects for Nursing in the 1990's*. London: King's Fund Institute.
Benner P (1984) *From Novice to Expert*. San Francisco: Addison-Wesley.
Billingham K (1989) Working in partnership with parents. *Health Visitor* **62**: 157-159.
Billingham K (1994) Questions of Leadership. *Health Visitor* **67**: 7, 240.
Butterworth T (1988) Breaking the boundaries. *Nursing Times* **84** (47): 36-39.
Butterworth T (1992) Clinical supervision as an emerging idea in nursing. In T Butterworth and J Faugier (Eds) *Clinical Supervision and Mentorship in Nursing*. London: Chapman & Hall.
Cowley S (1993) Skill mix: value for whom? *Health Visitor* **66**(5): 166-168.
Dalziel Y (1992) Health provision: the community development approach. *Health Visitor* **65**: 228-229.
Darbyshire P (1993) In the hall of mirrors, reflective practice. *Nursing Times* **89**(49).
Davies J (1990) Against the odds. *Nursing Times* **86**(44).
English, I (1993) Intuition as a function of the expert nurse: a critique of Benner's novice to expert model. *Journal of Advanced Nursing* **18**: 387-393.
ENB (English National Board) (1992) *Annual Report*. London: ENB.
Farrington A (1993) Intuition and expert clinical practice in nursing. *British Journal of Nursing* **2**(4): 228-233.
Ford P and Walsh M (1994) *New Rituals for Old: Nursing Through the Looking Class*. Oxford: Butterworth and Heinemann.
Hart E (1991) Ghost in the machine. *Health Service Journal* December, 20-22.
Jarvis P (1992) Reflective practice and nursing. *Nurse Education Today* No 12.
Kohner N (1994) *Clinical Supervision in Practice*. London: King's Fund Centre.
Luker K and Kendrick M (1992) An exploratory study of the sources of influence on the clinical decisions of community nurses. *Journal of Advanced Nursing* **17**: 457-466.
Marks L (1991) *Home and Hospital Care: Redrawing the Boundaries*. London: King's Fund.
McGee P (1992) What is an advanced practitioner? *British Journal of Nursing* **1**(1): 5-6.
McMurray A (1992) Expertise in community nursing. *Journal of Community Health Nursing* **9**(2): 65-75.
NHSME (1993 a) *New World, New Opportunities*. London: DOH.
NHSME (1993 b) *A Vision for the Future*. London: DOH.
Oakley A (1992) *Social Support and Motherhood*. Oxford: Blackwell.
Orme L and Maggs C (1993) Decision making in clinical practice: how do expert nurses, midwives and health visitors make decisions? *Nurse Education Today* **13**: 270-276.
Reid, B. (1993) 'But we're doing it already' Exploring a response to the concept of reflective practice in order to improve its facilitation. *Nurse Education Today* No. 12.
Robinson J (1993) *Problems with Paradigms in a Caring Profession in Nursing: Art and Science*. London: Chapman & Hall.
Rolls L (1991) *Team Development*. London: Health Education Authority.
Salvage J (1990) The theory and practice of the New Nursing. *Nursing Times* **86**: 4, 42-45.
Schon D (1993) *The Reflective Practitioner*. London: Maurice Temple Smith.
Shaw J and Bosanquet N (1993) *A Way to Develop Nurses and Nursing*. London: King's Fund Centre.
Snyder M (1993) Critical thinking: a foundation for consumer-focused care. *The Journal of Continuing Education in Nursing* **24**: 5, 206-210.
Williams J (1993) What is a Profession? Experience Versus Expertise. In A Beattie, M Gott, L Jones and M. Sidell (Eds) *Health and Wellbeing: A Reader*. Basingstoke: Macmillan Open University.
Wright S (1992) Advances in Clinical Practice. *British Journal of Nursing* **1**(4): 192-194.

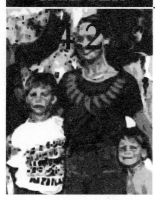

CLINICAL CARE AT HOME

Lesley Coles

KEY ISSUES

■ Technology and its effect on nursing in the home

■ Hidden nursing

■ Clinical leadership

■ Nursing concepts

INTRODUCTION

Let us not go over the old ground, let us rather prepare for what is to come (Marcus Tullius Cicero, 106–43 BC)

The International Council of Nurses (ICN) in joint consultation with the World Health Organization (1989) emphasizes that the demand for nursing care is likely to increase over the next decade due to:

• Ageing populations
• Life extending technological advances
• Demands for sophisticated surgery
• Increased levels of severity of illness in hospital

These measures call for the implementation and evaluation of innovative nursing practice – a need to build upon the best of what has gone before in order to achieve a new, dynamic shape to community nursing practice.

This chapter sets out to explore some of the major changes impacting upon society and nursing today. It is intended to challenge thinking and offer a critical view of where community nursing may see itself in the twenty-first century.

Technology and its Effect on Nursing Care in the Home

The twentieth century has been characterized by a rapid expansion in scientific knowledge and skills resulting in social and technological change unprecedented within our existence. One consequence of these developments has been the emergence of professional specialization and a much greater differentiation within the workforce (Lane, 1985). Yet fundamental to this thinking is the need to explore some of the frameworks within which modern social issues are represented and can be interpreted.

Rationalization and Nursing

The classical sociological theorist Max Weber (1947) (cited in Hewa and Hetherington, 1990) emphasized the shift away from the traditional views of thinking influenced by the dominant teaching of the Catholic Church as being a turning point for Western society. The subsequent demystification of many bodies of knowledge led to the belief that most problems could now be solved by logical application of rational thought, rather than divine intervention. One consequence of this process was the emergence of a paradox, that Weber himself referred to as 'the iron cage', whereby the achievement of goals through rational action may result in the destruction of fundamental social values.

Hewa and Hetherington (1990) utilize this thinking within their examination of the crisis confronting the nursing profession in Western society today. They present the view that 'The crisis in nursing is a reflection of the attack on fundamental values by growing instrumental rational systems of action – that is, the penetration of a mechanistic approach to health and medicine' (Hewa and Hetherington, 1994: 183). In essence, they submit that much of nursing's work has lost meaning and become devalued simply because the profession's desire to legitimize non-technologically orientated work cannot succeed in the scientifically dominated paradigm that exists today. The struggle to preserve basic human values and promote social and humane aspects of life, in a health care system that appears to be increasingly devoid of compassion, leaves nursing effectively trapped between the two competing paradigms.

Specialism within Nursing

The UKCC (1994) has identified community health care nursing as an area of specialized nursing practice, and clearly sees this new discipline as being rooted in practice and a key contributor to the health and care of people and their communities in the future. Yet it is still unclear as to what constitutes a nursing specialism, how it is defined, and more importantly, how it will evolve. If we are to accept the Weberian framework, it is not difficult to see why the development of many nursing specialties has often paralleled progress and developments in medicine. Indeed, Bowman and Thompson (1990) support this view, stressing how the medically dominated model common in the United Kingdom, whereby patients are categorized into convenient disease orientated groups, cannot help but influence the growth of clinical nurse specialists. However, they are adamant that 'the title "nurse specialist" should be reserved for those whose work is without doubt fixed in nursing' (Bowman and Thompson: 48). Yet, despite this commitment and the growing evidence that there has been an ongoing development of nursing knowledge, the rationalization, validity and value of that knowledge is still questioned within the dominant paradigm of science and medicine.

From this perspective, it is perhaps easier to see why nursing appears to be on an endless quest for some form of identity under the guise of progress, using labels such as nurse practitioner, advanced practitioner and nurse consultant. This may be inevitable as nurses seek to establish areas of 'expertise'. More significantly, the powerful influence of the paradigm of science and medicine may be seen to be 'winning' as the number of clinical nurse specialists entering the workforce increases. According to Humphries (1994: 3), clinical nurse specialists in particular are 'at the mercy of the prevailing forces within wider society' and it may prove difficult, if not impossible, to resist the forces of rationalization and medical dominance, especially if they are compounded by the current political climate of centralization and de-professionalization. Of greater concern, or even more worrying, is the idea that if divisions appear within the profession itself, nursing may lose its identity and cohesion at a crucial time.

Expansion of Technology and Expert Systems

Nowhere can this conflict be more evident than in the expansion of technology at the consumer's bedside and in their own homes. Advances in keyhole surgery, the development of specialized support systems such as patient controlled analgesia and the monitoring of conditions by computerized systems promote technology as the main focus and rationally accepted form of intervention. The growing pace of technological advance coupled with the need to operationalize 'skills' in a quality, cost-effective environment, makes it difficult not to foresee nursing hands simply becoming extensions of that technology, in a cold, computerized society of the future.

The development of 'high technological centres offering intensive and specialized care' (DOH, 1993a: 7) threatens to dehumanize and mechanize the delivery of care on an unprecedented scale. The danger of a proliferation of 'expert systems', designed with the utilization of rational knowledge and the saving of time paramount, and without the need to possess the attributes of 'experience' and 'intuition', threatens to erode human values even further, thereby strengthening the bars of Weber's 'iron cage'. As individuals are returned to their homes with or without a mass of micro technology, the challenge for community nurses may be to re-humanize and work alongside their patients in a very different partnership than we currently understand. Community nurses may well be 'a human counter-weight for sick people in an increasingly technical area' (DOH, 1993a: 7), if they are given the opportunity.

Hidden Nursing Issues

The current health care reforms, previously touched upon in this chapter, and discussed in more detail in Chapter 1.1, have produced pressure to demonstrate consumer-orientated, cost-effective care within a competitive market. Yet one of the most difficult questions facing many community nurses today is how to define and quantify what it is they actually do. The exploration of the nature of nursing (Watson, 1988; Benner and Wrubel, 1989) and the drive to quantify nursing workload has frequently appeared to be poles apart. Yet, increasingly there appears to be an emergence of agreement that much of the practice of nursing remains 'unseen' or 'secret'. This has led to the more commonly recognized term, 'hidden nursing'.

Wolf (1989) suggests that much of the activity captured under the umbrella of 'hidden nursing' is obscured due to the fact that it is often ignored, taken for granted, and/or devalued. Categories of hidden nursing have been explored revealing such concepts as: caring; comforting; body work; death work and dirty work. Yet it could be argued that these are primarily focused on direct patient care and use of nursing skills.

According to Benner and Wrubel (1989), the way nurses utilize highly specialized knowledge of science and technology today, in effect ignores many of the intangible elements of caring and clinical judgement inherent within our professional practice; 'hidden' nursing remains hidden, even to the profession. Yet, examination of Benner's (1984) framework of seven domains of work reveals that these elements are apparent in all domains.

Within the context of community nursing, therefore, it is perhaps more appropriate to examine those elements which are deemed to capture professional caring and clinical judgement at an expert level and within the primary health care setting. They include such activities as:

- Administering and monitoring therapeutic interventions and regimes of other health professionals.
- Monitoring and ensuring the quality of health care practices of the entire health care team.
- Organizational and work role competencies related to building, coordinating and maintaining team care.

Bureaucratic Contexts

Taking this viewpoint, recent work by McWilliam and Wong (1994) suggests that there is now a need to focus on nursing's unrecognized professional contribution to care from within just such a context, focusing particularly upon the bureaucratic nature of that arena. In other words, how is the context-related essence of nursing's work shaped and influenced by working alongside other professionals from within an organizational structure?

Using a sample of hospitalized older patients discharged to their own homes with ongoing care needs, findings indicated that, 'Nurses routinely worked with several persistent characteristics of a bureaucratic context' (McWilliam and Wong, 1994: 154) and that this work often went unrecognized. Hidden nursing work generated in this way fell into three headings identified in Box 4.2.1.

Primary Health Care Teams

These findings bear a striking resemblance to many of the issues raised by district nurses working in primary health community care teams, and deserve further development. Hypothesizing on some of this thinking and placing it within the context of primary health care, with its ever constant drive to provide and ensure quality patient care which challenges all health professionals involved, it could be theorized that community nurses are in fact assuming what the authors describe as, 'the hidden work of compensating for such system characteristics on behalf of all involved' (McWilliam and Wong: 154). In effect, they may be acting in the capacity of what Thomas (1983) refers to as 'the glue' which keeps the system together.

This could be interpreted in the community setting as district nurses and other community nurses applying their scientific, intuitive and tacit knowledge to the irrational events of life in an attempt to keep the service running, whilst at the same time appearing to ignore any approaches to rationalize what it is they are actually doing.

Box 4.2.1. Hidden nursing work in bureaucratic contexts

Working with the characteristics of bureaucracy

- Facilitating centralized control
- Mending fragmented work
- Overcoming anonymity

Compensating for the characteristics of bureaucracy

- Coordinating the work of others involved
- Troubleshooting
- Acting as the physician's handmaiden

Providing leadership within the bureaucratic context

- Educating colleagues and caregivers
- Serving as a primary source of information
- Acting as a patient's advocate

In an attempt to unravel some of this thinking further, it is important to acknowledge that one of the most striking features present is that many nurses generally fail to recognize the importance of the work created by the *context* within which they are working. Consequently, this leads to such work being further undervalued, 'hidden' or 'kept secret' by the profession itself and, ultimately, from other health care professionals. This could lead to the commonly held belief that much of nursing's activity is indefinable and therefore simply defies ready solutions.

The 'Handmaiden Role'

The challenge of recognizing some of this thinking is that by contextualizing nursing activities it may now be possible to view professional and ideological conflicts from an entirely different perspective. Take, for example, the 'handmaiden' role of the nurse. Here again it is possible to engage in the work of McWilliam and Wong (1994) and speculate as to the implications for community nurses. The suggestion is that this aspect of nursing often occurs naturally as a result of the humane and fundamental work of nurses, and is therefore a necessary and complementary role to medicine. However, this important relationship is often revealed within a context dependent situation such as primary health care teams, as an area of overt professional conflict. The challenge is frequently depicted as a nursing versus medicine issue, which often results in confrontations over power issues relating to gender, management and profession. These involve hardened attitudes and clashes of philosophies which have become embedded within our historical and cultural backgrounds. It is easy to see how they can detract from the real issue: that of collaborative patient care.

The tendency in many of these scenarios is that in the struggle to determine boundaries, nursing becomes enmeshed in its own inward thinking and falls into the trap of trying to define health care and the processes and outcomes of the professional role through the lens of its own discipline (Hegyvary, 1992, cited in McWilliam and Wong, 1994). By adopting this strategy, it could be argued that nurses are ignoring the very reality of the environment that they inhabit; that of patient care being set within a multi-professional context by which success and failure may only be measurable by multidisciplinary effort.

'Hidden nursing' has some exciting challenges to community nurses, not least of which is the opportunity to explore some of the concepts identified by Wolf (1989). Indeed, the concept of care is revisited later in this chapter. However, more important is the need for community nurses to recognize and acknowledge how working within primary health care teams can help shape and determine nursing's contribution to the broader context of health care. By focusing upon and documenting community nursing's contribution to the processes of multidisciplinary care in this way, new approaches to working may evolve. Expression of this work may in turn make community nursing more 'visible' and 'valued'. Consequently the impact upon care outcomes may be more easily recognized, thereby enhancing nursing's position in the purchasing and providing arenas of tomorrow.

Clinical Leadership

There has been much discussion on clinical leadership within the context of health care reforms (DOH, 1993b) and the profession (UKCC, 1994), yet like many other issues relating to professional practice, it is important not only to define leadership, but to contextualize it within the scope of health care provision now and in the future.

Previous views of leadership have described it as involving 'interaction between members of a group that initiates and maintains improved expectations and the competence of the group to solve problems or attain goals' (Bass, 1981: 584). More recently Naisbett and Aburdene (1990) describe leadership as a democratic process that respects individuals, encourages self-management and moves people in some direction. For community nursing this definition may offer appeal, particularly in terms of 'innovative clinical activity which can be evaluated and shared with colleagues' (DOH, 1993b: 13). Yet for many community nurses this may be an impossible goal, due in part to the confusion between leadership and management, and the interaction of these two elements within a cost-effective, consumer led health care market.

Leadership versus Management

In order to try and clarify some of these issues Bennis (1989: 19) offers a simple yet challenging (poignant) viewpoint: 'Leaders are people who do the right thing; managers are people who do things right'. This perhaps highlights the dichotomy being experienced by many at this time: that of management being seen in terms of cold inhuman engineering of society by technological advance and cost saving exercises, whilst nursing is endeavouring to explore some of the fundamental expressions of human life and compassion through intuition and artistry (Benner, 1984; Watson, 1988).

Ideologies and Assumptions

It is worth exploring at this point the growing importance of the prevailing socio-political ideology that promotes the belief that consumers of health care are in a position to exercise choice and express judgements concerning those choices (DOH, 1990). Historically, an accepted assumption has been that disease and illness could only be managed effectively by expert health professionals in a traditional paternalistic approach. The ideological shift away from this thinking has been progressive and reinforced from many directions, making it difficult to disengage and assess where individuals and the profession really stand. Nursing literature has widely promoted the importance of nurse–patient relationships in its attempts to define what it is nurses do. Indeed, it has been expressed by Salvage (1990) as a key aspect in what has been termed 'new nursing'. Equally, in terms of leadership emphasis has been placed on the transformational role of nurses, highlighting the qualities of empowerment and partnership. But what do these terms really mean? And, what are the implications for the future?

Empowerment and Autonomy

Empowerment has been defined as 'to authorise or enable' (Oxford English Dictionary). Many nurses when asked for a definition see it as a process by which people are able to both experience and exercise autonomy or control over their lives. The language of nursing has become littered with such commonplace terms as 'self care' and 'partnership' and we talk glibly of empowering individuals who are faced with a negative health experience. Yet Ashworth et al. (1992) argue that there is a fundamental need for clarification of the nature of this participation. Overall, the literature reveals concerns ranging from the use of empowerment as an opportunity for professionals and technocrats to improve their power base (O'Neill, 1989), to the use of fashionable rhetoric by professionals as a guise to modify individual behaviour (Grace, 1991). There is also the assumption, hidden amongst these complex issues, that increased autonomy for the nurse will result in more empowerment for the patient (Wuerst and Stern, 1991) – a challenging question and point to ponder.

Partnership and Participation

According to Griffiths (1988) the essence of community care is the placing of responsibility as near to the individual and his carer as possible. However, it is well recognized (Graham, 1992) that the United Kingdom policy aimed at developing 'care in the community' actually means 'care by the community'. This has had, and will continue to have, a tremendous impact on the informal carer population, and the responsibilities they are expected to carry (Wright, 1986; Henderson, 1986).

Bowers (1987) describes community nursing as occupying the 'pivotal' position in supporting and working in partnership with these individuals, yet argues that nurses do not appear to adopt an active enough role. Twigg (1992) acknowledges that although community nursing services recognize the importance of carer support as an appropriate aim, their focus of involvement is threatened by the pressures of technical medical tasks and crisis intervention. More positively Carlisle (1994) describes actions such as spending time talking to patients and involving them in decision-making as interactions which convey respect and enhance the partnership in care notion. Ive (1990) stresses the importance of empathy within the relationship, which again may enhance nurses' ability to assess and direct care on a more equal footing. Yet Nolan and Grant (1989) clearly identify a failure on the part of community nurses to provide relevant information and advice to carers which, they suggest, is vital in promoting a sense of control and consequently a degree of informed choice. Despite this, the idea of community nurses fostering the notions of partnership with resultant client empowerment remains a dominant feature throughout this debate and deserves further exploration.

Nursing Ideology

One underlying assumption stems from the very nature of nursing itself, and some of the issues explored earlier in this section. It could be argued that the 'new nursing' ideology of holism and active patient participation actually assumes that negotiation and patient choice are central tenets to the provision of high quality nursing care. Within this context, it is equally possible to assume that from the patients' perspective, they actually want to take an active role, and it is this assumption that has been promoted by some under the guise of consumerism within the current political climate.

Exploration of the literature in an attempt to try and unravel some of these issues is difficult as the evidence is scant and vague. Biley (1992) comments that evidence appears inconclusive on patients' opinions regarding involvement in decision-making, yet work by Brearley (1990) suggests that patient participation may in fact be beneficial. Similarly in a study exploring the concept of collaboration in care in an acute setting, suggests that 'some patients may not wish to become involved' (Waterworth and Luker, 1990: 975). However, a significant factor here may be the setting or context within which the study was conducted. The authors clearly identified the socializing role of hospitalization as having a possible influence, highlighting the complexities of such notions as conformity, compliance and passive acceptance through fear of repercussion. More significant, however, is the suggestion that 'promotion of individualized care is not necessarily synonymous with active patient involvement, as advocated in the literature' (Waterworth and Luker: 975).

Autonomy and Accountability

It would appear from the evidence that the extent to which people wish to negotiate and share in the decision-making processes of their care is a matter partly determined by personal choice and partly determined by the 'environment' they inhabit. This is particularly important for district nurses, in that the expression and interpretation of concepts such as compliance and conformity is often very different in a community setting.

However, from the nursing perspective one overriding feature is that of empowerment and autonomy of the practitioner themselves (Chavasse, 1992; Wuerst and Stern, 1991; Trnobranski, 1994). The attributes of autonomy and accountability are sanctioned within the Nurse's Code of Conduct (UKCC, 1992), yet it is debatable to what extent they are realized in practice. Gibson (1991) argues that empowerment refers to inequalities of power between individuals and between strata in society, and from this stand nurses should press for changes in the delivery of health care.

Political Perspective

There is a need to explore the political dimension of empowerment and autonomy and acknowledge the tensions that exist within the post 1990 National Health Service, as government policy continues to exercise a strong command and control culture within an environment of increasing fragmentation. It is argued that this is a deliberate policy strategy aimed at weakening the power bases of professionals within the current health care setting. Higgins (1994), centralizing her argument around this clash of cultures, speculates upon the future outcomes for the health reforms, arguing that ultimately command and control will increase, measures will be taken to reduce fragmentation, and planning will be strengthened. Projecting this into the late 1990s, the increase in centralization and political control will in effect further destabilize professional power bases, thereby making the notion of an autonomous practitioner an unrealistic expectation.

In the light of this thinking, community nurses need to consider adopting 'a more critical stance to the notion of "empowerment" ' (Skelton, 1994: 415) and not simply assume that there is an automatic causal relationship between increased professional autonomy and improved patient empowerment. This may involve a much greater understanding of the way alliances are forged and the action taken by nurses as they explore new ways of working effectively with patients and families. As Wertheimer (1993) suggests, participation is not just about services, how they are offered and how they are used, it concerns people's lives.

Nursing Concepts

Throughout this chapter nursing has often been depicted as a profession wrestling with the competing forces of politics and medicine, humanity and technology, whilst at the same time struggling to answer the question 'Is nursing an art or a science?' The relationship between nursing and science has occupied much time and energy, and although nursing theorists have questioned the scientific approach to nursing research, few have acknowledged the primacy of nurturing and caring in nursing.

The Phenomenon of Caring

The phenomenon of caring has been explored, notably by Leininger (1981) and Dunlop (1986), but to date, Benner and Wrubel (1989) may have conducted the most extensive study of this area. Yet it has been argued by Phillips (1993) that the concept of caring has simply become fashionable and the focus for the 1990s. Within the emotional and gender related connotations of the word 'caring', she explores the notion that its seemingly high profile in nursing literature is possibly a reaction against the increased use of technology in nursing. In this context, she warns of the dangers of recreating the view that caring is 'basic' or 'low-tech' work, is of low value and often seen as the role of women.

James (1992) examines this thinking further and calls for conceptual clarity when analysing nursing care and social care, arguing that the terms 'care' and 'caring' are so over used that they are in danger of becoming meaningless. Whilst the debate over nursing care and social care seems set to remain, James (1992) reminds us of the need to examine the rhetoric and the practice of 'care', and her work alerts nursing to the pervasiveness of 'care' in our lives as one aspect of a much broader social process. Her message is clear, 'If we intend to make "caring" central to our professional identities, to make it part of our contribution to health outcomes, then we need to examine our motives for doing so and the intended and unintended consequences of our claims' (James, 1992: 97).

Linked closely to the concept of caring is that of support. Although research in this area appears sparse, work by Davies and O'Berle (1990), based upon the experiences of expert nurses in the field of palliative care, has begun to reveal some of the complexities of this important function of nurses.

Palliative care is an emerging, and interesting nursing specialty in that the context of its work has firm historic roots within religious orders, and the rise of Christianity where caring for the body has been seen as a devalued, lower-order skill. Yet, it could be argued that palliative care has seen a substantial rise in its acceptability, by channelling its energy into this very area of so-called 'soft nursing'. By challenging the twentieth century taboo of death, they have also challenged the intensive use of technology, which dehumanizes and attempts to remove death from the normal order of life events. Palliative care nursing may have revealed another dimension of nursing previously untapped.

Supportive Dimensions of Care

During refinement of their work, O'Berle and Davies captured the imagination of other nursing groups, with the result that in 1992, whilst examining the application of their model in different contexts of clinical practice, they revealed even more tantalizing questions. Was the model one of 'support', 'caring' or 'nursing'? Equally, are 'support' and 'caring' synonymous or two different constructs? More important, however, was the authors' view that further research of the supportive care model is vital, as it appears to have 'practical utility as a tool for articulating the complexities of nursing care' and there is a need to 'determine whether it can be applied to all areas of nursing and whether support can be differentiated from caring' (O'Berle and Davis, 1992: 766).

The Supportive Care Model

This last section of the chapter sets out the basic components of the 'Supportive Care Model' (Box 4.2.2) as a framework for community nurses to examine and explore.

Box 4.2.2. The Supportive Care Model

The model comprises six interwoven dimensions:

- Valuing
- Connecting
- Empowering
- Doing for
- Finding meaning
- Preserving integrity

Valuing and Preserving Integrity

Within the model, valuing is considered a contextual dimension, i.e. the context within which all the nursing activities take place, and may include the base or foundation of nursing activities. It involves the nurse's belief in the inherent worth of individuals as recipients of care together with their strengths and capabilities.

The core concept of the model is preserving integrity, which involves nurses, valuing their own worth and questioning their behaviours and reactions. At the same time preserving integrity is patient-centred and acknowledges the wholeness of the patient.

Together, *valuing* and *preserving integrity* provide the context and the focus for nursing.

Connecting, Empowering, Doing For and Finding Meaning

These are considered to be the action components of nursing care. *Connecting* highlights the building of relationships: making the connection, sustaining the connection and breaking the connection. Breaking the connection is a little researched area of care, especially from the community nurse's perspective, yet demands energy and strength from nurses and patients if it is to be successful.

Empowering, within this model is seen as strength giving or energizing, rather than tangible or task-orientated. It can include such terms as 'facilitating', 'giving approval', and 'defusing' (allowing family members to vent anger/negative feelings). It is therefore much more in line with the definition of empowerment forwarded by Wertheimer (1993) earlier in this chapter.

Doing for is focused upon the physical care of the patient, but also includes the aspects of taking charge (e.g. controlling symptoms), and team-playing (e.g. negotiating the system on behalf of patients and families). Essentially, *doing for* is concerned with using resources extrinsic to the patient, whilst *empowering* seeks to activate their own intrinsic resources.

Finding meaning involves helping patients and families make sense of the situation they find themselves in. This may involve individuals and families developing insight and perspective on the illness they are experiencing, and how it is affecting their lives. It may include acknowledgement of impending death or a long and painful illness, and the use of reflection to help individuals reach an understanding of how best to deal with the presenting situation.

The components of supportive care are seen as overlapping circles, indicating that all aspects are interwoven and difficult to separate; indeed, in practice it may be difficult to tease out individual characteristics. For example, *doing for* can be an *empowering* action in itself. However, too much *doing for* can rapidly become *disempowering* if the nurse is unable to acknowledge the patient's ability and will to 'do' for themselves. This highlights the importance of the contextual component of valuing and the core concept of preserving integrity.

Recent refinement of the model has highlighted an interesting interpretation of the current societal, political and technological pressures influencing nursing. The authors argue that many of the technological interventions that have become so much a part of nurses' work are essentially related to the *doing for* domain. However, by concentrating on this element of nursing, it is suggested that *doing for* is being removed from the integrity of the whole and will therefore lead to less time being allocated to the other dimensions. The consequences of this are staggering. If *doing for* moves outside the nurses' value system, the first compromise is that of the relationship between patient and family. This may in turn damage the patient's own personal integrity. Similarly, removal of any of the so-called action components could ultimately jeopardize the integrity of the nurse *and* the patient, with the result that care itself now falls outside the valuing context.

CONCLUSION

When nurses appear trapped within a health care system which rewards technical competence over human care, is it not surprising that they appear frustrated, emotionally exhausted and in search of an independent, measurable identity? The only constant at this time of uncertainty is the future itself. No matter what it may hold, it is there, waiting for us all. How we deal with it will be one of our greatest challenges. Perhaps part of that challenge is the strength not to look back at what was before, but to expand and look forward to the contribution of other health professionals in helping to define the nature of nursing in the very different world of the twenty-first century.

SUMMARY

■ This chapter examines the expansion of technology within community nursing, its relationship to rationalization and the development of specialist nursing. This section seeks to raise the issue of the human/technological interface within community nursing.

■ Hidden nursing engages the reader with the challenge of identifying and making visible areas of nursing care which may influence the broader context of health care in the future. It offers the work of McWilliam and Wong (1994) as a framework for seeking to make the community nursing contribution to care more visible.

■ The chapter explores clinical leadership within the context of shifting ideologies and professionalism. It examines issues such as autonomy, accountability and empowerment and challenges the reader to examine current assumptions surrounding these frequently used terms.

■ The final section of the chapter returns to the original challenge of technological advances versus the art of nursing in a political arena where rationalization dominates. The supportive care model (O'Berle and Davies, 1992) offers a framework to explore not only the phenomenon of caring, but a way of understanding some of the issues confronting community nurses in the future.

DISCUSSION QUESTIONS

♦ How can community nurses enable people to become more empowered in their own lives?

♦ How realistic is the notion of professional autonomy and how can it be recognized in practice?

♦ How do community nurses define the terms 'support', 'caring' and 'nursing care'?

♦ If you implemented the Supportive Care Model in your clinical practice, how would you evaluate its effectiveness and measure nursing outcomes?

FURTHER READING

Leadership and empowerment

Humphries D (Ed) (1994) *The Clinical Nurse Specialist: Issues in Practice*. Macmillan Press.
Examines the development and future of Clinical Nurse Specialists.

Leddy S and Pepper J (1993) *Conceptual Bases of Professional Nursing*, 3rd edition. Chapter 16: Leadership. Lippincott.
Concepts, current perspectives on leadership and the nurse as leader.

Skelton R (1994) Nursing and Empowerment: concepts and Strategies. *Journal of Advanced Nursing* **19:** 415–423.
Examines nursing's position and understanding of empowerment.

Home Care and Technology

Milio N (1991) Telematics in the Future of Health Care Delivery: Implications for Nursing, Section 1 – Health Care: Issues and Trends, Chapter 7, in *Readings in Community Health Nursing*, 4th edn. Lippincott.
Presents an overview of technology, with a number of possible future scenarios to speculate upon.

Moons M, Kerkstra A and Biewenga T (1994) Specialized home care for patients with AIDS: an experiment in Rotterdam, The Netherlands, *Journal of Advanced Nursing* **19:** 1132–1140.
Explores the move of 'high-tech' care into the home situation.

REFERENCES

Ashworth PD, Longmate MA and Morrison P (1992) Patient participation: its meaning and significance in the context of caring. *Journal of Advanced Nursing* **17:** 1430–1439.

Bass BM (1981) *Stogdills Handbook of Leadership*. New York: The Free Press.

Benner P (1984) *From Novice to Expert: Excellence and Power in Clinical Nursing Practice*. Reading, Massachusetts: Addison-Wesley.

Benner P and Wrubel J (1989) *The Primacy of Caring: Stress and Coping in Health and Illness*. Reading, Massachusetts: Addison-Wesley.

Bennis W (1989) *Why Leaders Can't Lead; the Unconscious conspiracy Continues*. San Francisco: Jossey-Bass.

Biley FC (1992) Some determinants that affect patient participation in decision making about nursing care. *Journal of Advanced Nursing* **17:** 414–421.

Bowers B (1987) Intergenerational caregiving: Adult care-givers and their aging parents. *Advances in Nursing Science* **9**(2): 20–31.

Bowman G and Thompson P (1990) When is a specialist not a specialist? *Nursing Times* **86**(8): 48.

Brearley S (1990) *Patient Participation: The Literature*. London: Scutari Press.

Carlisle C (1994) Caring for carers: the district nurse's role. *District Nurse Direct* 1,3 Winter.

Chavasse JM (1992) New dimensions of empowerment in nursing – and challenges (guest editorial). *Journal of Advanced Nursing* **17**(1): 1–2.

Davies B and O'Berle K (1990) Dimensions of the supportive role of the nurse in palliative care. *Oncology Nurses Forum* **17**(1): 87–94.

DOH (1990) *Working with Patients*. London: HMSO.

DOH (1993a) *The Challenges for Nursing and Midwifery in the 21st Century*. DOH.

DOH (1993b) *A Vision for the Future; The Nursing, Midwifery and Health Visiting Contribution to Health and Health Care*. NHSME, DOH.

Dunlop MJ (1986) Is a science of caring possible? *Journal of Advanced Nursing* **11:** 661–670.

Gibson CH (1991) A concept analysis of empowerment. *Journal of Advanced Nursing* **16**(3): 354–361.

Grace VM (1991) The marketing of empowerment and the construction of the health consumer: a critique of health promotion. *International Journal of Health Services* **21**(2): 329–343.

Graham H (1992) *Women, Health and the Family*. Harvester Press.

Griffiths R (1988) *Community Care – Agenda for Action. A Report to the Secretary of State for the Social Services*. London: HMSO.

Hegyvary ST (1992) Outcomes research: integrating nursing practice into the world view. In McWilliam CL and Wong CA (1994) Keeping it secret: the costs and benefits of nursing's hidden work in discharging patients. *Journal of Advanced Nursing* **19:** 152–163.

Henderson J (1986) By the Community – an ideological response to the crisis in the Welfare State. In C Phillipson, M Bernard and R Strang (Eds) *Dependancy and Interdependancy in Old Age – Theoretical Perspectives and Policy Alternatives*. London: Croom Helm.

Hewa S and Hetherington RW (1990) Specialists without spirit: crisis in the nursing profession. *Journal of Medical Ethics* **16:** 179–184.

Higgins J (1994) *The Fragmenting NHS*. Public Lecture, Southampton University, 11th October 1994.

Humphries D (1994) *The Clinical Nurse Specialist: Issues in Practice*. London: Macmillan Press.

Ive V (1990) Informal carers. *Journal of District Nursing* **8**(11): 16–20.

James N (1992) Care, work and carework: A synthesis? In J Robinson, A Gray and R Elkan (Eds) *Policy Issues in Nursing*. Buckingham: Open University Press.

Lane B (1985) Specialization in nursing: some Canadian issues. *Canadian Nurse*, June 24–25.

Leininger M (1981) *Caring: An Essential Human Need* Proceedings of the Three National Caring Conferences. In BL Cameron (1993) The nature of comfort to hospitalized medical surgical patients. *Journal of Advanced Nursing* **18**: 424–436.

McWilliam CL and Wong CA (1994) Keeping it secret: the costs and benefits of nursing's hidden work in discharging patients. *Journal of Advanced Nursing* **19**: 152–163.

Naisbett J and Aburdene P (1990) *Megatrends 2000: Ten new directions for the 1990s*. William Morrow: New York.

Nolan MR and Grant G (1989) Addressing the needs of informal carers: a neglected area of nursing practice. *Journal of Advanced Nursing* **14**: 950–961.

O'Berle K and Davies B (1992) Support and caring: exploring the concepts. *Oncology Nurses Forum* **19**(5): 763–767.

O'Neil M (1989) The political dimension of health promotion work. In C Martin and DV McQueen (Eds) *Readings for a New Public Health*. Edinburgh: Edinburgh University Press.

Phillips P (1993) A deconstruction of caring. *Journal Of Advanced Nursing* **18**: 1554–1558.

Salvage J (1990) The theory and practice of 'New Nursing'. *Occasional Paper Nursing Times* **86**(4): 42–45.

Skelton R (1994) Nursing and empowerment: concepts and strategies. *Journal of Advanced Nursing* **19**: 415–423.

Thomas L (1983) *The Youngest Science* in McWilliam CL and Wong CA (1994) Keeping it secret: the costs and benefits of nursing's hidden work in discharging patients. *Journal of Advanced Nursing* **19**: 152–163.

Trnobranski PH (1994) Nurse patient negotiation. *Journal of Advanced Nursing* **19**: 733–737.

Twigg J (1992) Carers in the service system. *Carers: Research and Practice*. London: HMSO.

UKCC (1992) *Code of Conduct*, UKCC.

UKCC (1994) *The Future of Professional Practice – the Council's standards for Education and Practice following Registration*, UKCC.

Waterworth S and Luker K (1990) Reluctant collaborators: do patients want to be involved in decisions concerning care? *Journal of Advanced Nursing* **15**(8): 971–976.

Watson J (1988) *Nursing Science and Human Care: A Theory of Nursing*. New York: NLN.

Wertheimer A (1993) *User participation in community care: the challenge for services*. In (ed.) V Williamson, *Users First: The Real Challenge for Community Care*, University of Brighton, East Sussex, pp. 9–17.

Wolf ZR (1989) Uncovering the hidden work of nursing. *Nursing and Health Care* **10**: 462–467.

World Health Organization/International Council of Nurses (1989) *Perspectives for the Future*. Geneva: WHO/ICN.

Wright FD (1986) *Left Alone to Care*. London: Gower.

Wuerst J and Stern P (1991) Empowerment in primary health care: the challenge for nurses. *Qualitative Health Research* **1**(1): 80–99.

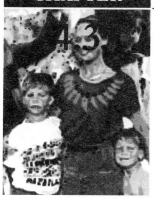

SHIFTING THE BOUNDARIES IN PRACTICE NURSING

June Smail

KEY ISSUES

- Professional identity – the developing role in practice nursing
- Policy shifts – the general practitioner contract, the implications of banding, fundholding and clinical audit
- Change and opportunities

INTRODUCTION

This chapter reviews the sources of influence over the development of practice nursing in the UK, particularly with regard to education and to government policies affecting the role and function of general practice. Consideration is given to the potential for integration of nursing resources within primary care settings and to the role of audit in the overall improvement of clinical practice.

Developing Role and Professional Identity

Practice nursing is a fundamental part of community nursing, its purpose primarily being the provision of care in general practice settings. The role itself is undergoing a period of great change and development, in common with other areas of community nursing, and in response to changing patterns of health, to the special needs of vulnerable groups and health policy developments.

The existence of practice nurses was acknowledged officially by the Department of Health, in a staff training memorandum (DHSS, 1975) although Bowling and Stilwell (1988) noted that there were nurses working in general practice as early as 1910. Practice nursing as a distinctive element of community nursing became established following the implementation of the General Practitioner Charter (1966), which radically altered the way in which general practitioners (GPs) were paid, providing incentives for having improved premises and more staff. Among these changes in GPs' terms of service, GPs were allowed a 70% reimbursement to employ a nurse to work in the practice.

The increase in the numbers of practice nurses was relatively slow for the first ten years – in 1977 there were about 1500 (Stilwell, 1991). The numbers increased rapidly and more than trebled between 1984 and 1990 from 3891 to 13 280 (Department of Health, 1990b). The most recent and reliable research carried out on the numbers of practice nurses in post was undertaken by the Social Policy Research unit (Atkin and Lunt, 1993). This census of practice nurses currently employed in England and Wales suggests that there are 15 183 in post, representing 9500 whole time equivalents.

Practice nurses represent about 20% of all nurses working in primary health care (Atkin and Lunt, 1993) and their importance is acknowledged in recent policy documents such as the National Health Service Management Executive's (1993) report, *New World, New Opportunities* and the Audit Commission's (1993) report on the role of family health service authorities (FHSAs).

The role of the practice nurse has developed in a rather haphazard way as it has adapted to the changes in general practice and primary health care. The literature and anecdotal evidence suggests that the three main issues central to the concern of practice nurses in developing their role and professional identity have been:

- Lack of appropriate training with professional and academic accreditation.
- Lack of commitment and support from some district health authorities and professional nursing bodies.
- Lack of support and encouragement from some employing GPs.

Practice nurses have often felt isolated in the past, and this was particularly the case when they were not included in a comprehensive study in England of community nursing, its role and practice within the primary health care team (Cumberlege, 1986). However, it is acknowledged that the terms of reference drawn up for the 'Cumberlege' working group did not include practice nursing in its remit.

The Edwards Report in Wales (1987) did recognize the potential of the practice nurse and stated:

> The role of the practice nurse working in the health centre or surgery is a developing one. We see these nurses eventually as specialist nurse practitioners taking their full place in the team and trained to the level of other specialist nurse practitioners. To achieve this, they may need to undertake further education and training. (Edwards 1987: para. 11.27).

The report also stated that practice nurses should be regarded as full members of the primary health care team (PHCT).

Prior to the 1990 GP contract, practice nurses had been employed by GPs to provide a nursing service in the practice which included investigative procedures, wound care, advising on minor ailments, health education and dietary advice, immunization, counselling, family planning advice and cervical cytology and chronic disease management. The English National Board review (Damant, 1990) concluded that the role and function of the nurse in general practice is underpinned by a range of complex processes, as set out in Box 4.3.1.

As the practice nurse's role has expanded, there has been considerable debate within the nursing, midwifery and health visiting profession as to how it should develop. Cooksley (1994) pointed out that the vast increase in the number of practice nurses has given rise to several contentious issues: professional rivalry, role threat and role confusion. This new and expanding role crosses role boundaries within the PHCT and can result in role overlap with other professional groups, such as district nurses and health visitors. Concern has also been expressed that the practice nurse's role is vulnerable to role confusion, as a result of ambiguity over whether their role extension is merely medical delegation. However, during the last ten years, practice nursing has made significant progress towards a professional identity, with the key issues now being autonomy, accountability and decision-making (Castledine, 1991).

- Problem-solving and decision-making processes, within limits of time, environment, the nature of decisions that practice nurses are empowered to make by their employers, and their access to a varying range of resources. An ability to recognize the potential complexity of the apparently 'simple' problem and the implications of omission and commission.

- *Interpersonal processes* with the accent on rapid relationship making skills and teamship; a counselling approach and the ability to hold constructive health conversations at different levels of complexity.

- *Professional processes*, nursing, autonomy and accountability with due regard for the rights, autonomy and individuality of the patient/client. Acting as the client's advocate/mediator.

- *Teaching and learning processes*, particularly in regard to health education, respecting the value systems and beliefs, self-motivation and personal development of others.

- *Clinical processes* in which knowledge of disease processes and their treatment are paramount and where safe practice is determined by an awareness of the extended role, human caring skills and value-free judgements.

- *Health promotion and maintenance processes* underpinned by epidemiology, neighbourhood knowledge, concepts of health which take account of the ageing process and an awareness of ethical considerations.

- *Management processes* in relation to self, time and enabling resources; the effectiveness and well-being of other members of the team. Marketing.

- *Research processes*, including the application of first principles of research to practice, the use of research findings, and the undertaking of research.

General Practitioner Contract (1990) (DOH and Welsh Office)

The new GP contract of 1990 outlining the terms and conditions for service for general practitioners had even greater implications for practice nurses and in particular their professional accountability. Increasingly their contribution to the PHCT was being acknowledged, as was their ability to provide quality clinical care including the management of chronic disease and health promotion within a general practice, health centre or surgery. The new contract, which was imposed by the government, specified more precisely the services GPs were required to provide for their patient and the terms of service were amended to make clear that health promotion and illness prevention fell within the definition of general medical services. Among the services eligible for financial entitlement were minor surgery, reaching targets in immunization and cytology screening, child health surveillance and health promotion clinics. It was evident that GPs could not achieve these targets without an increase in professional support.

There was a clear warning to GPs within the GP contract and the Red Book 'Statement of Fees and Allowances' (DOH, 1990a) that in delegating treatments and procedures to another person they must be sure of their competence to carry them out. To meet the increased workload of the GP contract, Robinson *et al.* (1993) found that 50.7% of respondents to a GP survey had created a new practice nursing post, 83.1% had expanded the role of existing nurses and 89.7% wished to see further expansion of the practice nurse's role. Of the responding general practitioners (2013), 90% were satisfied with the role of the practice nurse within their practice. Changes in the practice nurse's role following the 1990 GP contract were also surveyed in this study. Employing practice nurses to run health promotion clinics, three yearly health checks, new patient registration checks and assessment in the over 75 year olds, was cited most frequently by respondents, as the main changes in the role.

The government changes introduced at this time were also intended to increase patient information and choice, make practices more responsive to patients' demands and put more emphasis on health rather than sickness. However, the emphasis on health checks on non-attendees to the surgery and on annual checks on over 75 year olds, seemed to ignore much researched evidence that this approach is an ineffective way to spend time. Recent research for example has shown that targeting all identified three year non-attenders aged 16–74 years for an invitation to a health check was found to be an inefficient way of promoting good health or identifying patients at risk (Thomas *et al.*, 1993). Griffiths *et al.* (1994) also found that those in most need were least likely to attend.

In addition, much criticism has been voiced about health promotion clinics which could be set up not because of a perceived and identified need, but for financial incentive. In 1993 the government responded to such criticism by making amendments to the 1990 Contract and introduced the 'Banding' system to replace payments for health promotion clinics with a view to promoting a more strategic approach to health improvement.

Banding and Health Promotion

The National Census of Practice Nurses (1993) showed that 91% of practice nurses had been involved with running health promotion clinics. As stated previously, these clinics were not necessarily set up in response to the health needs of the practice population and it is well known that people in affluent and healthier social classes are more likely to take up the offer for health checks.

Hart (1971) and Turner (1992) suggest that health promotion initiatives that fail to pay attention to low income and material disadvantage may increase inequalities by improving the health of high income groups and doing little to change the health of low income groups. The health promotion clinic system failed to recognize that health promotion must be viewed in a social and economic context. Nurses involved with health promotion should not just focus on the psychological effects of lifestyle on health, but include broader subject areas such as social influences and how best to encourage behaviour changes in individual circumstances. Local interventions to improve the health of the practice population must be multiprofessional and primary health care teams need to collaborate on improving the health of the communities they serve, so that an intersectorial approach can be fostered.

The banding scheme introduced by the government in 1993 is based on three bands which build on one another.

Band 1: A programme to reduce smoking in the practice population.
Band 2: A programme to minimize mortality and morbidity of patients at risk from hypertension or with established coronary heart disease (CHD).
Band 3: A programme to offer a full range of primary prevention for CHD and stroke.

In each case practices have to plan and implement a programme of care for the practice population. The higher bands build on and include the achievements of the lower bands. The target population for each band is age related and set down by the government and practices' need to identify priority groups and find ways to invite them to attend the surgery. Each practice has to set out the intended coverage level of the target population and show an increasing coverage each year up to a defined level.

Detailed protocols are necessary, to explain how these health promotion programmes will be run and the advice and interventions offered by members of the practice team. Each practice has to apply to the FHSA for approval of their health promotion programmes, in order to claim payment under the banding system. Payment is only made if the programmes are carried out as approved and every year the practice has to submit an annual report and reapply for health promotion payments to the FHSA. Tattersell *et al.* (1993) explain in detail the criteria required for the banding scheme and how this may be achieved by a practice. Much of the confusion about the value of the government's health promotion programmes lies not in the screening but in subsequent intervention and follow-up. The two primary care interventions which are of proven effectiveness are the treatment of hypertension and the provision of smoking cessation advice and support (Fowler and Mant 1990). Practice nurses have a key role to play in these interventions although Rollnick *et al.* (1993) found that their approach should be more sensitively matched to the patients' readiness to change. For example, while an action orientated smoking programme may help those ready to change, it does not work for those who are unsure about it.

The goal of the new banding system should be to reduce coronary heart disease by lifestyle changes in patients. As practice nurses are the main providers of the programme, there appears to be an increasing need in primary care for training in motivational skills. Many practice nurses have received training and become proficient in giving health promotion advice, but they have been less successful in persuading patients to adopt permanent lifestyle change to reduce risks of coronary heart disease as cited by Gibbons *et al.* (1993) and the Family Heart Study Group (1994).

A further commitment to health is described in the government White Paper *The Health of the Nation* (DOH, 1992), which sets out a strategy for England. The NHS Wales document *Caring for the Future* (1994), highlights ten priority health areas for action (Box 4.3.2).

Health improvements in the community will only be achieved by focusing on local health needs and priorities, building on the information available to general practices and the primary health care team and working with other agencies to improve health.

Box 4.3.2. Ten priority health areas (NHS Wales, 1994)

- Cardiovascular diseases
- Respiratory diseases
- Cancers
- Healthy living
- Healthy environments
- Maternal and child health
- Mental health
- Learning disabilities
- Physical disability and discomfort
- Injuries

Fundholding

In January 1989 the government published a White Paper on the future of the National Health Service (NHS) – *Working for Patients* (DOH, 1989a). The proposals set out represented some of the most radical changes to the NHS since its creation over 40 years ago. The government recognized that GPs were uniquely placed to improve patients' choice of good quality services because of their relationships with patients and hospitals. The legislation for fundholding was passed as the NHS, and Community Care Act 1990, and the 'firstwave' fundholders joined the scheme in April 1991.

As the GP provides more than 90% of his patients' care, the fundholding scheme was introduced to give general practices the opportunity to exercise direct control over NHS resources for the immediate benefit of their patients. Before being allowed to obtain fundholding status, practices had to meet the following criteria:

- Full partner agreement
- List size of more than 9000 patients (this was reduced in 1992 to 7000).
- Practice computerization

Once a practice has made the decision to become fundholding, a preparatory year is essential, in order for the practice to collect information on services to purchase, and the expenditure involved. The FHSA has to approve the expenditure, guiding and monitoring the practices through the period of preparation.

Initially practices could make purchases in the following three key areas

- Hospital and specialist care
- Prescribing
- Staffing

From April 1993, fundholding practices were able to purchase community services including district nursing, health visiting and community psychiatric nursing. These services have to be purchased from existing community units as GPs are not given the resources to employ community nursing staff directly. This may change as fundholding develops and responds to changing demands.

Tettersell *et al.* (1993) suggest that the ability of a fundholding practice to specify conditions about the nursing services it wishes to purchase will ultimately change the nature of the primary health care team, and working arrangements between GPs, practice nurses and attached staff. Practices will want an involvement in selecting and retaining particular nurses and will insist on greater flexibility of roles and the setting of shared team objectives. Artificial barriers between employed and attached staff are likely to be removed and the team approach to assessing health needs and service objectives for a practice population will be encouraged.

Many practice nurses working in fundholding practices have noticed the benefits from a closer working relationship with their community nursing colleagues, resulting in greater flexibility across professional specialisms, and more cost-effective care through genuine teamwork. As practice nurses have always been employed by a GP, fundholding has not been seen as a threat to their employment or professional status and the practice nurse will continue to be an integral and key member of the primary care team through fundholding.

Clinical Audit

Nurses are responsible for ensuring a high standard of care for their patients. In general practice the most effective audit is achieved when there is a fully integrated team approach to clinical audit. The concept of clinical audit has recently received widespread support from government, the Royal Colleges and professionals.

Medical audit advisory groups (MAAGs) were set up in response to the government's White Paper, *Working for Patients* (DOH, 1989a). The MAAGs are responsible for ensuring that medical audit is occurring in general practices throughout the country. The MAAG is essentially an advisory committee, but in most areas it has developed a facilitating role in helping practices to set up audit. More recently MAAGs have been required, by the government, to become multidisciplinary and to foster clinical audit in general practice. The structure of the majority of MAAGs in each FHSA area includes appropriate professional representatives from the Local Medical Committee, the Royal College of General Practitioners, the local practice nurse group, the Practice Manager Association and in some areas, the Community Nursing Unit or Trust.

The main functions of MAAGs as described by Houghton (1994) are:

- To advise FHSAs/commissioning authorities, GPs, practice nurses and all practice staff on practical and educational aspects of clinical audit.
- To work closely with FHSAs/commissioning authorities and other interested bodies to promote primary health care development.
- To facilitate multipractice and multidisciplinary clinical audit activities.
- To liaise with secondary care providers to promote collaborative and interface quality working.
- To formulate clinical guidelines for use in general practice.

A number of MAAGs in liaison with FHSAs and hospital specialists have produced clinical guidelines and audit tools on a variety of topics namely:

- Diabetes
- Asthma
- Hypertension
- Cervical cytology
- Health promotion clinics

The NHS Executive has more recently sent further information to MAAGs and FHSAs and others concerned with audit in general practice. MAAGs will need to ensure that by 1996 all practice teams understand the principles of clinical audit, have an identifiable structure for supervising audit within the team, have identified their strengths and weaknesses and have selected a prioritized ongoing programme of audit. The majority of practices should also have undertaken surveys of the opinions of their patients. Clinical audit should therefore:

1. Contribute to an improvement in the health status of the patient and practice population.
2. Encourage research based practice and clinical effectiveness.
3. Encourage personal and professional growth through facilitated teamwork.

Luft and Smith (1994) summarize clinical audit and quality assurance in general practice as serving to:

- bring the team together to discuss desired standards in the practice;
- set the desired standards of any current practice within that team;
- compare the actual present standard with the desired standard;
- interpret findings;
- bring about changes in care that are required to achieve the desired standard;
- reassess the desired standard – is it achievable? – and make changes if necessary.

The Welsh Nursing and Midwifery Committee Report on Practice Nursing (1992) recommended that FHSAs and employers should facilitate the involvement of practice nurses in all aspects of audit and make available training in audit methodology.

Educational, Clinical and Professional Developments

Practice nursing has responded to change frequently since its inception, more so than any other branch of community nursing. Many changes continue to take place and the shift from hospital to community based care will certainly ensure that nursing in general practice will continue to develop. The key components for the future development of practice nursing are listed in Box 4.3.3.

Educational

The education pathway for practice nurses has developed in an ad hoc manner. The first reported training courses were organized by the Royal College of General Practitioners in the early 1980s. In 1985 an outline curriculum for practice nursing,

Box 4.3.3. Practice nursing: key components

- Educational – implications of the UKCC's community education and practice standards – practice nurse teachers and trainers
- Clinical initiatives in general practice nursing
- Professional development – nurse practitioner role – nurse prescribing – nurse advisers/facilitators
- Political issues
  Government policies
  UKCC and National Boards for Nursing, Midwifery and Health Visiting
- Organizational
  Shared vision of care
  Merging of DHAs and FHSAs
  Opportunities – teamwork

which described a course of no less than 10 days was published by the National Boards, but was only available in a limited number of nursing colleges. As the numbers of practice nurses increased, many were demanding a more comprehensive educational programme which reflected the recordable or registerable pathway available for other community nurses. The ENB's Review of Education and Training for Practice Nursing (Damant, 1990) recommended a course which would ensure a qualification recordable on the professional register of the UKCC, although this recommendation was not implemented.

The Welsh National Board framework for continuing education was implemented in 1989, which allowed practice nurses to obtain a certificate or diploma in professional practice, using a modular route. Some FHSAs and local practice nurse groups began to meet their own educational needs by organizing study days and courses, often in conjunction with the local postgraduate centre and continuing medical education tutors. Many traditionally trained practice nurses have attended a variety of accredited National Board or other specific courses to meet their individual needs.

The UKCC has now recognized the role of the practice nurse and in its *Standards for Education and Practice following Registration* (UKCC, 1994), has identified practice nursing as a specialism within the Community Health Care Nursing (CHCN) programme. This sets the framework for future practice nurse education. However, during the transitional period there are important issues to be addressed. Existing health visitors, district nurses, and other community nurses who have undertaken a course of at least four months in length approved by the Council, will automatically achieve the CHCN qualification. Many practice nurses will need to undertake further training before becoming a CHCN. However, the training and experience already gained in practice nursing will receive accreditation through the accreditation of prior/experiential learning (APEL) process.

Teachers and Trainers

Programmes for the specialist CHCN qualification are required to be modular and flexible. The clinical practice component will need to be practice based and the nurses supported and assessed by practice nurse trainers. The value of practice nurse trainers is now acknowledged but criteria and standards for the role need to be established, in line with other community practice teachers.

Initiatives in Clinical Practice

The King's Fund report, *Developing Primary Care, Opportunities for the 1990s* (Taylor 1992) describes 14 primary care development projects, the success of a number being attributed directly to the role of practice nurses, namely:

- Enhanced diabetic care in South Glamorgan (Smail and Stott, in Taylor 1992).
- Management of chronic disease in general practice (O'Dowd, in Taylor 1992).
- Screening the health and welfare of people in York over 75 years (Harding and Guthrie, in Taylor 1992).

Jones and Lester (1993) reported findings relating to the changing role of the practice nurse in relation to older patients. Older people's utilization and perception of primary care was investigated initially in 1990, to obtain baseline measures, and again in 1992 to assess the content and nature of the change which had taken place. Almost twice the number of older patients consulted the practice nurse in the second year of the study and there had been a considerable increase in the reasons for consulting the practice nurse, ranging from flu injections and blood pressure checks to weaning off psychotropic drugs.

Jacobson and Wilkinson (1994) in their review of teenage health suggest that one method of providing more sensitive care is to create separate clinics for teenagers and a rethink of how to tailor the existing primary care framework to be more teenager friendly. In some areas practice nurses are already addressing teenage health by using innovative and patient centred methods including separate clinics, sometimes run in youth centres. It is important to consider how teenagers could feel more comfortable in the surgery, so that health professionals and teenagers can discuss issues in a mutually supportive and helpful atmosphere.

Professional Developments

The nurse practitioner's role has received much attention in recent years and some practice nurses see this as a definite career pathway. (See Chapter 4.6.)

Nurse prescribing is now back on the statute books and is to be piloted in eight fundholding practices in England. Initially it will only be district nurses and health visitors who are allowed to prescribe from a limited Nurses' Formulary. However, practice nurses already influence GP prescribing through their knowledge and use of certain items.

Some of this development has been assisted by the appointment of nurse advisers and primary health care facilitators in FHSAs, many from a practice nursing background. The amount of advice and support available to practice nurses is variable throughout the UK but at a recent conference in Wales, *Practice Nursing: The Way Forward* (1994), it was recommended that all FHSAs should employ a nurse adviser/facilitator with knowledge and experience in practice and community nursing. The Welsh Nursing and Midwifery Committee Report (1992) also recognized the developing role of practice nursing and the need for greater nursing support and advice at FHSA level.

Political Issues

For some time now the Royal College of Nursing has recognized the active participation of its practice nurse members. Indeed, the Practice Nurse Association is said to be the most active of all the membership groups, participating in the formulation of college policy and being represented on Community Nursing Committees. Practice nurses are also represented on many local committees, including local medical committees (LMCs), MAAGs, FHSAs, nursing and midwifery committees, education committees and a variety of others. Three practice nurses were recently elected to the UKCC (April 1993) representing Wales, England and Scotland.

The National Boards for Nursing, Midwifery and Health Visiting are also recognizing the influence of practice nurses and addressing their educational needs. Damant *et al.* (1994) stated:

> It is this enthusiasm, political awareness and assertiveness of nurses in general practice that has provided the impetus for nursing in general practice to become established as a discrete area of practice and a potential force to be reckoned with politically.

Organizational Changes and Opportunities

Merging the DHAs and FHSAs as joint purchasing agents for community services has led to a far greater understanding of the roles and responsibilities of all community nurses. Much of the planning and purchasing of services is locality based and the health needs of a particular locality are assessed. The primary health care team is increasingly focusing on care at the local and community level and working with social services and voluntary organizations. Community nurses are being formally seconded to GP practices and services are gradually becoming 'needs-led' rather than 'service-driven'.

As fundholding is extended, GPs will become more interested in skill-mix and cost-effectiveness of community nursing services. Practice nurses, along with their community nursing colleagues, will need to develop marketing skills in order to communicate more effectively about the benefits of their services. They should continue to develop their knowledge, practice and decision-making skills, undertake research and audit the quality and outcome of their care.

CONCLUSION

Practice nursing has developed and expanded more rapidly than any other area of community nursing. Practice nurses are recognized as valuable members of the primary health care team. GPs acknowledge that without them it would be difficult to achieve their health gain targets, or carry out the amount of health promotion activity and chronic disease management in primary care which currently exists. The role, function and identity of practice nursing will continue to develop as the structure, organization and financing of the health service changes. The extension of GP fundholding, further developments of the commissioning/purchasing and provider roles, and changes in the provision of community nursing services will continue to have an effect on practise nursing. The way forward will be in greater collaboration and more effective teamworking with other community nursing colleagues, through shared team objectives and research based, audited practice.

SUMMARY

- Practice nursing has developed as a key discipline within the nursing profession.
- The role has changed and expanded rapidly in the last decade.
- Practice nurses are key members of the PHCT, employed by GPs to undertake the delivery of nursing care in general practice as self-directed practitioners.
- Practice nurses are responsible for developing clinical policies and ensuring high standards of care delivery.
- The Community Health Care Nursing (CHCN) programme sets the framework for future practice nurse education.

DISCUSSION QUESTIONS

- ◆ Consider potential sources of tension arising from attempts to achieve greater coordination between nursing disciplines associated with primary care. Suggest ways to promote the concept of a primary health care nursing team.

- ◆ What population based information might predict future developments in, or modifications to, practice nursing?

- ◆ Identity three priority groups within a practice population, highlighting significant health needs. Using research evidence suggest ways in which the impact of practice nursing could be gauged.

FURTHER READING

In *addition* to the books mentioned in the references, which are also relevant:

Hunt G and Wainwright P (1994) *Expanding the Role of the Nurse*. Oxford: Blackwell Scientific Publications.
This book considers the major issues influencing the expanding and developing role of the nurse and explores how they affect practice.

Jeffree P (1990) *The Practice Nurse, Theory and Practice*. London: Chapman & Hall.
This theory and practical skills textbook reflects the variety but also the importance of the practice nurse's role in preventative medicine and primary health care.

Ovretveit J (1993) *Co-ordinating Community Care – Multidisciplinary teams and Care Management*. Buckingham: Open University Press.
This book is about how people from different professions and agencies work together to meet the health and social needs of people in the community.

Pirie A and Kelly M (1993) *Fundholding, A Practice Guide*. Oxford: Radcliffe Medical Press.
This book gives practical guidance on the fundholding scheme in general practice, the criteria required to obtain fundholding status and the data gathering exercise required by the FHSAs.

Pringle M *et al.* (1993) *Managing Change in Primary Care*. Oxford: Radcliffe Medical Press.
The challenges and opportunities presented by the NHS reforms require a capacity for change. This book will help doctors, nurses and practice managers develop skills and techniques necessary to identify strategic management problems and discover methods of solving them.

Savage J (1991) *Nurse Practitioners*. London: King Fund Centre.
This book brings together the views and experiences of experts from the UK and overseas on the nurse practitioner role. It is becoming clear that the nurse practitioner offers new opportunities to meet existing and future needs, through a more flexible model of nursing practice.

REFERENCES

Atkin K and Lunt N (1993) *Nurses Count: A National Census of Practice Nurses*. Social Policy Research Unit: University of York.

Audit Commission (1993) *Practice Makes Perfect: The Role of the Family Health Services Authority*. London: HMSO.

Bowling A and Stilwell B (1988) *The Nurse in Family Practice*. London: Scutari Press.

Castledine G (1991) Accountability in delivering care. *Nursing Standard* **5**(25): 28-30.

Cooksley M (1994) *Autonomous Practice Nurse or Doctor's Handmaiden*. B N Dissertation, University of Wales.

Cumberlege J (1986) *Report of the Community Nursing Review Neighbourhood Nursing – A Focus for Care*. London: HMSO.

Damant M (1990) *Report of the Review Group for the Education and Training for Practice Nursing*. London: English National Board for Nursing, Midwifery and Health Visiting (ENB).

Damant M, Martin C and Openshaw S (1994) *Practice Nursing, Stability and Change*. Mosby.

Department of Health (1989a) *Working for Patients*. London: HMSO.

Department of Health (1989b) *Funding General Practice*. London: HMSO.

Department of Health (1990a) *Statement of Fees and Allowances*. London: HMSO.

Department of Health (1990b) *A Definition of Practice*. London: HMSO.

Department of Health (1992) *The Health of the Nation – a Summary of the Strategy for Health in England*. London: HMSO.

DHSS (1975) *Nurses Employed Privately by General Medical Practitioners*. London: HMSO.

Edwards N (1987) *Nursing in the Community. A Team Approach for Wales*: Welsh Office.

Family Heart Study Group (1994) British Family Heart Study: its design and method, and prevalence of cardiovascular risk factors. *British Journal of General Practice* **44**: 62-67.

Fowler G and Mant D (1990) Health checks for adults. *British Medical Journal* **300**: 1318-1320.

Gibbons R, Riley M and Brimble P (1993) Effectiveness of programme for reducing cardiovascular risk for men in one general practice. *British Medical Journal* **306**: 1652-1656.

Gledhill E (1994) Professional responsibility editorial. *Practice Nursing* **5**: 15. 9.

Griffiths C *et al.* (1994) Registration health checks: Inverse care in the inner city? *British Journal of General Practice* **44**: 201-204.

Hart JT (1971) The inverse care law. *Lancet* **1**: 405-412.

Houghton G (1994) *Audit Trends*. Department of General Practice, University of Leicester 2 (2.) 59.

Jacobson L and Wilkinson C (1994) Review of teenage health care: time for a new direction. *British Journal of General Practice* **44:** 420–423.

Jones D and Lester C (1993) The changing role of the practice nurse in relation to older patients. *University of Wales College of Medicine Report.*

Littlewood J (1987) *Recent Advances on Nursing, Community Nursing*. Edinburgh: Churchill Livingstone.

Luft S and Smith M (1994) *Nursing in General Practice*. London: Chapman & Hall.

NHSME (1992) *Guidance on the extension of the Hospital and Community Health Services elements*. London: DOH.

NHS (1993) *New World, New Opportunities*, Nursing in Primary Health Care. London: HMSO.

NHS Wales (1994) *Caring for the Future*. Welsh Office.

Patnick J (1994) Practice nurses win praise for boosting screening rates. *Nursing Times* **90**(42): 6.

Robinson G, Beaton S and White P (1993) Attitudes towards practice nurses – survey of a sample of general practitioners in England and Wales. *British Journal of General Practice* **43:** 25–29.

Rollnick S, Kinnersley P and Stott NCH (1993) Methods of helping patients with behaviour change. *British Medical Journal* **307:** 188–190.

Roy S (1991) Nursing in the Community NHS Management Executive.

Royal College of Nursing (1992) *Powerhouse for change* London: RCN.

Smail J and Stott N (1992) Enhanced diabetic care in South Glamorgan. *University of Wales College of Medicine Report.*

Stillwell B (1991) The rise of the practice nurse. *Nursing Times* **87**(24): 26–28.

Taylor D (1992) Developing Primary Care Opportunities for the 1990s. London: *King's Fund Institute* Research report 10.

Tettersell M, Sawyer J and Salisbury C (1993) *Handbook of Practice Nursing*. London: Churchill Livingstone.

Thomas K *et al.* (1993) Case against targeting long term non-attenders in general practice for a health check. *British Journal of General Practice* **43:** 285–289.

Turner T (1992) A healing nation? *Nursing Times* **88:** 18–19.

United Kingdom Central Council (1994) *Standards for Education and Practice following Registration*. London: UKCC.

Welsh National Board (1989) *Framework for Continuing Education*. WNB.

Welsh Nursing and Midwifery Committee (1992) *Practice Nursing*. Welsh Office.

Welsh Office (1994) *General Practice Nursing in Wales: The Way Forward*. Welsh Office.

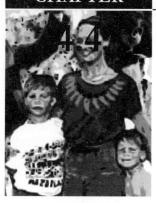

HEALTH VISITING AND PUBLIC HEALTH

Sarah Cowley

KEY ISSUES

- The meaning and purpose of 'public health'
- The development of the 'new public health'
- The links between public health, health promotion and primary health care
- The principles of health visiting will provide a framework to explain how public health permeates practice
- Some barriers to nursing work in public health, and emerging opportunities will be considered

INTRODUCTION

The NHS and Community Care Act 1990 marked the formal recognition of a public health role which had been advocated by Acheson (1988). The intention was that, in future, health care should be purchased to meet explicitly identified needs of the population being served. The responsibility for identifying these population needs was given to medical Directors of Public Health; as the new purchasing authorities became established, they were all required to appoint someone to take that role. However, the contribution of nurses to the public health and in the purchasing of health care was neither specified nor explored in any detail when this legislation was first proposed.

Some of the more recent publications and developments have sought to redress this early omission; of particular note are three policy documents. The nursing contribution to purchasing remains a source of some ambivalence and uncertainty, but the NHS Executive (NHSE) has stated a commitment to promoting this role (NHSE, 1994a). The Standing Nursing and Midwifery Advisory Committee (SNMAC) provided detailed information about how this can occur in practice through the public health role and contribution made by all nurses; particular importance is attached to the function within health visiting and school nursing (SNMAC, 1995).

The third document came from the United Kingdom Central Council for Nursing Midwifery and Health Visiting (UKCC). They detail the educational preparation required for qualification in community health care nursing, and likewise emphasize the importance of public health throughout this new specialist discipline (UKCC, 1994). They, too, single out health visitors and school nurses as having a particularly important contribution in this sphere, and propose the new title of 'public health nursing: health visiting'. This chapter will use the term 'public health nurse' when referring to activities or issues that concern any community nurses involved in public health, and the term 'health visiting' for that specific area of practice alone.

Public Health

Public health has been defined as 'the science and art of preventing disease, prolonging life and promoting health through the organized efforts of society' (Acheson, 1988). Reflecting a belief that the wellbeing of individuals is intimately linked to the health status of the whole society and community in which they live, public health focuses on three areas in particular:

- Contagious diseases are a major interest, not just because of the impact on the afflicted individual, but because of the potential to infect others.
- Health issues which may have an impact on the functioning of society, likewise, are singled out for particular attention.
- Using insights drawn from epidemiology, public health efforts are concentrated especially on vulnerable groups and those believed to be 'at risk' in some way.

Ashton and Seymour (1988) describe four distinct phases of public health, culminating in the current 'new public health' approach, which brings together the functions which separately characterized the first three: environmental change, personal preventive measures and therapeutic interventions. The priorities of public health are not fixed, but change according to the health status of the whole population being served. This contrasts with the familiar approach in which health care professionals consider as supreme the needs of an individual client or patient, and reach decisions to suit that person alone. Thus, although it may function by providing attention to individuals, public health is essentially concerned with populations and groups within society, and about the way health services are organized and delivered.

Public health nurses have individual clients on their caseload, but their responsibility lies with the health of the wider community (Gordon, 1991; McMurray, 1993). Inevitably, this leads to conflicting priorities in caseload management at times. The principles of health visiting (CETHV, 1977) will be used below as a framework through which to explain the actual practice and some of the dilemmas facing public health nurses.

This practice differs somewhat from the approach of public health medicine, not least because these doctors have no personal contact with a caseload of clients; however, their purchasing remit gives them a formally defined sphere of influence denied to public health nurses. Differences in approach and responsibilities have always existed between practising health visitors and those who control the service; this accounts for some of the current barriers and opportunities for developing public health work. These will be considered briefly before explaining the emergence of the 'new public health' and the principles of health visiting.

Organizational Arrangements

The history of health visiting shows that practitioners have never held full control over their service. It began with a non-stigmatizing, universal and practical ideal, providing a paid occupation for the working class women who pioneered the work, and an unpaid public health role for the middle class Victorian ladies who initiated and directed the service (Davies, 1988; Dingwall, 1977). However, once the cost of the occupation was established as a legitimate call on the public purse in the early years of this century, control was handed to the Medical Officers of Health (MOHs) and the service became increasingly individualistic, focused on infant welfare, then linked with midwifery and nursing in the years between the wars.

Both community nursing and medical public health functions were the responsibility of local authorities until 1974, when they were absorbed into a national health service which had previously been solely concerned with hospitals. General practitioners were not included in this merger; they continued to function as wholly self-employed and autonomous contractors to the health service, until the changes heralded by the NHS and Community Care Act 1990 offered them a new, broader option. Under that Act, general practitioners were afforded an opportunity to become 'fundholders', and to purchase hospital services to meet the needs of the people registered on their caselist. In 1993, this option was extended to include the purchase of certain community nursing services (NHSME, 1992). School nurses were not included, but community psychiatric and learning disabilities nurses could be contracted to accept referrals from the general practitioners.

However, the work of district nurses and health visitors was to be contracted in its entirety, as part of a move to establish a 'primary care led NHS'; this thrust has continued and extended (NHSME, 1993; NHSE, 1994b). Health visitors expressed concern about the potential loss of their public health role since general practitioners have no clear public health remit; as fundholders, their responsibility is to meet the identified needs of individuals registered at their practice. It was suggested that around 10% of a health visitor's time might be occupied in public health duties; the guidance advised that this amount of time should be built into the contracts (NHSME, 1992).

As a result, there was considerable soul-searching about which elements of a health visitor's work might be considered 'public health' or not, until the SNMAC report reaffirmed that these practitioners are 'public health workers in the entirety of their role' (SNMAC, 1995: 16). It is not yet clear how this will be translated into future contracts, and there remains a concern that separating health visitors from their peers who work elsewhere in the area, and placing them firmly under the direction of medical practitioners, may diminish the effectiveness and scope of their public health role.

The New Public Health

A report prepared for the Canadian government about the health of the nationals of that country (Lalonde, 1974) is generally recognized as the catalyst for the 'new public health', which Ashton and Seymour (1988) regard as the current phase of public health endeavour. The new public health aims to reap the combined benefits of environmental change, of personal preventive measures and of therapeutic interventions. Lalonde showed that all causes of death and disease could be attributed to four discrete and distinct elements as follows:

- inadequacies in current health care provision;
- lifestyle or behavioural factors;
- issues related to the environment, and
- bio-physical characteristics.

The Lalonde Report came at a time when the prevailing medical model was being widely criticized for focusing narrowly on scientific explanations, aetiologies and clinical disease while ignoring far more complex health-harming social issues like unemployment, homelessness and low income (Bunton and Macdonald, 1992). As well as a regeneration of public health, it has been associated with a changing approach from traditional health education to health promotion, and with a world-wide focus on primary health care as a mode of service delivery (Bunton and Macdonald, 1992; World Health Organization (WHO) 1977, 1986a).

These three approaches (public health, health promotion and primary health care) are all generally recognized as closely linked and interdependent; they share many common beliefs and it is not really possible or desirable to separate them completely from each other. Health visiting, which began its own process of regeneration in the same period of time, also shares a holistic, humanistic philosophy and broad, socially based belief in the value of health. It is, likewise, inseparable from the processes of public health, health promotion and primary health care. The principles of health visiting (CETHV, 1977) which justify this statement, and the implications of these for contemporary practice will be explored further below.

The Principles of Health Visiting

In 1974, as the Lalonde Report was being published in Canada, community nursing services in the United Kingdom were moved from the control of local authorities, and absorbed into the organizational structure of the National Health Service (NHS). Hitherto, the NHS had only been concerned with hospital services, and this move led to considerable soul-searching and much examination of the work of health visitors by its practitioners.

One move was initiated by the Council for the Education and Training of Health Visitors (CETHV) which, at that time, regulated the profession. This body convened a series of workshop meetings to examine the principles that guide the teaching and practice of health visiting. They concluded that the work was underpinned by a firm belief in the value of health, and that it involved four guiding principles (CETHV, 1977). These are:

- The search for health needs
- The stimulation of an awareness of health needs
- The influence on policies affecting health
- The facilitation of health enhancing activities

Robinson (1992) suggests that, while they are expressed as 'principles', they are best seen as a characterization of the role and functions of the occupation in the wider social context. In some respects, the document was very forward-looking, referring to a need for health promotion, questioning narrowly defined approaches to health education and drawing attention to the difficulties faced by people living in poverty and deprivation. The document stimulated much interest (CETHV, 1980, 1982), but the UKCC did not carry the debate forward when it replaced the CETHV in 1983.

However, a new working group was convened in 1991; they re-examined the principles in the light of contemporary practice, and of the reorganized NHS. They concluded that the principles not only remained relevant, they provided a potentially vital and important framework to underpin practice (Twinn and Cowley, 1992). There were some amendments and additional provisos which needed clarifying from the original document. In particular, a less individual focus and wider awareness of structural issues needed to be explicitly incorporated within the understanding of the principles.

The Value of Health

The working group acknowledged their views were influenced by the World Health Organization (1986a, 1986b) and Seedhouse (1986) as well as the original CETHV

(1977) document. Reiterating a commitment to health as a value which is worth pursuing for its own sake, they highlighted seven major beliefs which underpin the principles:

- Everyone has a fundamental right to the best possible state of health. In accepting this, health visitors take on a responsibility to address current inequalities and inequities in health care.
- Health promotion is important because having a positive sense of health enables people to make full use of their physical, mental and emotional capacities, so they can reach their full potential for achievement.
- Achieving health means that people have the power to shape their own lives and those of their families. This implies active participation in health from individuals, families and groups, and emphasizes the importance of empowering as a form of health promotion.
- Health care services should be readily accessible and acceptable, and involve full community participation. This is the basis of primary health care, which needs a full, equal partnership between professionals and the people they serve.
- Health is a positive concept, encompassing social and personal resources, as well as physical capacities. Resources which contribute to positive well-being may be personal and internalized, or may arise externally from the social and family context in which the individual lives. Health promotion, therefore, involves finding ways to create resources for health.
- Health cannot be separated from the socioeconomic and cultural context in which it is experienced. This is why health visitors focus at different times on individuals, families and communities.
- Health must be regarded in broad, holistic terms, encompassing whole individuals, within their personal situation. This has implications for the extent to which people are able to exercise personal choice, and to which they can be held solely responsible for their state of health.

Although the principles had always been listed sequentially, in practice they often appear interlinked and inseparable. In view of this, a diagram was devised which demonstrated their circular and integrating nature and allowed some of the more recent terminology to be incorporated (Figure 4.4.1). It also helps to demonstrate the link to health promotion and to primary health care. The way the principles integrate health visiting practice and public health will be explained as they are each explored below.

The Search for Health Needs

When first identified, this principle was regarded as important because those who are most in need are often the most poorly served by health professionals. This point has since been demonstrated by numerous surveys (e.g. Black, 1993; Phillimore *et al.*, 1994; Townsend *et al.*, 1988; Wilkinson, 1994); it is a public health issue because it prevents the health status of the whole population reaching its optimum potential.

The universal focus of the service, which may not be achieved where only pre-school surveillance is emphasized, is considered essential. This is partly because it places health visitors in a position to uncover unmet and hidden needs, then enable people to recognize that health care may help improve their situation. Also selection increases the likelihood of stigma. SNMAC (1995) underline the importance of having a clear knowledge of the health needs of the whole population served, not of individual care needs alone.

The potential for intrusiveness and suspicion, and the variable understandings of

Figure 4.4.1. Pictorial representation of the relationship between the principles of health visiting and the practice.

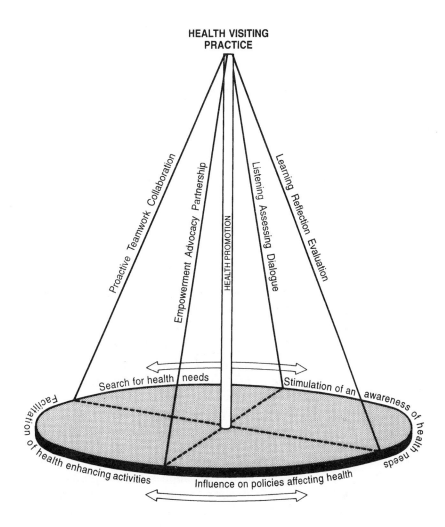

HEALTH VISITING PRACTICE

Proactive Teamwork Collaboration

Empowerment Advocacy Partnership

HEALTH PROMOTION

Listening Assessing Dialogue

Learning Reflection Evaluation

Search for health needs

Stimulation of an awareness of health needs

Facilitation of health enhancing activities

Influence on policies affecting health

the term 'health need' are well acknowledged (CETHV, 1977; Twinn and Cowley, 1992). However, these drawbacks are not inevitable, as demonstrated in a qualitative study of health visiting practice (Chalmers, 1993). It showed that the 'search' may be client initiated and may focus on needs which are 'easily seen', as well as on hidden needs which are suspected by the client or health visitor, or which may be uncovered during the process of discussion.

At times it may be important to investigate further; as when it is suspected that children may be in need of protection, for example. It has been suggested that the general surveillance of all preschool children focuses unfairly on working class families; health visitors are accused of 'policing families', perpetuating a middle class approach to child-rearing and acting as agents of social control on women (Abbott and Sapsford, 1990).

However, the Children Act 1989 clearly acknowledges the role of health visitors and school nurses as 'casefinders' of children who need protection, as between them they have contact with the whole child population. They are often the only professionals involved with vulnerable families, especially those who are not formally registered and receiving social work (Appleton, 1994). Dingwall and Robinson

(1993), likewise, invoke the terminology of 'policing', but claim it is essential for safeguarding the rights of children.

Browne (1995) points out that young children are, by European standards, particularly likely to be murdered by their adult caretakers in the United Kingdom. Child maltreatment is among the top five common causes of death, with preschool children being most at risk, and two or three fatal injuries occurring each week. Child abuse, therefore, rates as a major public health concern. It illustrates the recurring ethical dilemmas which face public heath nurses in carrying out the search for these particular needs within families and in their caseload, and in responding to repeated accusations that health visitors answer middle class 'moral panics' by targeting the working classes.

Stimulation of An Awareness of Health Needs

When this principle was first discussed, much emphasis was placed on helping people to become aware of their own health needs (CETHV, 1977). In the more recent discussions (Twinn and Cowley, 1992), it was suggested that this focus needed to be extended to three different levels of action:

- To clients: individuals, families and communities
- To health service managers in provider units and in commissioning/purchasing authorities, and finally
- To politicians and policy-makers

Establishing an awareness of health need is an essential first step in engaging clients in discussions about their own health; it is crucial in securing a proactive, health promoting service rather than one which simply reacts to demand to treat established needs. 'Awareness' encompasses different levels of knowledge, belief, understanding and psychological acceptance of health needs; it is influenced by personal experience, social and cultural background, individual agendas for action and political stance (Cowley, 1991).

SNMAC (1995) emphasize the important public health focus on health promotion, which involves enabling people to increase control over and improve their health. There is heavy pressure on health visitors to target clearly identified and acknowledged health needs (Audit Commission, 1994), and to move away from the more holistic and opportunistic approach which formerly characterized their work (Cowley, 1995). However, tightening the rhetoric around the way health needs are measured and constructed may reduce the ability of health visitors to respond to the needs they witness daily.

Edwards and Popay (1994), for example, considered the contradictions that arise for health visitors and other community workers, who freely acknowledge that their clients' greatest needs arise from poverty, and a lack of social support. However, the ability of the professionals to befriend, listen and offer social support may be limited by the acceptability of that as a 'proper response' to perceived health need, in the eyes of service managers and purchasers. Edwards (1995) showed how men who were isolated as well as living in poverty could be offered help with housework or babysitting if they found it hard to cope, but women (especially young single mothers) would be denied such relief lest they became 'dependent'. Instead, they would be offered education to improve their 'parenting skills'. This approach serves to distract attention from the stressful situations in which the women are obliged to live, but affords health visitors an opportunity to achieve easily measurable outcomes for their work. To avoid this 'perverse incentive', there is an urgent need to stimulate the awareness of politicians and policy-makers about the real health needs of the population.

Influence on Policies
Affecting Health

This principle was regarded as the most controversial when it was first identified, since it was suggested that nurses should not be involved with 'political' activity (CETHV, 1977). The inescapably political nature of health and the health service is more openly acknowledged now (Twinn and Cowley, 1992), but the extent to which health visitors might expect to be paid for such involvement is still subject to debate. The principle emphasizes collective and collaborative action, which is regarded as essential in public health (SNMAC, 1995). Again, this principle needs to be directed at various different levels. Twinn and Cowley (1992) suggested that:

- The 'influence' should be extended to include local, national and international levels of policy.
- The notion of 'policy' should be extended to encompass strategies and approaches to practice at a local as well as a national level.

Formally collated profiles of the health needs within a caseload, locality or practice list are increasingly viewed as essential (Audit Commission, 1994; Goodwin, 1992; NHSME, 1993; SNMAC, 1995) and a means of integrating the process of needs assessment with an influence on planning of services (Cernik and Wearne, 1992; Cowley *et al.*, 1995). Because of their daily involvement with their caseload, health visitors have access to information about health and the influences on health in the local area or the population served by a particular practice or primary care team, which may not be available on statistics drawn from a wider area. Health visitors' ability to record, report and synthesize this 'everyday' information for managers and purchasers explains how the notion of public health runs, as SNMAC (1995) suggest, through the entirety of their work.

A new and important way of influencing local policies involves the marketing of health visiting services to local purchasers, who may be commissioning health authorities, or general practice fundholders. As explained above, it is increasingly common for community services to be organized through primary health care teams and the purchasing function of general practitioners is expanding (NHSME, 1993; NHSE, 1994b).

Health visitors can influence the kind of care purchased by general practitioners (Goodwin, 1994), who appear more likely than commissioning health authorities to be aware of the range of health visiting practice, and to value their particular skills (NHSE 1994c). Support from general practitioners is very important, but their lack of a clear public health responsibility remains a matter of concern because of the potentially distorting effect on health visiting practice.

At a broader level, some health visitors have taken up the challenge to influence policies by joining the public health departments of larger commissioning health authorities, or developing a role in purchasing (NHSE, 1994a). The roles undertaken by these nurses are still developing; their functions are interpreted differently from one area to another, but are an important way of influencing health service policies across a wide area. The varied titles given to nurses in purchasing may make them difficult to identify, but practitioners who seek them out may find they provide a valuable channel through which to transmit locally derived information to health commissioners (Connolly, 1995; Goodwin, 1995; NHSE, 1994a).

Nationally, the influence on policies affecting health is carried out mainly through professional organizations, who promote campaigns and publish papers about health related issues. The commonest organizations for health visitors to join are the Health Visitors Association (HVA) or the Royal College of Nursing (RCN). While their policies differ in some important respects, they are both national organizations that are well placed to collaborate with other pressure groups; they provide a forum through which practitioners may comment or campaign without jeopardizing their own position as employees.

The Facilitation of Health-enhancing Activities

The principle of 'facilitation' has implications for the usual orientation of health visiting. It implies and assumes that the kind of 'doing-for' activities which characterize the nursing care of acutely sick or dependent individuals would be unusual in health visiting, which is directed at people who are well. This principle is, perhaps, the one which most clearly illustrates the combination of activities which comprise the 'new public health', as it contains elements of environmental change, of personal preventive activities and of therapeutic endeavour.

Examples of therapeutic endeavour include identifying vulnerable families or children in need of protection, then providing suitable interventions in the form of intensive family visiting (Appleton, 1994, Browne, 1995). The therapeutic effectiveness of health visitors in identifying and responding to postnatal depression is also well established (Holden *et al.*, 1989).

Personal preventive activities have traditionally been promoted using the approach which Twinn (1991) characterizes as 'directive, individual advice-giving', perhaps exhorting parents to stop smoking or bring their children for immunization. While the effectiveness and ethical basis for 'telling people what to do' remain highly questionable, individual, personal support may empower by promoting psychological development (Twinn, 1991; Williams, 1995). The structured visiting approach used with first-time parents living in deprived areas for the Child Development Programme has been shown to be highly effective in ameliorating long-term disadvantage in health (Barker and Anderson, 1988; Barker, 1992).

Fundamentally important to this principle is an acknowledgement of the harmful impact of the unhealthy environments in which many people are obliged to live. Some of the most exciting new approaches in health visiting, and those which are most recognizable as 'public health initiatives', are directed at environmental change. Boyd *et al.* (1993), Packham and Stanton (1994) and SNMAC (1995) all give practical examples to show how seeking the views of local people about what prevents them from engaging in health-enhancing activities can prove fruitful, and help to direct activities towards relevant issues. This may involve practitioners in helping establish campaigns for improvements to street lighting, to play facilities for children or to public transport. Neighbourhood groups may start shopping cooperatives or press the local housing authority to improve their provision for families with young children.

The challenge is to establish a link to health, and to find ways of evaluating these public health and community development projects, as purchasers of the service need to be convinced that investing in such collective approaches will yield clearly measurable health-related benefits. Current health service information systems are unhelpful as they tend to relate only to individuals and single episodes of care (Cowley, 1994).

General practitioners are held to account for achieving measurable targets, but they have no formal responsibility for the health of any member of the public who is not registered on their list. Moreover, they are encouraged to compete with other practices in the local area. Thus, approaches which involve collaboration across a whole community may be viewed as a 'poor investment' for the business of the general practice. This barrier to developing public health initiatives within primary health care may reduce, if it becomes more common for fundholders to contribute to locality-wide purchasing consortia (NHSE, 1994b), instead of focusing solely on the needs of a single practice case list.

There is a debate about the extent to which these three different approaches (environmental change, personal preventive activities and therapeutic endeavour) can all be carried out by the same health visitor, or whether they are best met by a locality, neighbourhood or primary care team that includes practitioners who 'specialize' in particular ways of working. While Billingham (1991) favours the latter approach, the SNMAC (1995) report accepts that there are various ways of achieving the same ends; each area should select the way which suits its own administrative arrangements and needs.

CONCLUSION

This description illustrates how the principles of health visiting link the work to public health. In the current organizational scene, health visitors will only be paid for their work if they can market their services, and demonstrate their effectiveness. It is much easier to demonstrate effective outcomes when dealing with specific disorders, behaviour change and individual clients, as these are all readily accounted and acknowledged in existing health service expectations and information systems. This 'easy focus' contradicts the public health requirement to focus on whole communities as well as individuals, and to maintain a priority attention on promoting health.

However, there is a formal requirement now, which has never existed in the past, for health authorities and general practices to ensure their services are responsive to identified health needs. Health visitors have access to a wealth of information about local health needs, and the public health skills to collate and interpret these data into community, caseload or general practice list profiles. Paradoxically, the apparently threatening imperative for health visitors to market their ability to collate this information, and their service as a whole, offers a powerful opportunity to influence policies affecting health.

Nevertheless, health care contracts provide a means of ensuring close and authoritarian control on day-to-day approaches to practice. Prevention is increasingly formulated in medical terms, and general practitioners are held to account for achieving measurable targets in relation to their own practice list; they have no formal responsibility for wider public health issues.

While the policing of practice by the market orientated NHS creates new pressures and difficulties for practitioners, the associated 'customer' focus provides new solutions, by emphasizing the importance of listening to the views of consumers. Health authorities and general practice fundholders are required to ensure the quality of services they commission, and consumer views are highly regarded in evaluating this. Health visitors are already used to forming informal contracts with their clients, and can show how community based approaches, which begin by seeking opinions from the public they serve, can promote participation and empowerment as a form of health promotion. This is one powerful way of to ensure that future provision is geared to the genuine needs of the population, constructed in a way which is acceptable and helpful to them as consumers.

The shift of community health care into general practitioner led primary care teams may lead some health visitors to feel professionally isolated if they have no immediate peers at their work base, and are directly accountable to the medical practitioners who contract for their services. However, becoming more closely involved in these teams offers health visiting practitioners a new opportunity to extend awareness of public health issues in that situation. By developing practice within the framework of the principles of health visiting, and networking across the different levels of local and national policy, practitioners can continue to make an important and real contribution to the public health.

SUMMARY

- Health visiting developed from the public health movement in the mid nineteenth century. Recent changes to their education and the role and responsibilities expected of health visitors within the 'new NHS' indicate they are returning to these roots and origins.
- The notion of 'public health' is outlined and explained in relation to health visiting, which shares the same holistic, humanistic philosophy and broad, socially based belief in the value of health.
- Parallel developments within the public health and health visiting movements are traced from the start until the 'new public health' emerged in the late 1970s, when health visiting was also entering a period of regeneration.
- The principles of health visiting are used as framework to explain how the entirety of health visiting practice is concerned with public health. Practical examples are offered to illustrate the extent and diversity of the role.
- Some challenges which have recurred since the advent of health visiting are noted. The chapter concludes by noting new opportunities and strengths which health visitors can call upon in finding ways to address these difficulties.

DISCUSSION QUESTIONS

- The ideals of public health suggest that a population-wide focus is necessary to avoid stigmatizing and development of a victim-blaming approach. The ideals of systematic management and care-planning suggest that targeting individuals with identified needs increases clarity and efficiency. Consider some strategies that health visitors might adopt which address the conflicting demands of these two ideals.

- Health visitors have long focused attention on the most disadvantaged sections of society. How might a public health focus be used in the self-empowerment of these groups?

- Draw up a profile of health needs in a particular defined population (e.g. health visiting caseload, geographical area, whole school community or general practice list) and decide which are the most pressing public health issues within it.

- Within a defined locality, identify the names of people, groups and networks through which the influence on policies affecting health can best be achieved. Consider ways of developing these networks and links with the individuals identified.

FURTHER READING

Standing Nursing and Midwifery Advisory Committee (SNMAC) (1995) *Making it Happen. Public Health: The contribution, role and development of Nurses, Midwives and Health Visitors*. Department of Health. London: HMSO.
An influential Department of Health publication which details the background, sets out the basic concepts for public health nursing and offers a multitude of practical examples.

Council for the Education and Training of Health Visitors (CETHV) (1977) *An Investigation into the Principles and Practice of Health Visiting*. London: CETHV.

Twinn S and Cowley S (Eds) (1992) *The Principles of Health Visiting. a Re-examination*. London: United Kingdom Standing Conference/Health Visitors' Association.
The principles of health visiting, and the more recent re-examination of these are encompassed in these two publications.

Gillam S, Plamping D, McClenahan J and Harries J (1994) *Community Orientated Primary Health Care*. London: King's Fund.

Laffrey S and Page G (1989) Primary health care and public health nursing. *Journal of Advanced Nursing* **14**: 1044–50.
Ways of integrating public health principles into primary health care, and the similarities and differences in the concepts, are explored in these two publications.

Davies C (1988) The health visitor as mother's friend: a woman's place in public health, 1900–1914. *Social History of Medicine* **1**(1): 39–59.

Dingwall R (1977) Collectivism, regionalism and feminism: health visiting and British social policy. *Journal of Social Policy* **6**(3): 291–315.
Anyone interested in the social history of the occupation and its links with public health should read these two papers which detail the difficulties faced by the pioneers of the health visiting movement. Many of these problems continue to the present day.

REFERENCES

Abbott P and Sapsford P (1990) Health visiting: Policing the family? In P Abbott and C Wallace (Eds) *The Sociology of the Caring Professions*, pp 120–152, Basingstoke: Falmer Press.

Acheson D (1988) *Public Health in England*. London: HMSO.

Appleton J (1994) The concept of vulnerability in relation to child protection: health visitors' perceptions. *Journal of Advanced Nursing* **20**(6): 1132–1140.

Ashton J and Seymour H (1988) *The New Public Health*. Milton Keynes. Open University Press.

Audit Commission (1994) *Seen but not heard: Co-ordinating community child health and social services for children in need*. London: HMSO.

Barker W (1992) Health visiting: Action research in a controlled environment. *International Journal of Nursing Studies* **29**(3): 251–259.

Barker W and Anderson R (1988) *The child development programme: an evaluation of process and outcome*. Early childhood Development Unit, University of Bristol, Bristol.

Billingham K (1991) Public health and the community. *Health Visitor* **64**(2): 40–43.

Black D (1993) Deprivation and health. *British Medical Journal* **307**: 1630–1631.

Boyd M Brummell K Billingham K and Perkins F (1993) *The Public Health Post at Strelley: An Interim Report*. Nottingham Community Health Trust, Nottingham.

Browne K (1995) Preventing child maltreatment through community nursing. *Journal of Advanced Nursing* **21**(1): 57–63.

Bunton R and Macdonald G (1992) *Health Promotion: Disciplines and Diversity*. London: Routledge.

Cernik K and Wearne M (1992) Using community health profiles to improve service provision. *Health Visitor* **65**(10): 343–345.

Chalmers K (1993) Searching for health needs: the work of health visiting. *Journal of Advanced Nursing* **18**: 900–911.

Connolly M (1995) Commissioning community health services. *Health Visitor* **68**(2): 70–73.

Council for the Education and Training of Health Visitors (CETHV) (1977) *An Investigation into the Principles and Practice of Health Visiting*. London: CETHV.

CETHV (1980) *The Investigation Debate*. London: CETHV.

CETHV (1982) *Principles in Practice*. London: CETHV.

Cowley S (1991) A symbolic awareness context identified through a grounded theory study of health visiting. *Journal of Advanced Nursing* **16**: 648–656.

Cowley S (1994) Counting practice: the impact of information systems on community nursing. *Journal of Nursing Management* **1**: 273–278.

Cowley S (1995) In health visiting, the routine visit is one that has passed. *Journal of Advanced Nursing* **22**(2): 276–284.

Cowley S Bergen A Young K and Kavanagh A (1995) Exploring needs assessment in community nursing. *Health Visitor* **68**(8): 319-321.

Davies C (1988) The health visitor as mother's friend: a woman's place in public health, 1900-1914. *Social History of Medicine* **1**(1): 39-59.

Dingwall R (1977) Collectivism, regionalism and feminism: Health visiting and British social policy. *Journal of Social Policy* **6**(3): 291-315.

Dingwall P and Robinson K (1993) Policing the family? Health visiting and the public surveillance of private behaviour. In A Beattie, M Gott, L Jones and M Sidell *Health and Well-Being: a Reader*. Basingstoke: Macmillan.

Edwards J (1995) Parenting skills: views of community health and social service providers about the needs of their clients *Journal of Social Policy* **24**: 237-259.

Edwards J and Popay J (1994) Contradictions of support and self-help: views from providers of community health and social services to families with young children. *Health and Social Care in the Community* **2**(1): 31-40.

Goodwin S (1992) Community nursing and the new public health. *Health Visitor* **64**(9): 294-296.

Goodwin S (1994) Purchasing effective care for parents and young children. *Health Visitor* **67**(4): 127-129.

Goodwin S (1995) Commissioning for health. *Health Visitor* **68**(1): 16-18.

Gordon P (1991) What and to whom are the responsibilities of nursing service providers and practitioners for patients in the community? In *Nursing in the Community - A Consensus Conference in the South East Thames Region*. London: South East Thames Regional Health Authority.

Lalonde M (1974) *A New Perspective on the Health of Canadians*. Minister of Supply and Services, Information Canada, Ottawa.

McMurray A (1993) *Community Health Nursing: Primary Health Care in Practice*. London: Churchill Livingstone.

Holden J, Sagovsky R and Cox J (1989) Counselling in a general practice setting: controlled study of health visitor intervention in treatment of post-natal depression. *British Medical Journal* **298**: 223-226.

NHS Executive (1994a) *Building a stronger team: the nursing contribution to purchasing*. Leeds: NHS Executive.

NHS Executive (1994b) *Developing NHS Purchasing and GP Fundholding*. London: NHS Executive.

NHS Executive (1994c) *Health Visitor Marketing Report*. London: NHS Executive.

NHSME (1992) *Guidance on the extension of the hospital and community health service element of the GP fundholding scheme from 1st April 1993 (EL [92] 48)*

London. National Health Service Management Executive (NHSME).

NHSME (1993) *New World, New Opportunities*. London: NHSME.

Packham S and Stanton J (1994) Community development approaches to health needs assessment. *Health Visitor* **67**(4): 124-125.

Phillimore P Beattie A and Townsend P (1994) Widening inequality of health in northern England. *British Medical Journal* **308**: 1125-1128.

Robinson J (1982) *An Evaluation of Health Visiting*. London: CETHV.

Robinson K (1992) Knowledge and practice of working in the community. In K Luke and J Orr (Eds) *Health Visiting: Towards Community Health Nursing*, 2nd edn Oxford: Blackwell Scientific Publications, pp 16-42.

Seedhouse D (1986) *Health: The Foundations for Achievement*. Chichester: John Wiley.

Standing Nursing and Midwifery Advisory Committee (SNMAC) (1995) *Making it Happen. Public Health: The contribution, role and development of Nurses, Midwives and Health Visitors*. Department of Health. London: HMSO.

Townsend P Davison N and Whitehead M (1988) *Inequalities in Health: The Black Report and The Health Divide*. Harmondsworth: Penguin.

Twinn S (1991) Conflicting paradigms of health visiting: a continuing debate for professional practice. *Journal of Advanced Nursing* **16**: 966-973.

Twinn S and Cowley S (1992) *The Principles of Health Visiting: A Re-examination*. London: United Kingdom Standing Conference/Health Visitors' Association.

United Kingdom Central Council for Nursing, Midwifery and Health Visiting (UKCC) (1994) *The future of professional practice - the Council's standards for education and practice following registration*. London: UKCC.

Wilkinson R (1994) Divided we fall. *British Medical Journal* **308**: 1113-1134.

Williams J (1995) Education for empowerment: implications for professional development and training in health promotion. *Health Education Journal* **54**(1): 37-47.

World Health Organization (WHO) (1977) *Primary Health Care*. Geneva: WHO.

WHO (1986a) *Ottawa Charter for Health Promotion* WHO Canada reproduced as an Appendix in A Dines and A Cribb (Eds) (1993) *Health Promotion: Concepts and Practice*, pp 205-210. Oxford: Blackwell Scientific Publications

WHO (1986b) *Targets for Health for All*. Copenhagen: WHO.

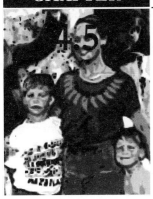

SHIFTING BOUNDARIES IN PAEDIATRIC COMMUNITY NURSING

Jim Richardson

KEY ISSUES

- The focus of care for sick children
- The historical background to paediatric nursing in the community
- Influences on current paediatric nursing practice
- Influences on the education of paediatric nurses
- Forms of organizing child health care in the community
- Means of fostering efficient and effective teamwork between the professionals involved in providing child health care in the community

INTRODUCTION

In recent years there has been an acknowledgement that wherever possible sick children should be cared for within their own homes. Hence the majority of sick children will be cared for by the family supported by primary care and nursing services including the community paediatric nurse. The acutely ill child or the child with very complex nursing needs is likely to receive care from a specialist paediatric community nurse (PCN).

As the focus of care for sick children is firmly rooted in the family it is important for PCNs to identify how roles, responsibilities and relationships within the family have been affected by the child's illness. This needs to be coupled with an assessment of the parents' potential ability to cope with the demands and stresses of caring for their child and the likely impact on siblings. Only when these have been identified, negotiated and acknowledged can areas of responsibility between the parent(s) and the nurse be defined.

A Glimpse at the History of Children's Health Care

Health care for children has evolved as society's conception of children and their rights has developed. It is a relatively recent development that children are recognized as developing, dynamic individuals in their own right. The characteristic needs of children as dependent but growing people are increasingly recognized and these needs translated into rights. Modern thinking about children and their rights is expressed in the United Nations Convention on the Rights of the Child. Although much has been done to ensure that these rights are protected in the United Kingdom, through legislation such as the Children Act (1989), there remains a great deal to be done (Newell, 1991).

Traditionally, until this century, children's care was firmly situated within the family, perhaps with the assistance of lay helpers such as servants. Children were seen for what they were not – they were not adults and were the property of parents to be cared for or disposed of as parents wished. The mortality of children at the turn of the century was enormous with infectious disease being the most lethal. This susceptibility to infection, for which there was no effective treatment, meant that due to fear of contagion children were not welcome in the early hospitals. This, along with a beginning realization of the strong bond between mother and child which could be damagingly disrupted by admission to hospital, meant that early child health care was developed on the basis of the dispensary, an outpatient clinic.

Until relatively recently the poor and vulnerable in society had no assistance or assistance which was so grim that it was to be avoided if at all possible. Large families in the absence of family planning and poor social conditions such as housing, employment and food supply conspired to undermine child health and contributed to enormous child morbidity and mortality. In extreme situations children were seen as expendable and might even be abandoned by parents. This situation led to the establishment of the foundlings' hospitals by religious orders, philanthropic social reformers and charities. Quite naturally these institutions led to the founding of the first children's hospitals. The development of these hospitals was encouraged by the advances in medical understanding of the causes and cures of disease in childhood. It was in the context of the development of these first children's hospitals that the first formal training courses for paediatric nurses were established.

Despite the success of immunization in reducing the effect of some of the infections of childhood the effective treatment of other conditions had to wait for further improvements in social conditions and the general health state of the population along with the development of antibiotics. Since childhood illnesses were often perceived as being a result of contagion, sick children were cared for in quarantine conditions in hospital. Parents were excluded despite the earlier warnings of Armstrong (1767) that: 'if you take a sick child away from the parents or nurse, you break its heart immediately'.

Factors Influencing the Development of Paediatric Nursing

Children's hospitals, as bureaucratic institutions, were rigid in their organization, hierarchy and routines and right into the recent past families were unwelcome guests in the majority of children's wards. The damaging effects on children of separation anxiety superimposed on the natural fear and anxiety caused by illness were not recognized. James and Joyce Robertson in the 1970s were able to illustrate this quite chillingly in their films of withdrawn, frightened but compliant children in hospital wards. Treatment for conditions such as tuberculosis could involve a hospital stay of many months resulting in a very damaging rupture between child and family.

Health care professionals were slow to recognize the value of the full involvement of families in the care of sick children. By the first half of the twentieth century the care of the acutely ill child had been transferred from the family to the doctor and nurse. At this time parents were largely excluded from the hospital setting in which care was provided. This is in sharp contrast to the philosophy underpinning the parent/professional partnership approach in today's care of sick children.

Other important factors in the evolution of the child health services in the UK are changes in the demography and the changing pattern of health in our society. Children in the UK are undoubtedly healthier than ever before but new patterns of ill health are being seen. More children are living with the consequences of chronic illness, genetic disorders and serious injury. Advances in the technology of medicine and nursing are allowing children to live longer with disorders which would have been rapidly lethal even a decade ago. Childhood cancers are a good example of this and very recently children with AIDS related disease have joined this group of children. Health problems related to affluence such as obesity and dental caries are also undermining child health.

When child health is seen as the foundation for future adult health the significance of what seem to be minor deviations in health status in childhood gain in importance (Hall, 1991). The increased pressures of a rapidly changing modern society also have their effect on child and family health and indicators of minor psychological and psychosomatic illness are important predictors of child health. Social and psychological distress are mirrored, for example, in the ever increasing reports of cases of child abuse and neglect.

The availability of paediatric community nursing services has a long history in the UK. The first recorded service was in Rotherham in 1954 (While, 1991). Despite this, progress in expanding such schemes has been slower than might have been expected given the weight placed on community services by successive British governments. As While (1991) points out, although we have seen a 250% increase in home care schemes during the 1980s this still only represents an increase from 7 schemes in 1981 to 23 in 1987.

The damaging psychological effect of separating a sick child from his or her family was highlighted in the Platt Report as long ago as 1959 (DHSS, 1959). The publicity resulting from the publication of this report gave rise to a growing realization by families of the unsuitability of the existing provisions for the care of sick children. In response to this unease the National Association for the Welfare of Sick Children in Hospital (NAWCH) was established. The aims of NAWCH, a pressure group, were summarized in a charter which still expresses the benchmarks of good practice in child and family health care. NAWCH had, and continues to have, a profound affect on paediatric nursing education and practice. From the outset NAWCH stressed that parental involvement should be central to the care of children in hospital: hospitals could no longer merely tolerate parents during very restrictive visiting hours. Gradually facilities began to appear for parents to stay with their child in hospital and parents and health professionals began to define what their respective roles should be in caring for sick children.

Families involved in the care of their sick children have increasingly been expected to articulate and define how that care should be organized and delivered. However, Dearmun's research findings show that there is still a lot of work to be done (Dearmun, 1992). Against this backdrop modern models of paediatric nursing seek to reflect a parent/child/professional relationship. In relation to this Casey (1993) defines the child's health care needs as:

- Family care – the care which satisfies the child's normal everyday needs. This care is normally carried out by the child or family but may be performed by the nurse if the family is not present or is unable to carry it out.
- Nursing care – this satisfies the 'enhanced' care needs often brought about by ill health and may be carried out by nurses while they teach the family how to perform this care. The nurses later provide support and encouragement while the family continues to care.

With the recognition that the optimum place for the care of the acutely ill child is in their own home within the context of the family, the family has to be seen as a potential resource in improving and promoting a child's health and well-being. Health care professionals increasingly realize the effect that child health has on the family and the effect of the family on child health. Paediatric nursing activity is becoming more orientated towards identifying and augmenting families' own strengths and coping strategies in dealing with childhood ill health. Of course, there will be times when families are unable or unwilling to care for their sick child. This response must also be identified and if possible reduced. Families will obviously vary in the degree to which they feel able to undertake care which will satisfy the needs of the sick child. As this ability changes with time and according to circumstances this forms the basis of the negotiation between nurse and family as to who provides what in terms of care for the child. Areas of responsibility may need to be defined or in some instances a transfer of responsibility may be required.

In the past, paediatric nurses, have perhaps been naive, and certainly paternalistic, in 'taking over' responsibility for the care of sick children. Cunningham-Burley and Maclean (1991) have demonstrated in their research the degree to which families', and in particular mothers', efforts form the mainstay of child health care out of sight of the professionals.

Acknowledging this, 'NAWCH' has recently changed its name to Action for Sick Children. This name change they believe, more accurately reflects the move in emphasis from hospital care for childhood illness to care occurring in a range of settings including the child's home.

These trends have resulted in registered sick children's nurses, who had previously tended to work with acutely or chronically sick children in a hospital setting, finding themselves employed more often in community settings. This has exposed the weaknesses in the educational preparation of children's nurses and has fuelled educational innovations.

The contribution which the paediatric nurse can offer to a community child health service is still in the process of being defined. The Royal College of Nursing (RCN) published a guide for general practitioners in 1993 (RCN, 1993a) which outlined the contribution which could be made to community services by health visitors, district nurses, community psychiatric nurses and community learning disabilities nurses. Unfortunately, this otherwise valuable document failed to mention paediatric community nurses at all. A considerable reaction by children's nurses led to the RCN publishing a similar guide to the contribution of paediatric community nurses (RCN, 1993b). This oversight is perhaps indicative of the stage of evolution of paediatric community nursing as a distinct professional group and should not detract from the value of the document which resulted.

The role and function of the paediatric nurse is therefore developing in line with the demands of an evolving service and an increasingly informed consumer group. A central issue which has to be confronted is the part played by the interaction in the relationship between the paediatric nurse, the sick child and the family. Without a clear understanding of respective roles and responsibilities care plans cannot be achieved.

Central characteristics of the role of the paediatric nurse and factors affecting that role were identified in a qualitative research study by Long (1991) (Box 4.5.1.).

These categories and influences were yielded through interviews with registered nurses working in a paediatric area in hospital. It is interesting to speculate what differences might be found in the responses of comparable nurses working in community settings or those of the children and families who are recipients of the

Box 4.5.1. The role of the paediatric nurse

Characteristics

- Advocacy
- Psychological care
- Screening
- Awareness
- Interpersonal skills
- Ethical considerations

Influences

- Problems peculiar to children
- Family dynamics
- Care by the family
- Other workers

services of these nurses. These categories do, however, begin to allow us to examine what paediatric nurses actually do and what their contribution to child health might be. However, a good deal remains to be done in sharpening these definitions but this process will be helped by evaluation of the evolving roles of children's nurses.

Campbell and Clarke (1993) have also identified important elements of the specialist care offered by paediatric nurses (Box 4.5.2).

Influences on the Education of Paediatric Nurses

A major change which is having a profound effect on the role definition of the paediatric nurse is the innovations of the Project 2000 educational reform. Paediatric nurses have had to struggle to maintain their profession's equal status with colleagues qualified in adult nursing. The supplementary register for the Registered Sick Children's Nurse was only included in the terms of the Nurses' Registration Act in 1919 after much heated debate. Again, when the Project 2000 programme was designed there were those who favoured the universal 'generic' adult nurse option as the initial educational qualification with children's nursing being offered as a post-registration course. This argument has been won and paediatric nurses have parity with that of colleagues who have undertaken the other branch programmes.

The important features of the Project 2000 qualification from the point of view of a discussion about the paediatric nurse's contribution to community child health nursing are as follows. The course of study is orientated towards higher education.

Box 4.5.2. Features of paediatric nursing care

- Recognizing the family as the constant in the child's life,
- Facilitating parent–professional collaboration
- Sharing unbiased and complete information with parents
- Providing emotional and (obtaining) financial support
- Recognizing family strengths and individuality
- Understanding developmental and emotional needs of infants, children and adolescents
- Encouraging parent-to-child support
- Assuring that health care is flexible, accessible and responsive to family needs

The skills of identifying appropriate knowledge and synthesizing and defending an informed view are highly valued. In order to strengthen and consolidate the knowledge base of the profession, research skills are promoted. These skills assist the nurse to systematically identify need for nursing care and the best strategies for effectively and efficiently satisfying these. The modern children's nurse should also be an efficient 'consumer' of the research work of others. This will allow the results of valid research to inform the practice of children's nursing.

An initial Common Foundation Programme (CFP) of studies is undertaken by all students seeking registration. This course introduces the student to issues of health and health promotion across the lifespan. The sciences underpinning nursing practice are introduced at this point. The concept of health is central to these studies and is helping the new nurse to adopt a more versatile and flexible approach to what the consumer might be assisted to achieve in terms of their own health. The emphasis in practice placements tends to be on community settings which encourages the student to see people as consumers of health services in the context of their rich and varied lifestyles. This emphasizes the idea that nursing activity is no longer solely concerned with the care of the sick. Health promotion and improvement is for everyone.

The Branch Programme for the children's nursing student consolidates the learning of the CFP and continues the process of identifying and assisting to satisfy health needs both in good and poor health. Central to the ideology of the child branch is the emphasis on the child and family as consumer. The strengths and weaknesses of the family, in the whole constellation of forms in which it occurs, are recognized for their influences on the health of the child and that of the family as a whole. The family is the child's primary carer and its efforts in this task are augmented by paediatric nursing intervention. Of course, regard must be paid to those situations in which the family's situation and responses might be damaging to a child's health and strategies produced for improving this situation.

A significant new feature of nurse education resulting from the Project 2000 pattern is the emphasis placed on community and primary care experience for nursing students. This move is in line with current National Health Service (NHS) policy which seeks to place primary and community health care at the centre of NHS service delivery. Against this background of rapid reorganizations in the way health care is delivered it is important that the nurse is equipped to work in flexible ways and in differing settings. It is desirable that nurses do not simply work with, and adapt to, change but also themselves become the catalyst for change in improving the health of the community. The foundations for such methods of working are laid in the careful use of epidemiological principles such as the identification of health needs of individuals, families and communities.

Through the new curricula for nursing students the concept of culture is being emphasized. This is not simply concern for individuals or groups with exotic or unusual lifestyles or value systems but has been expanded to include issues such as gender, social class, professional group membership, age group and regional origin. As British society is now multicultural, attention must also be focused on the specific needs of children from ethnic minority groups.

In the past some nurses and others may have been inclined to be somewhat resigned to the fact that, for example, poor housing or low income has a damaging effect on people's health. In this context children are particularly vulnerable to such disadvantage. But community nurses, social workers and other groups are beginning to find new and creative ways to help mitigate some of these damaging factors.

Emphasis is being placed on working with colleagues in other professional groups in order to produce the most versatile responses to improve health. In this context nurses are becoming stronger and more confident in the knowledge of the contribution they can make. Working in collaboration with others, key objectives and action plans can be jointly determined. Through the application of health needs assessment it is clear that the professionals, indeed the individual professional, who is in the best position to make an effective contribution to care, can be identified. The paediatric community nurse brings to this situation the skills of identifying needs not simply of a child but also of the family. Learning disability nurses have pioneered a form of service where a key worker coordinates the activities of health and social welfare professionals very effectively.

New developments in post-registration education promise to increase the opportunities for nurses to improve their skills and expertise in community settings. The UKCC Post-registration Education and Practice proposal, when implemented, could improve educational support for paediatric nurses as programmes of clinical support and supervision should be in place (see Chapter 3.1).

It is generally recognized that in order to function effectively the paediatric community nurse requires educational preparation not simply in the area of paediatric nursing but also in the specialist field of community care. Until now the provision for this specialist education has been very variable. Paediatric nurses had to be registered as general nurses in order to gain access to a course leading to a community qualification such as district nursing and health visiting. Once admitted to these courses the students often found that scant regard was paid in the curriculum to the needs of the future community paediatric nurse (Whiting, 1994). Fortunately, new more applied and appropriate courses are being developed (Gastrell, 1993) but at the time of writing these remain the exception. This perhaps explains Whiting's (1989) research findings that 51.1% of the paediatric nurses working in the community at the time that the research was conducted, held a recognized district nursing qualification whilst 8.9% were health visitors. This situation needs to be urgently addressed if we are to achieve a highly qualified paediatric nurse workforce with recognized qualifications capable of producing the creative and flexible service required by families both in hospital and community settings. The proper use of appropriately skilled health professionals will also meet current demands for the best use of finite resources.

Factors Influencing Consumer Expectations of Paediatric Nursing

The importance of strong, flexible educational pathways will be appreciated when we consider that the continued expansion of paediatric community nursing provision will presumably be dependent on a parallel disinvestment in institutional hospital paediatric services. This will leave a group of traditionally prepared RSCNs who will require further education in order to allow them to move towards employment in community settings.

Philosophies underpinning health care provision for children and their families have proliferated since the 1950s. This is reflected in the large number of reports and guidance documents which have been published. The Department of Health's guide, *Welfare of Children and Young People in Hospital* (Department of Health, 1991), summarizes and confirms many of the recommendations of the Platt Report (Department of Health and Social Security, 1959) and the Court Report (Department of Health, 1976). This document provides guidelines for good practice in paediatric hospital care and was intended to define minimum standards for purchasers and providers of child health services. These included an unequivocal commitment to the ideal of children being cared for by an appropriately qualified paediatric nurse workforce. Unfortunately, these are merely guidelines and as such not mandatory standards. Indeed, the fact that these standards for child health care are not being consistently applied is pointed out by the Audit Commission's report on children's health services (Audit Commission, 1993).

Since these documents represent standards for good practice in the hospital care of children and their families it would make good sense to apply similar standards to community child health care. In fact, a parallel document to the *Welfare of Children and Young People in Hospital* which would address community health services for children was announced in 1991 but is still not published in 1994. The Audit Commission (1994) has addressed the coordination of community child health and social service provision for children and found a similar range of deficiencies to those found in the hospital setting.

While these reports are undoubtedly valuable they all share the tendency to perpetuate the divide between 'sick' children and 'well' children. There is an argument for beginning to consider health services for children as a whole which would address the promotion, safeguarding and improvement of the health of *all* children in our community. In relation to this the organization 'Caring for Children in the Health Services' has published an influential document, *Bridging the Gaps*, which describes a study that examined ways to improve the bridge between primary and secondary child health services (Thornes, 1993). The principles and standards outlined in this study indicate means by which a more integrated child health service might be achieved. If implemented these proposals would go some way towards removing the artificial boundaries between primary and secondary child health service and will assist in the process of shifting the focus from hospital provided services towards care offered in the primary, community setting.

The British Paediatric Association (BPA) has also produced a series of papers outlining the tasks, and suggesting means of tackling these in order to achieve an ideal community child health service (BPA, 1992a). Proposals for clear directions for the integration of child health services were outlined in BPA (1991) and examples of innovative projects working to achieve integrated services in BPA (1992b). These documents are important because they define the range of frameworks within which paediatric community nurses may find themselves working.

One of the major issues to be broached in the process of encouraging the growth of community child health nursing services is that of convincing purchasers of health of the value and utility of such a service. Numerous studies have evaluated the benefit for children and families of avoiding hospital admission where possible (Atwell and Gow, 1985; Campbell *et al.*, 1988, While and Wilcox, 1994). With the current emphasis on day surgical treatment as an effective option in the care of children, attention must be paid to the fact the such a service cannot be expected to operate efficiently and to the satisfaction of consumers without a community paediatric nursing service (Thornes, 1991). NAWCH/Action for Sick Children have defined a range of standards of child health care which are useful in outlining for commissioners of health care the minimum standards which can be expected of health care providers.

Paediatric community nurses themselves have an important task in clarifying the value of their own contribution to the health care provision offered in the community. One aspect of this task will be in carefully defining what their role and function actually is. It is essential that it is clearly indicated how this will complement and enhance the functions of the other major professional nursing groups working in community child health: health visitors and school nurses. These professional groups have clearly defined roles and it will be important in the first instance to avoid role disputes and territoriality between professionals. The Project 2000 diplomate paediatric/child health nurses are an entirely new professional group and time will be required to identify the place and means of achieving their optimal contribution to child health care both in the community and in hospital. This process will require time, patience and much open, frank debate between professionals both at a national and a local level (Richardson and Edwards, 1993).

Forms of Organization of Paediatric Community Nursing Services

With an increased focus on community health service provision and the rise in importance of services tailored to meet local needs, greater variability in the format and composition of services will be inevitable. The multidisciplinary team of health and social welfare professionals should provide services for each individual family which are led and implemented by whoever is perceived as having the best fit of professional skills and judgement most suited to the demands of the situation. This means that the needs of the child and family should determine the focus of nursing activity. This sort of thinking is supported by the scenario painted by a group of nursing leaders in a recent discussion document, the 'Heathrow debate' (Department of Health, 1993). This paper suggests that in order to provide optimal health services there should be a considerable blurring of boundaries between professionals.

> In reality, there is likely to be a reallocation of tasks between nurses and others, including other professionals. (DOH, 1993: 12)

This argument strengthens the case for greater flexibility, creativity and increased professional cooperation and collaboration to find and implement the forms of health service most suited to the consumers.

There are currently several models suggested for the provision of paediatric community nursing. All are worthy of consideration and in their own way have something to offer.

Outreach

This model provides home nursing services by hospital based nursing personnel. This form of care organization tends to focus on acute illness and allows for the provision of highly technical expert care. This form of provision may be most appropriate for children with complex medical and nursing needs. A drawback of this form of service as it is currently practised is that the nurses offering such care are often not qualified as community health nurses and hence may be tempted to try to reproduce a hospital environment in a community setting.

Inreach

Primary care based professionals might assume responsibility for ensuring consistency of care for the chronically ill or disabled child and their family during short-term hospital admissions. Emphasis would lie on supporting the family to continue to perform the caring role and on educating hospital personnel with regard to the child's, and family's particular needs. This form of care organization is commonly seen in continuity of care programmes in midwifery practice.

Paediatric Community Nursing Teams

Groups of nurses qualified in both paediatric nursing and community health nursing might provide care in settings where there are large numbers of children requiring nursing care at home such as in urban areas (Gow and Ridgway, 1993).

- Specialist paediatric nurse in a generic community health team – this model may be expected to become more popular as the team approach to providing health care for discrete populations becomes more general. Paediatric community nurses may find a role in existing primary health care teams as skill mix innovations are explored.
- Child health nurse as practice nurse – the increasing emphasis on general practitioner led primary care may offer opportunities for paediatric community nurses to demonstrate their skills in particular circumstances.

These options represent only a few of the organizational options which might be used. Creativity and ingenuity will no doubt produce local solutions to local needs which will be variations on these themes.

A number of highly specialized community paediatric nurses, such as community paediatric oncology nurses, paediatric diabetic nurses, cystic fibrosis nurses, asthma nurses are already in post. They have an important contribution to make but in some instances their activities have been disjointed. However, the growing influence of fund holding general practitioners as purchasers of health care may influence the way such roles are absorbed within primary care settings. In this context children's nurses themselves have an important role to play in ensuring that commissioners of health care are aware of the health gains made possible by the professional activities of children's nurses. To do this they will need to clearly articulate their contribution to care.

CONCLUSION

This chapter has discussed a range of issues which are affecting the provision of community child health services. As has been seen, the situation is characterized by dynamic change. Children's nurses will have to work with professional colleagues, not simply to adapt to this change but also to be themselves agents of positive change. Child and family health can only be improved in partnership with parents who are, after all, the main carers of children. The skills required by paediatric community nurses, if they are to practise at a specialist level, require high quality education and preparation for the task. Children should be admitted to hospital only if the care they require cannot be provided at home (RCN, 1993b).

SUMMARY

- As the focus of care for sick children is rooted in the family it is important for paediatric community nurses to identify how roles and responsibilities within the family have been affected by the child's illness.
- The facilitation of parent/professional collaboration in the care of the sick child is essential.
- Health care has evolved and is evolving against a backdrop of societal awareness of the 'needs and rights of children'.
- Families involved in the care of sick children are usually articulate and expect to define how they would like 'care' to be organized and delivered.

■ New developments in pre- and post-registration programmes of education for nurses looks set to improve specialist educational support for paediatric community nurses.

■ Suggested models for the provision and organization of paediatric community nurses are discussed, albeit briefly. These suggested models provide food for thought as to how this specialist branch of community nursing can best be organized and delivered.

DISCUSSION QUESTIONS

◆ What cultural, social and ethnic factors would you need to consider when negotiating family centred care of the sick child at home?

◆ When planning the care of a sick child at home, describe ways in which the application of a particular perspective would contribute to your plan.

◆ How might paediatric community nurses seek to influence the commissioning of locally based community nursing services?

◆ Based on your knowledge of your local community spend some time considering a model of organizing paediatric community nursing services which might satisfy local needs. Try to define those groups of children and families who would use this service and how their access to the service could be made as easy as possible. What kind of links would your proposed service need to make with other health and social care professionals and providers of, e.g. hospital services? With what other professionals and agencies might community paediatric nurses work to improve child health and welfare in the area?

Glossary

In this chapter the terms 'paediatric nurse', 'children's nurse' and 'child health nurse' have been used interchangeably. These all relate to first-level registered children's nurses; they can be regarded as synonyms. Some feel that the title paediatric relates to a more traditional RSCN role while child health nurse describes a more modern, versatile role.

FURTHER READING

Baggot R (1994) *Health and Health Care in Britain*. London: Macmillan.
A topical description of the system of health care provision in the UK today as well as an analysis of current changes to that system and their likely effects.

Jones A and Bilton K (1994) *The Future Shape of Children's Services*. London: National Children's Bureau.

A proposal for child and family centred multidisciplinary, inter-agency approach to child health, social welfare and educational services.

Ottewill R and Wall A (1990) *The Growth and Development of the Community Health Services*. Sunderland: Business Education Publishers.
An interesting and detailed account of the develop-

ment, functions and objectives of the widest range of community health services.

Ovretveit J (1993) *Coordinating Community Care: Multidisciplinary Teams and Care Management.* Buckingham: Open University Press.
A very detailed, challenging analysis of the range of team work possibilities in community health care.

Pickin C and St Leger S (1993) *Assessing Health Need using the Life Cycle Framework.* Buckingham: Open University Press.
The basic ideas of health assessment and epidemiological method are introduced in this text which also examines areas of health need typical of each life stage.

Soothill K, Mackay L and Webb C (1995) *Interprofessional Relations in Health Care.* London: Edward Arnold.
Interprofessional relations in health care examined from a range of perspectives. Topical and sometimes provocative.

Stanhope M and Lancaster J (1992) *Community Health Nursing: Process and Practice for Promoting Health*, 3rd edn. London: Mosby Year Book
Although North American, this exhaustive and authoritative text introduces and discusses a vast range of the important issues in primary health care nursing. The focus is firmly on health promotion.

REFERENCES

Armstrong G (1767) *An essay on the diseases most fatal to infants.* Cited in Miles, I (1986) The Emergence of Sick Children's Nursing. Part 2. *Nurse Education Today* 6: 133-138.

Atwell JD and Gow P (1985) Paediatric trained district nurse in the community: expensive luxury or economic necessity? *British Medical Journal* **291:** 227-229.

Audit Commission (1993) *Children First: A Study of Hospital Services.* London: Audit Commission.

Audit Commission (1994) *Seen but not Heard: Co-ordinating Community Child Health and Social Services for Children in Need. Detailed Evidence and Guidelines for Managers and Practitioners.* London: Audit Commission.

Barlow S and Swanwick M (1994) Supplementary benefits. *Paediatric Nursing* **6**(3): 16-17.

British Paediatric Association (1991) *Towards a Combined Child Health Service.* London: British Paediatric Association.

British Paediatric Association (1992a) *Community Child Health Services: an information base for purchasers.* London: British Paediatric Association.

British Paediatric Association (1992b) *Management Models in Established Combined or Integrated Child Health Services.* London: British Paediatric Association.

Campbell S and Clarke F (1993) *The ethos of paediatric intensive care.* In B Carter (Ed) (1993) *Manual of Paediatric Intensive Care.* London: Chapman & Hall.

Campbell IR, Scaife JM and Johnstone JMS (1988) Psychological effects of day case surgery compared with inpatient surgery. *Archives of Disease in Childhood* **63:** 415-417.

Casey A (1993) *Development and Use of the Partnership Model of Nursing Care.* In EA Glasper and A Tucker (Eds) *Advances in Child Health Care.* London: Scutari Press.

Cunningham-Burley S and Maclean U (1991) *Dealing with children's illness: mothers' dilemmas.* In S Wyke and J

Hewison (Eds) (1991) *Child Health Matters.* Buckingham: Open University Press.

Dearmun A (1992) Perceptions of parental participation. *Paediatric Nursing*, **4** (7): 6-9.

Department of Health and Social Security (1959) *The Welfare of Children in Hospital: Report of the Platt Committee.* London: HMSO.

Department of Health (1976) *Fit for the Future: Report of the Court Committee on Child Health Services.* London: HMSO.

Department of Health (1991) *Welfare of Children and Young People in Hospital.* London: HMSO.

Department of Health (1993) *The Challenges for Nursing and Midwifery in the 21st Century: the Heathrow Debate.* London: Department of Health.

Elfer P and Gatiss S (1990) *Charting Child Health Services: a Survey of Community Child Health Services provided by Health Authorities in England, Scotland and Wales.* London: National Children's Bureau.

Gastrell P (1993) Diploma courses for PDNs. *Paediatric Nursing* **5**(10): 13-14.

Gottlieb B (1993) *The Family in the Western World.* Oxford: Oxford University Press.

Gow P and Ridgeway G (1993) *The Development of a Paediatric Community Service.* In EA Glasper and A Tucker (1993) (Eds) *Advances in Child Health Nursing.* London: Scutari Press.

Hall DMB (Ed) (1991) *Health for all Children*, 2nd edn. Oxford: Oxford Medical Publications.

Hendrick J (1993) *Child Care Law for Health Care Professionals.* Oxford: Radcliffe Medical Press.

Kurtz Z (Ed) (1992) *With Health in Mind: mental health care for children and young people.* London: Action for Sick Children in association with South West Thames Regional Health Authority.

Long T (1991) Towards a definition of children's nursing. *Paediatric Nursing*, November, 12-15.

National Association for the Welfare of Children in Hospital (1984) *Charter for children in hospital*. London: NAWCH.

Newell P (1991) *The United Nations Convention and Children's Rights in the United Kingdom*. London: National Children's Bureau.

Phillips T (1994) *Children and Power*. In B Lindsay (Ed) *The Child and Family: contemporary nursing issues in child health and care*. Baillière Tindall: London.

Richardson J and Edwards J (1993) Integrating services in community child care. *Nursing Standard* **8**(7): 32-35.

Royal College of Nursing (1993a) *Buying Community Nursing: a Guide for GPs*. London: Royal College of Nursing.

Royal College of Nursing (1993b) *Buying Paediatric Community Nursing: an RCN Guide for Purchasers and Commissioners of Health Care*. London: Royal College of Nursing.

Shaw I and Shaw G (1993) Demography, nursing and community care: a review of the evidence. *Journal of Advanced Nursing* **18**: 1212-1218.

Thornes R (1991) *Just for the Day: Children admitted to Hospital for Day Treatment*. London: National Association for the Welfare of Children in Hospital (on behalf of Caring for Children in the Health Services).

Thornes R (1993) *Bridging the Gaps*. London: Action for Sick Children (on behalf of Caring for Children in the Health Services).

United Nations (1990) *The Convention on the Rights of the Child*. Geneva: United Nations. (Available through HMSO)

While AE (1991) An evaluation of a paediatric home care scheme. *Journal of Advanced Nursing* **16**: 1413-1421.

While AE and Barriball KL (1993) School nursing: history, present practice and possibilities reviewed. *Journal of Advanced Nursing* **18**: 1202-1211.

While AE and Wilcox VK (1994) Paediatric day surgery: day-case unit admission compared with general paediatric ward admission. *Journal of Advanced Nursing* **19**: 52-57.

Whiting M (1989) Home truths. *Nursing Times* **85**(14): 74.

Whiting M (1994) Meeting needs: RSCNs in the community. *Paediatric Nursing* **6**(1): 9-11.

Woodroffe C, Glickman M, Barker M and Power C (1993) *Children, Teenagers and Health: the Key Data*. Buckingham: Open University Press.

World Health Organization (1985) *Targets for Health for All: targets in support of the European regional strategy for health for all*. Copenhagen: World Health Organization, Regional Office for Europe.

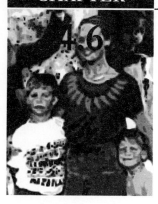

THE NURSE PRACTITIONER IN THE COMMUNITY

Mark Jones

KEY ISSUES

- What factors led to the development of the nurse practitioner role in the United States and in the United Kingdom?

- How is the role of the nurse practitioner defined?

- How does a nurse become a nurse practitioner?

- How do nurse practitioners improve quality of care?

- What are the future opportunities and threats for the nurse practitioner?

INTRODUCTION

Health Care Change and Innovative Practice

The final decade of the twentieth century will be remembered as a time of rapid change of health care systems on a global scale, as nations seek to find an answer to the seemingly impossible question of providing a universal, comprehensive, and cost-effective health care service to all their citizens. This quest brings a number of differing solutions, and perhaps the changes occurring either side of the Atlantic are among the best examples of alternative means being pursued in order to achieve this ideal.

Since the introduction of the health care 'reforms' of the early 1990s, the UK health care system has moved steadily towards a 'managed market' form of health care, epitomized in the so-called 'purchaser–provider' split, with provider units, be they hospitals, community trusts, ambulance services, or whatever, competing for business as purchasing authorities, who in turn are altering their guise almost daily, strive to find the most cost-effective option for health care provision.

Five thousand miles away, the United States struggles with the desire to bring every citizen into a universal health care system, through a combined strategy of Federal legislation requiring employer financed health insurance, and an increased involvement from central government through enhanced state subsidies to health care programmes providing for the elderly and poor - Medicare and Medicaid. It seems strange that in America today there is the strongest push ever from Federal government to provide for universal health care through central control (White House Domestic Policy Council, 1993), when the UK system is moving away from principles of socialized medicine to those of letting the market decide and provide.

Additional complexity to these changes in health care is added when we consider the move away from emphasis on high dependency acute hospital care as the epitome of a modern health care service. The developments following the Tomlinson Report (1992) on health services in London, whereby long established large teaching hospitals are closing, and a new realization of the importance of public health and primary health care represent a whole new focus on priority provision of health services in the UK.

These issues are discussed in detail elsewhere in this text. Suffice to say this brief account demonstrates the level of change and potential for turmoil which exists within the health care field today. This turmoil and change of priority does, however, provide great opportunity for innovation. Today we seek innovation in the development of new means of health care delivery to individuals, groups and communities. The development of the nurse practitioner role is such an innovation.

Nurse Practitioner Development – the US Context

1960s America is widely recognized as the birthplace of the nurse practitioner movement and development of the role is well documented by the early pioneers – Ford *et al.* (1966), Ford and Silver (1967), Lewis and Resnick (1967). Loretta Ford, in particular, spearheaded development of the role, and through her efforts the first nurse practitioner educational programme was devised at the University of Colorado, Denver, in 1965. This programme was only 16 weeks long and oriented toward paediatric practice, but nevertheless provided the springboard for the nurse practitioner movement across all areas of health care.

Innovation usually arises from a need for change in order to address a problem. The beginnings of the US nurse practitioner can be traced back to a time of change and refocused priority on part of the American population, the nursing profession, and the health care system (Leff, 1978; O'Hara Devereaux, 1991).

Changing Demand

In 1960s America, health care consumers were calling for accessible, affordable, and sensitive health care (Jolly, 1992), with renewed emphasis on the promotion of health in addition to the treatment of illness (Bennet, 1984; O'Hara Devereaux, 1991). Spurred on by changing morbidity patterns with more people dying of preventable disease, the US health care system was already beginning to fear the escalation in costs associated with a concentration on 'hi-tec' medicine (Trnobranski, 1994).

The combination of excessive cost and new modes of delivery being considered, gave an ideal opportunity for the development of the nurse practitioner role. Particularly suitable settings for development were those where access to health care was difficult, either due to geographical location, or as a result of poor provision. Trnobranski (1994) sees the latter point as being especially relevant, again reflecting the financial dynamics of US health care, in that doctors chose not to set up business in poor communities (generally rural and inner city) as profit maximization potential was lacking. As a result, the early nurse practitioner role was created to enable the extension of the provision of medical care, as provided by doctors in other areas, to underserved communities. To do this, nurse practitioners began to be trained in diagnosis, prescription of treatment, and the performance of some medical tasks. For some nurse opinion leaders of the time this was seen as a retrograde step, undermining the nature of nursing (Skeet, 1978; Reeder and Mauksh, 1979), whereas others saw this is a legitimate extension of the nursing role (Shamansky, 1985).

In addition to changing perception of health care need amongst the American public, the nursing profession was also keen to grasp the opportunity of a move away from the dominance of the medical model to a broader view of primary health care emphasizing prevention in addition to cure. Jolly (1992) indicates this was a major step for US nursing. For the profession to gain from these changes in attitude they had to challenge the medical establishment. Jolly believes that the rapidly developing women's movement, with an exhortation of feminist principles and collective effort for better economic reward for women through the creation of new professional roles, gave nurses the encouragement they needed to become aware of the need to move from a position of being undervalued and lacking in autonomy, in order to grasp the opportunity of meeting the new health care challenges through the provision of comprehensive nursing care.

So, from an historical position of change in attitude toward health, and health care, the US nurse practitioner found a niche in the market, beginning with child health, which today has expanded into every conceivable specialty. In 34 of the 50 American states the concept of advanced nurse practitioner is enshrined in state legislation, and nurse practitioners exist in all the others (Pearson, 1994). As we will consider later, American nurse practitioners have proved themselves to be able to deliver high quality care of at least the same standard as a medical practitioner, whilst still practising in a nursing context, and what is more, their work is seen to be cost-effective (McGrath, 1990; Brown and Grimes, 1992).

In the USA nurse practitioners have arrived, staked out their territory, and are most definitely here to stay.

Nurse Practitioner Development – the UK Context

The concept of nurse practitioner was first recognized in the UK in the early 1980s as the work of two pioneers, Barbara Stilwell and Barbara Burke-Masters, and came to be discussed in the nursing press (Stilwell, 1984; Gaze, 1985). In general terms, it is possible to draw some parallels between US events and their emerging roles.

In her inner city practice in Birmingham, Stilwell offered an alternative, yet complementary, service to that of the general medical practitioner. She would see patients with undifferentiated diagnoses, irrespective of the ailment, undertake a health screening programme using a physical examination technique, with the provision of health education and counselling at every consultation (Stilwell, 1984).

Burke-Masters' early work was different in that she worked outside of a practice setting, among the homeless of inner-city London. She adopted a more medically oriented model in her approach, giving advice and 'prescribing' a wide range of drugs including antibiotics and tranquillizers, whilst referring directly to local medical consultants (Gaze, 1985; Burke-Masters, 1986).

In a similar way to US doctors deciding not to set up practice in poorer rural and inner city areas, Lewis and Wessely (1992) suggest, in a variation of Tudor Hart's 'inverse care law' (1971), that the more common the condition, or the less interesting the complaint, the less the professional interest from doctors. The motivator is different, but the resulting distribution of medical care is similar – more sparse and lower quality care in poorer areas.

Also, just as the USA experienced a paradigmatic shift from emphasis on acute to primary health care, Jordan (1993) suggests from a review of contemporary health policy literature, that as the UK moved into the 1980s the medical profession became increasingly unable to fill the gap in dealing with chronic disease and health promotion, and other health care professionals, notably nurses, began to claim this ground. Fawcett-Henesy (1990) continues this theme, suggesting that in the UK over the past twenty years there has been a virtual revolution in the way people wish to direct their own lives which is now permeating health care. The result is that people are now asking why it is that medical dominance exists when for most of human history the management of sickness, health, childbirth, child development, old age and death has been a matter for individuals and the communities in which they live without the imposition of some 'biomechanical rationale' (Fawcett-Henesy, 1990: 35).

The work of Stilwell and Burke-Masters reflected these issues, confirming Trnobranski's opinion (1994) that nurse practitioner development arises from the key prerequisites of deficit in provision, lack of appropriately qualified medical practitioners, and change in patient opinion concerning the health care they require.

Both Stilwell and Burke-Masters, through an extension of their nursing practice, sought to fill the gaps and claim the opportunity offered by the lack of a flexible, patient centred, health oriented service. The examples given by these practitioners, and emerging evidence from the USA, began to generate debate concerning the nurse practitioner role in the UK, to the extent that government reports recognized the benefit of such a development. In 1986, the report of the community nursing review group headed up by Julia Cumberlege, firmly supported the idea of an autonomous nurse practitioner practising with a range of advanced skills in order to bring a wider range of health care opportunity to the community (*Neighbourhood Nursing – A Focus for Care*: 1986).

Following on from this, in its evidence to the UK Health Departments' consultation on primary health care, the Royal College of Nursing identified three essential aspects of nursing provision:

- There should be direct access to nursing care for whoever chooses it, with services offered directly to people.
- Nursing assessment of patient problems should be available, using existing and extended skill, with provision of programmes of care and treatment which offer help in maintaining health and coping with illness.
- An autonomous nursing service which encompasses responsibility for accepting and discharging, and in some cases referring patients to other agents. (RCN, 1987).

These attributes built upon the principles developed within the nurse practitioner roles of Stilwell and Burke-Masters, and the evolution of the role was endorsed by the government in the subsequent primary care White Paper *Promoting Better Health* (DHSS, 1987), and later through the definition of the primary health care nurse as set out in the *New World New Opportunities* document (NHSME, 1993: 12 para. 3.6).

As in the USA, changes in health care need, perceptions of service required, and issues of access, can thus be seen as the stimulant for nurse practitioner development in the UK, albeit some twenty years later. The UK nurse practitioner role is now on the ascendancy, driven by our pioneers, experience from the USA, and government support. Nurse practitioners can be found in many areas including Accident and Emergency Departments, working in specific night duty roles, and working in surgical firms of general hospitals (Lowry, 1993; Dillner, 1993) although the main emphasis is in the primary health care setting (Iazzatti, 1992; Young and Perkin, 1993; Lindeke, 1993).

The work of Stilwell and Burke-Masters no doubt played a key part in UK nurse practitioner development. Unfortunately the latter's activity was rapidly curtailed as her 'prescribing' incurred the wrath of the British Pharmaceutical Society, who threatened to take legal action against her for dispensing prescription only medicines (Gaze, 1985). Stilwell, however, continued to develop her practice and went on to develop the first UK nurse practitioner programme at the Royal College of Nursing. The first course ran in 1990 with twenty students, and by 1994 some 300 students were registered.

What Makes a Nurse Practitioner? Towards a Role Definition

A UK Definition

The RCN Institute of Advanced Nurse Education (IANE) sees the nurse practitioner in primary health care as offering a complementary service to that of the general medical practitioner, offering 'direct access to clients seeking health care', and being able to 'undertake clinical assessments of any health problems likely to be encountered' and 'initiate treatment falling within her range of knowledge and skills'. The nurse practitioner also performs a similar gatekeeping role to the general medical practitioner demonstrated by the ability to 'admit people to the primary health care system, both by offering initial treatment herself, and by referral to others, including physicians' (RCN IANE, 1989).

The IANE definition goes on to describe the nurse practitioner as someone who:

- makes professionally autonomous decisions, for which she has sole responsibility;
- receives clients with undifferentiated and undiagnosed problems, diagnoses and prescribes treatment;
- screens clients for disease risk factors and early signs of illness;
- develops with the client an ongoing plan for health with an emphasis on preventative measures;
- provides counselling and health education.

Aside from these role descriptors, the definition also cites 'essential personal prerequisites for a nurse practitioner'. These include:

- professional confidence and self-awareness;
- a knowledge base of sufficient breadth and depth to form the basis of informed decision-making;
- a repertoire of skills which embraces those within physical, psychological, and social domains, especially diagnosing, prescribing, counselling and health promotion. (RCN IANE, 1989).

These descriptions are representative of a comprehensive and advanced nursing role, especially so far as physical assessment and diagnosis are concerned. However, it is the question of how these skills are obtained and demonstrated which now seems to cause most interest. Can one become a nurse practitioner gradually, or only after a de facto course providing all of the above attributes?

The previous analysis has indicated that in both the UK and USA, the nurse practitioner concept developed incrementally and opportunistically in times of change, although throughout its history many within the nursing profession have alleged that there is nothing particularly special about the nurse practitioner role, as any nurse could demonstrate such role expansion given time and experience. In the UK, the United Kingdom Central Council for Nursing, Midwifery and Health Visiting (UKCC) has gone as far as to say that the term nurse practitioner is 'ambiguous and misleading' and that it should not be used (UKCC, 1993). So what are the problems with role definition?

Incrementalism and Acquired Knowledge Versus Prerequisite Education

A key area of contention arises from the incremental nature of nurse practitioner development, with nurses pushing back the boundaries to their practice as need and opportunity dictated. As discussed, there were no formal courses in the USA until 1965, and even then they were very short in duration and limited in academic content. Similarly, in the UK, the first recognized course appeared only in 1990, yet the likes of Stilwell and Burke-Masters claimed the nurse practitioner title some years before.

Nurses have had the ability to extend their roles in order to provide a wider range of care, long before the term 'nurse practitioner' was used. In 1977 the Department of Health and Social Security issued a guidance letter in the names of the Chief Nursing Officer and Chief Medical Officer, endorsing the ability of nurses to accept delegated tasks from medical practitioners (Friend and Yellowlees, 1977), provided that they and the doctor concerned were sure that they were sufficiently competent to accept that delegation. Using this guidance, nurses could essentially purloin parts of medicine to add new skills to their existing repertoire (Robinson, 1993). As Davis (1992) indicates, the concept of role extension operated under the implied authority of a medical practitioner. This would seem to differ little from the position of the nurse practitioner pioneers in the USA who simply acted as an extension to the physician's ability to care for people in remote communities, and acquired the necessary medical knowledge on an ad hoc basis (O'Hara Devereaux, 1991).

Role Extension and Role Expansion

In order to overcome the criticism that role extension just means practising medical tasks under delegated authority of a medical practitioner, the nursing profession changed the terminology and sought to redefine the scope of practice speaking in terms of 'role expansion'. Robinson (1993) indicates that role expansion differs from role extension, in that it recognizes the true role of nursing as a separate therapeutic activity. The expansion theme was seen by nurses, and leaders of the profession as a means of developing a wider range of skills and ability without deference to the medical profession. In his text *Nursing Power and Politics* (1987) Trevor Clay, the then General Secretary of the Royal College of Nursing, explained that the 'expanded role is about holism', and that nurses can legitimately expand their role in order to meet the wider needs of patients rather than simply taking on medical tasks.

Defining the Scope of Practice

In 1992, the UKCC brought the concept of the expanded role into 'official' usage, through the publication of its *Scope of Professional Practice*. The *Scope* document is a radical text, in that it allows individual nurses to expand their role in whatever direction they see fit, acquiring skills from medicine, or anywhere else for that matter, provided that the nurse can rationalize the expansion as enhancing the delivery of nursing care, and is prepared to accept individual accountability for any actions undertaken within this context. It is interesting to note, however, that whilst it may be an accepted principle that safe practice cannot be assured as roles expand, unless there is a sound educational framework underpinning that expansion (Trnobranski, 1994), as with the extended role concept before it, the UKCC does not insist that nurses must attend courses to prepare them for such expansion, but relies on the ability of the individual to gauge their level of competence and seek to address any deficit. Given the UKCC's belief that the term nurse practitioner is ambiguous anyway this is an important point for nurse practitioner development, as any nurse could technically claim competency in the skills required to practise at this level.

Nurse Practitioner Practice Requires Specific Educational Provision

Against the incrementalist view toward nurse practitioner practice is that which sees nurse 'practitionering' as so complex in its incorporation of medical skills with excellence in nursing ability, that a specific preparation is required, and that it is not just the possession of skills but rather the way they are brought together and utilized which is the issue. Shamansky (1985) identifies the first attempt at defining the nurse practitioner by way of knowledge base acquired from a specific preparation, as that made by the US Department of Health, Education, and Welfare (albeit drafted by the American Nurses Association):

The nurse practitioner is:

A registered nurse who has successfully completed a formal program of study designed to prepare registered nurses to delivery primary health care including the ability to:

(a) assess the health status of individuals and families through health and medical history taking, physical examination, and defining of health and developmental problems;

(b) institute and provide continuity of health care to clients;

(c) provide instruction and counselling to individuals, families and groups;

(d) work in collaboration with our other health care providers and agencies.

(US Department of Health, Education, and Welfare (USDHEW), 1976: 3552-3556).

In the UK, the first definition of nurse practitioner practice emanated from the RCN IANE, again citing the need for specific educational provision:

The Nurse Practitioner requires an advanced comprehensive programme of education and training in theory and practice, which incorporates experience of dealing with clients under the guidance and mentorship of preceptors, and assessment of competence in key areas of the nurse practitioner role. (RCN IANE, 1989).

Resolving the Dilemma

The arguments for nurse practitioner preparation consisting of a specific course of study, generally centre around the fact that on the one hand basic nurse education programmes are lacking in the subject areas needed for this type of advanced practice, such as biological sciences, pharmacology, pathophysiology and physical examination technique (Diers, 1985; Akinsanya, 1987; Stilwell, 1985; Gould, 1990), and on the other that the scope of practice of nurse practitioners is essentially different from other nurses with expanded roles, such as clinical nurse specialists (Soehren and Schumann, 1994; Hockenberry-Eaton and Powell, 1991). It is seen to be difficult to pick up the necessary skills and incorporate them into one's practice in an ad hoc way, the specific educational pathway in which theory and practice are combined together being the preferred option.

Logic would seem to dictate, though, that given the fact many nurses are seeking to claim the title nurse practitioner, and current course places are limited, with funding also being a potential problem, methods must be found whereby individuals can measure the extent to which their role and practice meets the attributes of nurse practitioner, and if necessary obtain the additional education and practical skills required to make up any deficit through flexible approaches such as modular courses, distance learning, and workplace teaching and assessment. Work has yet to start in these areas, but until it does it will be difficult to define accurately what the title nurse practitioner actually means.

Irrespective of how one actually becomes a nurse practitioner, the key questions are whether those using the title can actually deliver an effective service, and whether that service is value for money.

The Effectiveness of Nurse Practitioners

The introduction of nurse practitioners has been examined in terms of changes in cost, accessibility, quality and productivity (Shamansky, 1985), with a multitude of data justifying their effectiveness, largely emanating from the USA, but more recently from the UK also.

The US Message

In 1978 Edmunds published an analysis of 471 books and articles considering the work of nurse practitioners, with a generalizable opinion that patients fully accepted them as care providers and that they delivered high quality care. Sox (1979) found through 21 studies of nurse practitioners matched against primary care physicians that there was no difference in the quality of care provided. Building on such earlier studies, and those which they in turn had investigated, the US Congressional Office of Technology Assessment (OTA) issued a report in December 1986 which became a benchmark for the success of American nurse practitioners, confirming they made a positive impact on quality of care, increased accessibility to health care services and cost reduction. In 1992 the American Nurses Association, bolstered by such success, and the continued need to be able to demonstrate the effectiveness of the nurse practitioner, published a meta-analytical survey of process of care and cost-effectiveness of nurses in primary care roles, nurse practitioners and nurse-midwives, which included the OTA data and an information synthesis of 248 further studies undertaken between 1987 and 1992 (Brown and Grimes, 1992).

The ANA study utilized rigorous research methods considering the type of patients cared for, time available for consultation, and site of delivery of care, in order to produce data on effectiveness in comparison with other health care providers. The study shows that nurse practitioners provided more health promotion activities than did physicians, scored higher on quality of care measures, spent longer with patients (24.9 minutes average against 16.5 for physicians) and achieved greater success in the resolution of pathological conditions and improving the functional status of patients (Brown and Grimes, 1992). Combined with the fact that the nurse practitioner also scored higher in terms of patient satisfaction and compliance with care programmes, nurse practitioner patients were hospitalized less, and that the average consultation cost was cheaper ($12.36 for the nurse practitioner against $20.11 for the doctor), it is easy to see why this survey is now a standard reference point for nurse practitioner success within the USA.

The UK Message

The work of Stilwell, and contemporary colleagues, Burke-Masters and Restall (1988), produces similar results to the US data, indicating that patient acceptability of the role is high, as are quality of care outcomes. As Stilwell indicates: 'For many patients this style of care seems to be a safe and appropriate alternative to consulting a physician' (1988: 74), other studies such as that by Tettersell and Salisbury (1988) paint a similar picture.

The only large-scale UK research is that undertaken by management consultants

Touche Ross on behalf of South Thames NHS Executive and Regional Health Authority (1994). This work analysed the development of nurse practitioner roles in 20 sites, drawn from general practice settings, hospitals, casualty units and community settings (including retail pharmacy).

The study showed that as nurse practitioners moved through their educational programmes (they studied at the RCN as part of the project), their role became clearly defined, their practice was safe, and that 83–84% of patients reported a high degree of satisfaction with their consultations, compared to 78% of GP and 69% of senior house officer consultations.

Cost-Effectiveness

Holleran (1993) underlined the fact that the desire to save money gives excellent opportunity for nurses to expand their roles. As can be seen from the ANA meta-analysis nurse practitioners have been shown to reduce costs on numerous occasions, and this is not just because they take home a lower wage than physician colleagues. For instance, McGrath (1990) showed that nurse practitioners reduced costs in a cardiology clinic where they were used as direct substitutes for doctors, simply because more patients were dealt with on an outpatient basis with the cost of increased clinic sessions being easily recovered from the savings on admissions. In addition, McGrath (1990) found that a major area in which savings could be identified was the early detection and prevention of medical problems through increased accessibility to health care services, particularly to low income individuals who visited the nurse practitioner but would not otherwise have sought medical attention.

The South Thames research study (Touche Ross, South Thames Region, and NHSE South Thames, 1994) concluded that in the absence of agreed outcome measures it was not possible to determine cost-effectiveness accurately. The study did show, however, that the nurse practitioners in the study saved doctors' time and are 'a potential benefit for the NHS that it can realize in some form or other', with the assumption that 'either the NHS would in the long run operate with fewer doctors or that doctors would use the time released for other health care services (e.g. longer consultations, more home visits)' (1994: 60).

Nurse Practitioners as the Cheap Option

The downside of the ability of nurse practitioners to demonstrate effectiveness is that they may be seen as the cheap option. Davis (1992) is clear that the future role of nurse practitioners will depend on the policy decisions and choices made by purchasing authorities, and Warden (1988) believes that the main reason for governmental interest in the nurse practitioner is because they come cheaper than doctors whilst still providing high quality care. This issue is also relevant to the ongoing commitment from government to reduce the number of hours junior doctors work, with nurse practitioners being considered as a replacement (Moyse, 1994).

On the face of it, one might ask whether it really matters if nurse practitioner development is boosted by these factors. However, proponents of the role suggest this approach is detrimental to the philosophy of the nurse practitioner – one of being a supplement rather than substitute for medical practice (Shamansky, 1985; Tettersell and Salisbury, 1988). Of even greater concern is the suggestion that acceptance of the role by patients could be undermined if nurse practitioners are seen as a cheap alternative to doctors. For example, Warden cites the case of the charity Age Concern's response that nurse practitioners would be a source of 'second rate care, especially for the elderly' (1988: 1478).

As mentioned above, the 1994 South Thames study showed the cost of employing nurse practitioners to be in the region of £23–25 500 before practice overhead costs. This exceeded the employment costs of SHOs, but was just over half the £41 900 target income of GPs, with hourly costs being £25.15 for a GP as opposed to £11–15 (depending on locality inside or outside of London) for the nurse practitioners.

Whilst these figures may on the face of it look encouraging, nurse practitioners, though, have to play the cost-effective card carefully and ensure that cost reduction is measured appropriately against quality of care, and the desire to maintain an image of valued professionals in their own right, rather than being seen as a lower cost alternative to medicine. This is but one of the challenges for the future.

Future Challenges

Role Compromise

We have touched upon this to an extent in discussing cost-effectiveness. However, there are other dimensions to the issue, such as the attraction of the nurse practitioner role being rooted simply in a desire to escape from the relative low-esteem of nursing and seek surrogate value through the acquisition of medical skills. Robinson feels there is a 'risk of seduction into the seemingly glamorous technical mini-doctor role' which nurse practitioners must resist by stressing the uniqueness of their nursing background (1993: 54). Similarly, Rogers is even more forceful in condemning the hidden agenda of nurses being tricked into leaving their own philosophy of care behind in favour of a mistaken attraction to the technology of medicine:

> Clichés such as 'expanded role', 'physician's assistants', 'pediatric associates', and multiple other meaningless verbosities provide subtle and not so subtle come-ons for the naive-nonsensical nomenclature designed to gull registered nurses into leaving nursing in order to play handmaiden to medical mythology and machines. (Rogers, 1972: 135)

Rogers summarizes in saying nurse practitioners must be vigilant not to lose sight of, or compromise, their nursing values so falling victim to the mini-doctor myth. Maintaining a pride in their nursing contribution and their ability to use medical skills as part of it, is essential: 'Medical knowledge, no matter how relevant to medical practice, is not a substitute for the nursing knowledge that is essential to nursing practice' (Rogers, 1972: 133).

Disputes over Role Demarcation

In addition to maintaining the connection with nursing, nurse practitioners need to consider the potential for demarcation conflicts with other professional groups, in particular the medical profession. Davis (1992) sees that the development of the nurse practitioner role confronts the issue of the doctor having achieved the ultimate status at the top of the health care power hierarchy by virtue of having exclusive specialist knowledge. Moyse also feels 'What may muddy the water is the long history of interdependence between the medical profession and nursing, and the former's insistence that they alone should set the agenda' (1994: 53). Even though in addressing the fears that nurse practitioners will take over medicine, Stilwell suggests that 'nurses have more significant paths to tread than those of medical science' (1987: 61); it may well still take some deft manoeuvring on their part to achieve Salvage's vision (1988) of the development of the nurse practitioner role binding together the professions of medicine and nursing in the provision of health care, allowing them to be mutually influential. Nurse practitioners will have to consider carefully the dividing line between them meeting needs which hitherto had not been met, and becoming competitors to established health care providers.

Autonomous Practice

Much is said about autonomy in the context of expanded nursing roles. However, whilst nurse practitioners may well make decisions about patient care and treatment which are theirs and theirs alone, barriers still exist to fully independent practice.

Firstly the link between professional accountability and individual liability needs to be recognized. Davis (1992) and Butterworth (1990) rightly point out that at present nurse practitioners are shielded from true responsibility in a relationship of vicarious liability with their employer, quite often a doctor. They are still accountable for their own practice, and can lose their registration, yet others will bear the financial burden. Nurse practitioners may no longer be able to expand their roles without facing the true consequences of autonomy, standing up in a courtroom defending their actions, and paying a sum of money commensurate to medical colleagues for their indemnity insurance, in case they are found to be at fault.

Secondly, the structure of the National Health Service is currently insufficiently flexible to support independent nursing practice. There is no mechanism for a group of nurse practitioners setting up their own practice to be paid for the work they do, unless they are employed by a general medical practitioner or an existing trust or community unit. This will change in due course, but nurse practitioners must be ready to compete for contracts to provide health care, and work in partnership with other providers to convince purchasers of their efficacy.

Finally, nurse practitioners need to secure additional rights underpinning their practice, prescriptive authority is a classic example. What is the point of equipping nurse practitioner students with an in-depth module on pharmacology as in the RCN course (RCN IANE, 1992) when 98% of the products they are allowed to prescribe can be bought over the counter? Other 'privileges' are equally important such as the right to admit patients to hospital and refer for tests and investigations.

CONCLUSION

The nurse practitioner movement has a history of success founded in the ability to react to a changing world of health care needs and means of providing for those needs. Nurse practitioners are able to demonstrate that they provide high quality care relevant to the needs of individuals and communities at reasonable cost. The future seems bright. However, issues of role demarcation, and the move toward true autonomy, will undoubtedly have to be dealt with before the nurse practitioner progresses from being the heretic of the past, the experimenter of today, to the norm of tomorrow.

SUMMARY

This chapter discusses:
- The historical development of the nurse practitioner role in the USA and the UK, identifying key factors contributing toward that development, such as: a 'new professionalism' permeating through the US and UK nursing professions (albeit separated by three decades), and dissatisfaction with a medical model approach to health care and a dawning realization that doctors do not, and never will have, all the answers.
- Defining the role of nurse practitioner. The chapter considers the question 'what is a nurse practitioner', drawing on role analysis from both the UK

and USA, and attempting to locate the nurse practitioner within the expanding role of the nurse as defined by the Royal College of Nursing and the UKCC.

■ Preparation for nurse practitioner practice. In addition to defining the role, we also consider the education required in order to fulfil it, whether any nurse can develop nurse practitioner skills incrementally, or whether a formal program of study is required as a prerequisite for nurse practitioner practice.

■ The future for nurse practitioners. This chapter probably poses as many questions as it provides answers. It is clear that issues of role demarcation, education requirements, scope of practice, employment situation and the omnipresent question as to whether nurse practitioner is the superlative nurse or a mini-doctor, will be the topics of debate for several years to come. The reader is left to decide the answers.

DISCUSSION QUESTIONS

◆ How do you become a nurse practitioner – by experience (incrementally), or by taking a defined course of study?

◆ Is the primary health care nurse practitioner role any different from that of an experienced practice nurse, district nurse or health visitor?

◆ Is the primary health care nurse practitioner a highly developed nurse or a mini-GP?

◆ How can nurse practitioners develop their work without compromising their ideals?

◆ Is it inevitable that nurse practitioners and doctors will come into conflict?

◆ Do you think the development of nurse practitioners will benefit patients and clients? If yes – why?, if no – why not?

FURTHER READING

Brown SA and Grimes DE (1992) *A Meta-Analysis of Process of Care, Clinical Outcomes, and Cost-effectiveness of Nurses in Primary Care Roles: Nurse Practitioners and Nurse Midwives.* Washington DC: American Nurses Association.
The full text of the ANA report is worth reading in that it gives a multitude of useful reference points so far as the nurse practitioner role, acceptance by patients and cost-effectiveness are concerned.

Fagin CM (1981) Primary care as an academic discipline. In IG Mauksh (Ed) *Primary Care, A Contemporary*

Nursing Perspective. New York: Grune and Stratton.
Discussion of the need for academic discipline and detailed knowledge base underpinning nursing practice in primary health care.

Maguire J (1980) *The Expanded Role of the Nurse.* London: King's Fund Centre.
Detailed discussion of the expanded role concept and its relevance to advanced nursing practice.

Stilwell B and Bowling A (Eds) (1988) *The nurse in family practice.* London: Scutari Press.

An overview of the development of the nurse practitioner in the global context. Also considers the differences between the nurse practitioner role and that of the practice nurse.

Towsend P, Davidson N and Whitehead M (1990) *Inequalities in health*. Harmondsworth: Penguin Books. More in-depth analysis of factors leading to inequality of access to and provision of health care in the UK.

REFERENCES

Akinsanya J (1987) The life sciences in nurse education. In B Davis (Ed) *Nursing Education: Research and Development*. London: Croom Helm.

Bennet MC (1984) The rural family nurse practitioner: the quest for role identity. *Journal of Advanced Nursing* **9**: 145–155.

Brown SA and Grimes DE (1992) *A Meta-analysis of Process of Care, Clinical Outcomes, and Cost-effectiveness of Nurses in Primary Care Roles: Nurse Practitioners and Nurse Midwives*. Washington DC: American Nurses Association.

Burke-Masters B (1986) The autonomous nurse practitioner: an answer to a chronic problems of primary care. *Lancet* **1**: 1266.

Butterworth T (1990) Patients' needs or professionalism? *Nursing Standard* **4** (21): 36–37.

Casteldine G (1993) Nurse practitioner title: ambiguous and misleading. *British Journal of Nursing* **14**: 734–735.

Clay T (1987) *Nursing Power and Politics*. London: Heinemann.

Cumberlege J (1986) *Neighbourhood Nursing – a Focus for Care. Report of the community nursing review*. Chair. Julia Cumberlege. London: HMSO.

Davis J (1992) Expanding horizons. *Nursing Times* **88**(47): 37–39.

DHSS, Secretaries of State for Social Services, Wales, Northern Ireland, and Scotland (1987) *Promoting Better Health: the government's programme for improving primary health care*. London: HMSO.

Diers D (1985) Preparation of nurse practitioners, clinical specialists and clinicians. *Journal of Professional Nursing* **1**(1): 41–47.

Dillner L (1993) Juniors' new deal meets its first deadline. *British Medical Journal* **306**: 807–808.

Fawcett-Henesy A (1990) Setting the scene for revolution. *Nursing Standard* **4** (21): 35.

Ford LC, Seacat MS and Silver GG (1966) Broadening roles of public health nurses and physicians in prenatal infant supervision. *American Journal of Public Health* **56**: 1097–1103.

Ford LC and Silver HK (1967) The expanded role of the nurse in child care. *Nursing Outlook* **15**: 43–45.

Edmunds MW (1978) Evaluation of nurse practitioner effectiveness. An overview of the literature. *Evaluation and the Health Professions* **1**: 69–820.

Friend PN and Yellowlees H (1977) *The Extending Role of the Clinical Nurse - Legal Implications and Training Requirements*. CMO(77)10/CNO(77)9. London: HMSO.

Gaze H (1985) Out in the cold. *Nursing Times* **81**(9): 18, 20.

Gould D (1990) How is your biology? *Nursing* **4**(11): 33–35.

Hockenberry-Eaton M and Powell ML (1991) Merging advanced practice roles: the NP and CNS. *Journal of Pediatric Health Care* **5**: 158–159.

Holleran C (1993) *Lessons for the future*. Nurse Practitioners the UK/USA experience. In *Proceedings of the First International Conference on Nurse Practitioner Practice*. London: Nursing Standard.

Iazzatti L (1992) Extended role allows growth. *Nurse Practitioner* **17**(3): 15.

Jolly U (1992) Primary health care nurse practitioners. *Journal of Advances in Health and Nursing Care* **2**(2): 53–58.

Jordan S (1993) Nurse practitioners, learning from the USA experience: a review of the literature. *Health and Social Care* **2**: 173–185.

Leff S (1978) The standard of care questions. *Nurse Practitioner* **72**: 34–36.

Lewis CE and Resnick BA (1967) Nurse clinics in ambulatory care. *New England Journal of Medicine* **277**: 1236–1241.

Lewis G and Wessely S (1992) The epidemiology of fatigue: more questions than answers. *Journal of Epidemiology and Community Health* **46**: 92–97.

Lindeke L (1993) An educator's perspective on the increased demand for NPs. Nurse Practitioners the UK/USA experience. In *Proceedings of the First International Conference on Nurse Practitioner Practice*. London: Nursing Standard.

Lowry S (1993) The pre-registration year. *British Medical Journal* **306**: 196–198.

McGrath S (1990) The cost-effectiveness of nurse practitioners. *Health Care Issues* **15**(7): 40–42.

Moyse G (1994) Growing gains. *Nursing Standard* **8**(25): 53.

National Health Service Management Executive (1993) *Nursing in Primary Health Care: New World New Opportunities*. London: HMSO.

O'Hara Devereaux M (1991) Nurse practitioners in North America. In J Salvage (Ed) *Nurse Practitioners Working for Change in Primary Health Care Nursing*. London: King's Fund Centre.

Pearson LJ (1994) Annual update of how each state stands on legislative issues affecting advanced nursing practice. *Nurse Practitioner* **11**: 17–18, 21–53.

Reeder S and Mauksh H (1979) Nursing: continuing change. In HE Freeman, S Levine and LG Reeder (Eds) *Handbook of Medical Sociology*. New York: Prentice Hall.

Robinson DK (1993) Nurse practitioner or mini-doctor? *Accident and Emergency Nursing* **1**: 53–55.

Rogers ME (1972) Nursing: to be or not to be. *Nursing Outlook* **20:** 42–46.

Royal College of Nursing of the United Kingdom (1987) *RCN Response to the Consultation on Primary Health Care Initiated by the UK Health Departments*. London: RCN.

Royal College of Nursing of the United Kingdom Institute of Advanced Nursing Education *Nurse Practitioner in Primary Health Care: Role Definition*. London: RCN IANE.

Royal College of Nursing of the United Kingdom Institute of Advanced Nursing Education (1992) *Health Studies Programme: Nurse Practitioner Diploma. (Syllabus)*. London: RCN IANE.

Salvage J (1988) Professionalisation – a struggle for survival. A consideration of current proposals for the reform of nursing in the United Kingdom. *Journal of Advanced Nursing* **13:** 515–519.

Shamansky SL (1985) Nurse practitioners and primary care research: promises and pitfalls. *Annual Review of Nursing Research* **3:** 107–125.

Silver HK, Ford LC and Stearly SG (1967) A program to increase health care for children: the pediatric nurse practitioner program. *Pediatrics* **39:** 756–760.

Skeet M (1978) Health auxiliaries: decision makers and implementers. In M Skeet and K Elliot (Eds) *Health Auxiliaries and the Health Team*. London: Croom Helm.

Soehren PM and Schumann LL (1994) Enhanced role opportunities available to the CNS/nurse practitioner. *Clinical Nurse Specialist* **8**(3): 123–127.

Sox HC (1979) Quality of patient care by nurse practitioners and physicians assistants: a ten-year perspective. *Annals of Internal Medicine* **91:** 459–468.

Stilwell B (1984) The nurse in practice. *Nursing Mirror* **158**(21): 17–22.

Stilwell B (1985) Evolution not revolution. *Senior Nurse* **4**(6): 10–11.

Stilwell B (1987) Different expectations. *Nursing Times* **83**(24): 59–61.

Stilwell B (1988) The Origins and Development of the Nurse Practitioner Role – a Worldwide Perspective. In B Stilwell and A Bowling (Eds.) *The nurse in family practice*. London: Scutari Press.

Stilwell B, Restall D and Burke-Masters B (1988) Nurse practitioners in British general practice. In B Stilwell and A Bowling (Eds) *The Nurse in Family Practice*. London: Scutari Press.

Tettersell MJ and Salisbury CJ (1988) Comparison of the work of a nurse practitioner with that of a general practitioner. *Journal of the Royal College of General Practitioners* **38:** 314–316.

Tomlinson B (1992) *Report of the Enquiry into London's Health Service, Medical Education and Research*. London: HMSO.

Trnobranski PH (1994) Nurse practitioner – redefining the role of the community nurse? *Journal of Advanced Nursing* **19:** 134–139.

Tudor Hart J (1971) The inverse care law. *Lancet* **1:** 405–412.

Touche Ross, South Thames Regional Health Authority and NHS Executive, S. Thames (1994) *Evaluation of Nurse Practitioner Pilot Projects*. London: Touche Ross.

United Kingdom Central Council for Nursing, Midwifery, and Health Visiting (1992) *Scope of Professional Practice*. London: UKCC.

United Kingdom Central Council for Nursing, Midwifery, and Health Visiting (1993) *Final Draft Report on the Future of Professional Education and Practice*. London: UKCC.

United States Congressional Office of Technology Assessment (1986) *Nurse Practitioners, Physicians Assistants, and Certified Midwives – Policy Analysis*. Washington DC: US Government Printing Office.

United States Department of Health, Education, and Welfare (1976) Nurse practitioner training: proposed grant program. *Federal Register* **41:** 3552–3556.

Warden J (1988) Letter from Westminster: rise of the nurse practitioner. *British Medical Journal* **296:** 1478.

White House Domestic Policy Council (1993) *The President's Health Security Plan*. New York: Times Books.

Young T and Perkin R (1993) *Growing Family – Preparation of the Paediatric Critical Care NP*. Nurse Practitioners the UK/USA experience. In *Proceedings of the First International Conference on Nurse Practitioner Practice*. London: Nursing Standard.

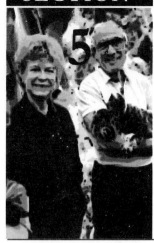

DILEMMAS AND CHALLENGES

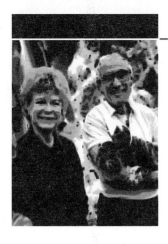

INTRODUCTION

This final section draws attention to some of the more significant implications of change within the overall health care system. Community nurses are not only encouraged to explore the concept of value for money in relation to health service provision but also to consider the complexity of health behaviour and the political and professional issues associated with providing community nursing across a social divide. Different perspectives are adopted to consider the consequences of various shifts in the strategic developments of the NHS; for example the shift from institutional to community care, the shift of emphasis to health promotion within a society where socio-economic conditions play an increasing role in the health status disparities between rich and poor, and the shift of role boundaries across the provision of health and social care.

The first chapter includes an historical overview and rationale for community care and highlights current issues and research priorities. This if followed by an explanation of how to balance the costs and benefits of health care with value for money in mind and the third chapter goes on to examine some of the practical issues which arise when 'health gain' targets are translated into action.

The fourth chapter considers the position of community nurses in a health service which underlines individual responsibility for health and well-being. The final two chapters provide an overview of the philosophy and process of marketing with special reference to health services and to the potential for improving communication about the distinguishing features of community nursing services and the benefits likely to accrue in a primary care or community setting.

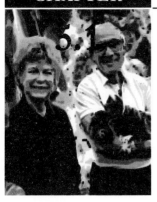

COMMUNITY CARE: OBSTACLES AND OPPORTUNITIES

Colin Pritchard

KEY ISSUES

- Current issues surrounding community care
- Progress and current issues
- Structure and resources
- The influence of internal markets
- The concept of affordability
- Unemployment

INTRODUCTION

Whilst interests in notions of community and society may rise and fall with political fashions, on reflection 'society/community' is as real as the air we breathe, and as such is so integral to our everyday existence that we never notice it, until it or we break down; the waterworks staff don't work; road sweepers don't sweep; shop keepers don't open; or because of our incapacity, we cannot earn, pay taxes, or fulfil the responsibilities expected by our society/community.

Humankind through 7000 years of recorded history, irrespective of hierarchy, have lived together in various types of societies, but all have the same essential mutually dependent and identifying experience of community. Strong or weakly defined, the community still provides the contextual framework for individuals to live out their lives. The 'boundaries' of such communities are defined by geography, family and martial state, gender, age, ethnicity, social class and employment status etc., and as such defines the norm for that individual.

Consequently in times of ill health, and distress, the actual or potential supportive strength of those various community or social networks becomes all important. And in times of crisis the person predominantly wishes to have as little change to their social context as possible, in order to maximize those community supports. Not surprisingly, therefore, the vast majority of people in trouble prefer to stay at home, or return home as soon as possible.

Let us consider age. Richard Titmus (1968) said, 'reality starts with history', so just consider how someone born at the beginning of the century perceives today. There are many service users for whom the First World War has considerable meaning, yet for the majority of practitioners this is an event as historical as the Napoleonic Wars. Yet when *your* grandmother was born, say 1914, it was the Poor Law, based upon

Queen Elizabeth's Act of 1601 and 'modernized' as 'recently' as 1832, which created 'workhouses' for destitute people, be the need physical or mental. It is worth noting that their secondary purpose was to be institutions which should be so austere as to deter people from using them only in the direst circumstances, and ensure that assistance should only be available for the 'deserving' rather than the 'undeserving' poor. Such institutions lasted in law until 1948 (National Assistance Act) yet the former workhouse buildings often had to be taken over, given a lick of paint, and called the old people's home or geriatric hospital.

The good old days 'when Britain really ruled the waves', were not so good, if you were old, poor, low paid, mentally or physically ill or handicapped etc., and older clients still retain some of their 'angst' about the stigmatizing experiences of *their* parents. There clearly have been major improvements, though there is evidence of a resurgence of some of the older attitudes.

The Coming of the Welfare State

About fifty years ago, Beverage, with all party support, described the five 'giants' which oppressed the spirit of the person and society: want, squalor, ignorance, disease and idleness – translated into poverty, poor housing, education, health care and full employment. Crucially Beverage and others saw that all five aspects were integrated, seeing the community as the normal context in which to deliver services, and seeing health in its widest sense, thus including employment, housing, education as well as preventative and curative treatments; demonstrating for the first time the indivisibility of health and social care.

The growth and development of the NHS is discussed fully elsewhere (Chapter 1.1) but suffice to say the NHS first needed to develop an integrated 'nationalized' hospital service. Local government remained responsible for the preventative elements which were epitomized by public health developments, social/health care of mothers and children, and the development of health visiting and domiciliary nursing services.

Not only were local authorities responsible for child protection with the advent of children's departments in 1948, but also for the development of mental health departments in 1959, responsible for the care and treatment of the mentally ill. By 1962 the clear notion of 'Care in the Community' was first articulated. With historical hindsight, we can see that the five 'giants' which needed slaying were tackled separately, with the result that independent departments inevitably created impermeable boundaries, to the detriment of the 'generic' service user. The average family would be in contact with education, child health, general practice, housing departments in ordinary times, and in times of crisis with hospitals, benefit agencies, employment services, police, probation, mental health and children's departments. This was recognized by the late Lord Seebohm, a man of particular vision, whose report led in 1970 to the integration of the majority of 'social' based services into the current Social Service Departments (SSD) whose rationale is to provide a one-door entry, of easy access to 'a personal social service for the citizen' (Seebohm, 1988).

Progress

Almost 25 years on there are very and not very effective achievements. Certainly there is evidence of a substantial but not total reduction in the extreme consequence of child abuse, i.e. dead children, which despite criticisms from some 'vested' interests, is irrefutable (Creighton, 1993; Pritchard, 1993a, 1993b).

Conversely, community mental health, whilst continuing as the central policy of care of the mentally ill (Department of Health 1992; Reed Committee, 1994), when compared with social service departments' child protection achievements, is disappointing. The reason why will be explored later, but sufficient to say, the *community* base of such care and protection is central. The proposed restructuring of local government, apart from the size, is not a political issue, for all agree there are to be benefits from greater unification leading to 'unitary authorities', bringing together education, social services and housing, under one area responsibility. Thus we will have five big 'care' systems which impinge upon the life of the citizen and family, united by the 'genericism' inherent in the person and family, but separated by fiscal and therefore organizational and practice boundaries; these are the health (both hospital and primary care), education (the only 'normative' service which includes *every* citizen), social care social services and probably housing), the benefits system (social and housing) and the criminal justice system (including police and probation). All are orientated towards serving a defined community. Let us now explore how well or otherwise the community services are faring in the pursuit of social justice.

Current Issues

There are essentially three interrelated, long-standing issues surrounding community care: these are the optimal structure, resources and accessibility. Difficulties in any of these areas can impact upon the practice and morale of the front-line professional.

Structure and Resources

We have already intimated something of the evolutionary and occasionally erratic developments of both NHS and Community Care agencies. Two amongst a number of themes are discernable and are reflected in the debate concerning mental health as seen in the last two pieces of legislation, the 1959 and 1983 Mental Health Acts, namely primacy of 'treatment', versus 'prevention' versus 'rights', though not it should be noted, rights to resources. The National Health and Community Care Act 1990 (NHCCA) also mirrors this different focus as the emphasis moves to 'patients' rights/charters', rather than an alternative, say a rolling proportion of the nation's wealth, gross disposable product (GDP), which would be extremely easy to legislate for and probably, if carefully explained, would be very popular.

The 1990 NHCCA emphasizes the indivisibility of prevention and treatment, and moves towards some form of combined authority so that primary and secondary care, i.e. community and hospital care, will become a joint responsibility. The only doubt will be the size and locus of control – local or central government. But since 1945 the search for an optimal structure for both community and hospital services has continued to attract controversy and suspicion. The local government changes of 1974 matched changes in the NHS, initially with a strong drive towards larger organizations and the expected benefits of size. At that time ignoring criticisms of those who would preserve the smaller local authority and the small 'cottage' hospital. The clinical argument has been undoubtedly won. The problem now is to whom in the chain of command should the district general hospital relate?

Figure 5.1.1 shows the NHS structure from 1948 to 1974, the internal 'reorganization' in 1982 and the 'reforms' of 1990 and 1992, with the division into 'purchasers' and 'providers'

The community care structures are broadly moving towards closer integration into 'one-door entry' for the citizen (Seebohm, 1988), with aspirations to have common boundaries with health. But arguments about size and economy of scale persist. The review of local government, ostensibly driven by decision-making at the smallest and lowest 'local' level, is likely to see new unitary authorities coalescing a number of presently separate services, but serving much smaller communities. Cynics, including the author, note that any evidence about optimal size for the delivery of services was expressly excluded from the remit of the review, just as the socioeconomic background of children was excluded from any definition of children with 'special needs' in the 1988 Education Act (Baroness Warnock, 1993). Whilst there can be more 'Chairs' of committees to share out in a larger number of authorities and thus 'more involvement of local democracy', the authorities may be too small to offer an alternative vision to central government. Critics argue that they will be too small to raise sufficient independent capital to have alternative styles of service or to develop an effective level of expertise. Today

Figure 5.1.1. The Health Management Structure (a) pre-1991 and (b) post-1991.

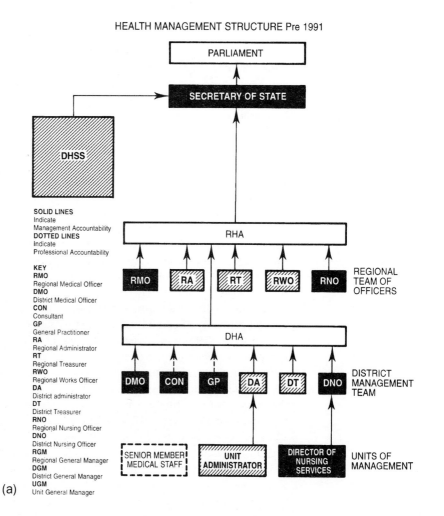

HEALTH MANAGEMENT STRUCTURE Pre 1991

it is almost impossible for local authorities to run an independent policy at odds with central government. It is feared that local government instead of being revitalized will be further disempowered and may be nothing more than an agent for central government.

Thus, as Parliament contains both executive and legislative powers, without a Bill of Rights, Freedom of Information Act and Rights of Assembly (which the present Criminal Justice Bill 1994 has largely removed), there is virtually no balancing or alternative power to Parliament. This may be an extreme view but the *essence* of democracy is that we should never trust power in the hands of any for too long, and without adequate safeguards, power corrupts, even the most altruistic. If you doubt this, consider who is *your* local tyrant, were they always so dominant? How many well-meaning nursing sisters, senior social workers, charge nurses, as well as politicians, were so very reasonable until they moved upwards and became removed from the pain and distress encountered daily by front-line staff? All in the human services need to remember we make our living out of other people's ignorance, pain and suffering. Unless we are undoubtedly part of their solution, we may have become part of their problem. Yet despite the rhetoric of citizens' rights and local involvement, emancipating the citizen from the toils of bureaucracy, freeing them from

Figure 5.1.1. *cont.*

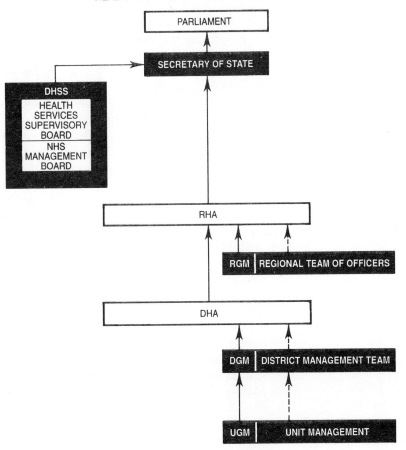

HEALTH MANAGEMENT STRUCTURE Post 1991

(b)   NB Regions will be disbanded in 1996

over-zealous professionals, *all* community based services be they in health, education, central or local government have never been more active and dominant. While using the language of progressive liberty, both citizens' and, in part, local government's, autonomy have been whittled away. Thus hard-won rights which British citizens were born to in the 1940s have in the name of efficiency disappeared almost imperceptibly.

The Influence of Internal Markets

With the introduction of internal markets, purchasers and providers can be viewed as a built-in scheme to seek reduction in costs, which coincides with the deprofessionalization of the caring services, especially in teaching, social work and nursing. This is presented as anti-elitism and anti-professionalism, and at the same time egalitarian, as it is intended to recruit people who have missed out educationally, but have qualified in the university of life! Some cynics might believe the rumours of cabinet conversations, that as such tasks are mainly done by women, do we really need all that training, when a good mother, a sensible middle-aged person, or in the case of delinquency a redundant SAS sergeant might well be best for dealing with what is increasingly called the 'underclass' (Lawson and Wilson, 1995). Thus we have National Vocational Qualifications, on the job training, and either supine or collusive quangos who under the guise of independence, carry out the political agenda of the government of the day.

Answers are fine but questions are more important, otherwise we do not learn. In accepting the intellectual and professional theories of the day without being disturbed, we reinforce our approach and seldom relearn. Examples in the mental and physical health field abound; one will suffice: classically the professors of obstetrics were outraged by Pasteur's request that they wash their hands between the examination of patients.

This is not to deny that colleagues who have journeyed along the National Vocational Qualification route can contribute. The danger is their 'training' is limited to the present, rather than being a professional 'education' which teaches a degree of independence. Protagonists for this approach talk about bedside skills and would separate out the 'high tech'. But on the highest of 'high tech' authority (Pritchard, 1995), those so-called basic skills, potentially easily ignored in a busy neurosurgical theatre, are what protects and keeps safe the patient.

In the community sector, the same potential difficulties regarding safe practice are occurring. More people holding National Vocational Qualifications, qualifications who are less likely to challenge, and cheaper to employ, are taking on those direct face-to-face contacts with the client, leaving the complex technical procedures and 'case management' to the more professionally trained staff. It is feared by some that there is a trend towards inadvertent 'ware-housing' with the subtle message for those dealing with social care and the vulnerable, the disturbed and disturbing, 'it's good enough for them'.

It has been reported, for example, that as part of the 'fight against crime', the training of probation officers may well be withdrawn from the university/higher education system, partly to avoid the pervasive influence of 'do gooders', and encourage the recruitment of former sergeants, to instill discipline into those of the 'yob orientation' (Howard *Conservative Party News*, 1994). Unfortunately life is not so simple because there is very strong evidence to show, first that more than 25% of people in prison were in care as children, and secondly, more than 40% of offenders have some form of mental health problem (Pritchard *et al.*, 1992; Stewart and Stewart, 1993; Hudson *et al.*, 1993). If government is serious and not just parading prejudice as policy, then such an approach might well lead to placing the public at risk, together with a further rise in prison suicides (Dooley, 1990).

Is this again too extreme? Probably not, because what needs to be appreciated is that those on the margins of society: the mentally ill, the homeless, the offender, the substance misusing person etc., often form a core group of people who cross *all* the community/health boundaries. Many have an inherited background of poverty and poor educational opportunity or achievement (Whitehead, 1990; Hudson *et al.*, 1993; Marshall and Reed, 1993; Scott, 1993); indeed when looking at acute admissions in London, it was found that more than 10% were homeless (Morrell *et al.*, 1994), and that HIV infection and risky lifestyle behaviour, along with homelessness, increases the incidence of tuberculosis amongst those on the margins of society.

Indeed, for some young adults, the only way to combat chronic and demoralizing poverty is to take the 'alternative market response', which includes delinquency, drug distribution and prostitution.

The Concept of Affordability

The slogan, 'Value for Money', rightly reminds us that we need to maximize all resources devoted to public expenditure. Indeed, the assertion of Prime Minister Thatcher (1987) is totally accepted, 'we can only have the services we can afford'. However, what we can and do afford, may not be the same, and there is evidence that the argument has not been properly explained. The key issues for consideration centre around the following question, which you may like to consider for yourself.

One way to explore such a question is to take the issue of health care and make some comparisons between various United Kingdom Government departments and with other countries of similar affluence. Used in this way the concept of affordability is useful and can be measured by contrasting what proportion of the annual gross domestic product (GDP), i.e. the nation's annual wealth, was and is devoted to health expenditure (Box. 5.1.1).

For example at the end of Mr Heath's government 1973/74, total GDP for that financial year was £75 billion pounds, an enormous sum of money. That year we spent £3.1 billion pounds, or 4.13%, of our GDP on the NHS However, in 1974 apart from Greece, Ireland and Portugal, we spent *less* of our GDP than *any* other developed nation in the Western world. Currently, as will be seen, it is *slightly* worse as only Denmark and Greece spend less than us (Box 5.1.2). Nevertheless, as a proportion of *all* government expenditure (portrayed as general government expenditure GGE) the £3.1 billion represented 9.7% of all GGE; thus virtually ten pounds in every hundred of public expenditure went to the NHS. That sounds better. But is it as much as we can afford? However, staying with 1973/74 as a baseline, the outgoing Labour government, five years later, had spent twice as much, £7.4 billion (less incidently than they spent on defence), which in cash terms was an increase of 139% more – but that £7.4 billion only represented 5.2% of GDP, which proportionally was only 27% more. The point of such detail is to show, if it needed demonstrating, just how easy it is without proper defined *baselines* to present and misrepresent financial statistics. Consider that at the end of the 1993/94 period, the nation spent £30.1 billion on the National Health Service, in cash terms

Box 5.1.1. Social and defence budgets as proportion of GGE and GDP 1973/4–1996/7 (£ billions)

Budgets	(Outturn of spending)			Estimated planned* spending		Index of change	
Years	1973/4+	1978/79	1983/84	1993/94	1996/97	73–94	73/4–96/7
Social security (£ bn)	6.5	16.4	35.2	61.0	67.8	938	1043
% of GGE	20.3	21.9	24.9	21.3	20.8		
% of GDP	8.7	9.4	11.4	10.1	8.9		
Index 1973–79 = 108			1979/94 = 116			1979/97 = 095	
Health (£ bn)	3.1	7.4	14.7	30.1	33.3	945	1065
% of GGE	9.7	9.9	10.4	10.5	10.2		
% of GDP	4.1	5.2	4.7	5.0	4.3		
Index 1973–79 = 127			1979–94 = 096			1979/97 = 083	
Education (£ bn)	4.5	8.7	13.4	30.5	Local authority plans not available	678	n/a
% GGE	14.1	11.6	9.5	10.7			
% GDP	6.0	5.0	4.3	5.1			
Index 1973–79 = 083			1979/94 = 102			1973–94 = 085	
Defence (£ bn)	3.6	7.5	15.5	23.4	22.8		
% GGE	11.3	10.0	10.9	8.2	7.0		
% GDP	4.8	4.3	5.0	3.9	3.0		
Index 1973–79 = 090			1979/94 = 091			1979/97 = 070	

* Local authority expenditure changes in system, 1991/92 last year identifiable on old procedure. Local authority planned expenditure not available after 1993/94. Therefore National calculation only possible to this period. Because of changes in accounting presentation, no longer possible to compare Housing expenditure over time.
Source: Extrapolated from HM Treasury Government Expenditure Plans (1974–1994/5–1996/97 in Pritchard (1992).

ten times as much under Mr Major than Mr Heath, or four times more than Mr Callaghan's government.

Indeed, health expenditure is planned to rise to the colossal sum of £33.3 billion pounds. Thus for every billion spent by Mr Callaghan, it is expected to spend four and a half times as much. At first sight, the phrase 'the NHS is safe in his hands – whilst I have breath left', appears to have financial confirmation. But, that £33.3 billion is only equivalent to 4.3% of GDP, as there is a *planned* reduction of GDP, devoted to the NHS, so that the 5.0% scheduled for the 1993/94 session, will fall to 4.3% GDP, and a real reduction of what we did and can afford. Thus we are intending to spend proportionally less of the nation's wealth on health than at any time since 1973/74. To be scrupulously fair, in 1987, Mrs Thatcher's government spent proportionately more of one year's GDP, than ever before or since, but GDP on health has fallen and continues to fall. In these simple terms, against Mrs Thatcher's own measurement, of 'what we can afford', we are clearly not affording as much as we used to, especially when we remain at the bottom end of the international league table, as seen in Box 5.1.2.

Box 5.1.2. Percentage of GDP devoted to health 1980–1991 (Index 100 = 1980)

COUNTRY and rank order		1980 (%)	1991 (%)	Index of change
1	USA	9.3	13.4	144
2	Canada	7.4	10.2	135
3	France	7.6	9.1	120
4	Finland	6.5	8.9	137
5	Sweden	9.5	8.6	091
6	Germany	8.5	8.5	100
8 =	Austria	7.9	8.4	106
8 =	Iceland	6.4	8.4	131
8 =	Australia	6.5	8.4	129
10 =	Netherlands	8.2	8.3	101
10 =	Italy	6.7	8.3	124
12 =	Switzerland	7.3	7.9	108
12 =	Belgium	6.2	7.9	127
14 =	New Zealand	7.2	7.6	106
14 =	Norway	6.6	7.6	115
16	Ireland	9.0	7.3	081
17 =	Japan	6.4	6.8	106
17 =	Portugal	5.9	6.8	115
19	Spain	5.6	6.7	120
20	United Kingdom	5.8	6.6	114
21	Denmark	6.8	6.5	096
22	Greece	4.3	5.2	121

NB: GDP calculated differently, based upon purchasing parities between countries, translated into constants of US dollars; thus percentages different from UK levels.
Source: Extrapolated from Department of Commerce (1993).

Box 5.1.1 provided some interesting intra-governmental budget comparisons, not least because a number of the 'social' budgets have to be taken together because self-evidently what is spent on say social services departments in local government, will have a direct bearing on what the NHS might need to spend.

Unfortunately, it is no longer possible to make direct fiscal comparisons over time on all budgets since 1992.

Some cynics would say that the changes – for example in social service and housing costs during the period 1990 and 1992, have been made deliberately confusing and difficult to make comparisons over time.

Unemployment

Why are the jobless figures relevant to health and community care? Simply because unemployment damages health, mental and physical; their morale and the quality of their lives and that of their children (e.g. Whitehead, 1990; Judd and Benzeval, 1993; Lawson and Wilson, 1994). Consequently there may well be greater pressures upon *all* public services, NHS and community; especially with regard to child protection, delinquency, homelessness, mental health and, we argue, HIV infection (e.g. Hudson *et al.*, 1993; Marshall and Reed, 1993; Pritchard *et al.*, 1992; Pritchard and Clooney, 1994).

It is worth noting that the 1979 level of unemployment of a million plus people would only be about 700 000 if calculated by today's system. Box 5.1.3 shows how the job prospects for the unemployed have changed.

Taking the end of the last recession as a baseline, January 1990, to January 1994, total unemployment rose by 71% to reach 2.89 million people. In 1990 for every vacancy in the United Kingdom there were approximately three unemployed people; by 1994 there were more than eight jobless people for every job.

Thus the gap between job vacancies and the number of unemployed has widened considerably in the four year period. Sadly, if the unemployment rate continues to fall at the very good rate of 30 000 per month, it will take until 1997/8 to get back to the state of January 1990. Further, the new recession of

Box 5.1.3. Regional unemployment and notified vacancies, January 1990–1995; ratio of vacancies* to jobless (thousands)

REGION	1990	1995	INDEX 1990–95
UK	1687.0	2503.4	148
Vacancy	600.2	454.8	076
Ratio Vac: Unem	2.8	5.5	196
1 South East	348.7	768.5	220
Vacancy	158.4	124.5	079
Ratio	1.6	6.2	388
Greater London	199.5	407.5	204
Vacancy	52.2	43.5	074
Ratio	3.4	9.4	276
2 East Anglia	36.0	71.9	200
Vacancy	21.3	13.8	065
Ratio	1.7	5.2	306
3 South West	96.8	184.2	190
Vacancy	48.0	32.1	067
Ratio	2.0	5.7	285
4 W. Midlands	156.5	227.1	145
Vacancy	52.2	36.6	070
Ratio	2.9	6.2	214
5 North	129.1	159.7	124
Vacancy	31.8	19.8	062
Ratio	4.1	8.1	198
6 East Midlands	99.5	162.1	163
Vacancy	35.7	32.7	092
Ratio	2.8	4.9	175
7 Wales	90.3	115.8	128
Vacancy	38.7	33.3	086
Ratio	2.3	3.5	152
8 Yorkshire and Humberside	167.3	222.5	162
Vacancy	36.3	33.6	093
Ratio	4.6	6.6	143
9 North West	243.2	276.0	113
Vacancy	70.2	55.2	079
Ratio	3.5	5.0	143
10 Scotland	219.2	223.7	102
Vacancy	69.6	56.4	081
Ratio	3.1	3.9	126
11 Northern Ireland	100.4	91.9	092
Vacancy	12.3	17.1	139
Ratio	8.2	7.5	091

*NB: Officially it is estimated every vacancy can be trebled to account for the non-reported vacancies; therefore the proportions of jobs to the jobless are a third of the Department of Employment's actual figures but are more realistic, though the Index of Change remains the same. (Greater London data is *included* in the Total South East Region data).

the 1990s has affected the country differently. In the 1970s and 1980s the biggest impact of lost jobs was in Northern Ireland, the North, Yorkshire and Humberside and the North West. To be jobless in Liverpool, Belfast, Manchester, Glasgow or Middlesbrough was distressing but these communities developed a degree of mutual support, so extensive were the job losses that the unemployed individual was less personally stigmatized, as was the case in more affluent areas which had 'plenty of jobs'.

However, as Box 5.1.3 shows, this recession damaged the four richest regions of Britain, for though the *level* of unemployment continued to be lower than 'traditional' unemployment areas, the worsening index of jobs to jobless was 293 in the UK; but widened to 481 in the South East, 442 in the South West, 428 in East Anglia and 347 in the West Midlands. Whilst the scourge of unemployment in Northern Ireland and Scotland had, for example, only widened by 104 and 169. This is not to deny the distress of any unemployed person within the United Kingdom, but it is suggested that to be jobless in Bournemouth, Cheltenham, Norwich, Warwick and Winchester creates a sense of isolation and stigma even greater than in the disadvantaged regions. The poor in the affluent areas are financially poorer, as national benefits stretch less far in supermarkets that are catering for the well off.

Finally, one other substantial change in the unemployed is that in 1990, Class A professionals constituted only 0.8% of the jobless; by 1994, this had risen to 2%, reflecting that it was Classes A, B and C2 who were most affected by the new recession, with indexes of 367, 206 and 201 respectively, which was far higher than the national increase (Bassett, 1994).

Consider the following brief national and international research findings on the unemployment and health link. Unlike the 1960s, by the late 1970s onwards there was a positive correlation between increases in suicide and unemployment in both genders (Pritchard, 1990) and particularly in young men in the UK (Pritchard, 1992a). Despite the USA being the most affluent country the world has ever known, the association between poverty of ethnic minorities and a range of psychosocial disadvantages is beyond question. (Lawson and Wilson, 1995).

It is feared therefore that when some of the targets within the 'Health of the Nation' (DOH, 1992), such as reduction of suicide or teenage pregnancies are not met, it will be the services which will be blamed not the lack of resources (Pritchard, 1995). The rationale for such a pessimistic forecast is found when examining the unit of resource.

CONCLUSION

We saw in the international comparison, that Britain had one of the lowest GDP expenditures on health in the world (Box 5.1.2). In Box 5.1.1 we saw how proportionately, since 1987, less GDP is being devoted to health than before and the decline is planned to continue (HM Treasury, 1994).

Yet at present, in terms of clinical outcome Britain still has amongst the best morbidity and mortality levels in the developed world. Indeed if we compared clinical outcomes, with pound for pound spent, our NHS and community care services must be amongst the most *effective* and *efficient*. Despite this, workers at all levels in the NHS and community care services are under considerable pressure to increase efficiency and to save money. Of course the cliché 'there can never be enough money to spend on health, it would be a bottomless pit' has some truth, but the evidence presented shows that we are not spending what we could, and comparatively, nothing like it. Rudolf Klein in the early 1980s saw that at the centre of the government's health policy was a single primary economic objective – to reduce public expenditure proportionate to the GDP (Klein, 1995). If this target could be achieved in health, one of central government's largest budgets, then the policy would be achievable. This has meant that the policy discussions on health have been obscured, some would say deliberately so. In essence, health and community care policy in the UK is economically, not health directed and driven.

SUMMARY

■ However defined, the community still provides the contextual frameworks for individuals to live out their lives.

■ The boundaries of communities are defined by geography, family and marital state, gender, ethnicity, social class and employment status and as such define the norm for that individual. Consequently, in times of ill health and distress the actual potential supportive strength of those various community or social networks become all important.

■ The three interrelated long-standing issues surrounding community care are to do with, structure, resources and accessibility.

■ The introduction of internal markets can be viewed as a built-in scheme to seek reduction in costs, which coincides with the deprofessionalization of the caring services. This is presented as anti-elitism and anti-profession-alization.

■ Those on the margins of society: the mentally ill, the homeless, the offender etc., often form a core group of people who cross all the community health boundaries.

■ International comparisons show that Britain has one of the lowest GDP expenditures on health in the world.

■ Yet, at present in terms of clinical outcome Britain is still amongst the best in terms of morbidity and mortality levels within the developed world.

DISCUSSION QUESTIONS

♦ Critically examine the position detailed on pp. 321–322 and consider whether it is merely an alternative rhetoric or a positive agenda for change.

♦ In what ways may the changes discussed here affect access to services and service provision?

♦ Consider whether spending on health and community care services is determined by what we as a nation can afford or, by political priorities.

♦ What factors would you consider when seeking to introduce skill mix into your work situation?

FURTHER READING

Klein R (1995) *The New Politics of the NHS*. Heinemann. A deceptively easy read on the development of the NHS; although the author approaches the topic from a non-practitioner perspective, the implications of his analysis are profound.

Lawson R and Wilson JW (Eds) (1995) *Poverty, Inequality and the Future of Social Policy*, New York: Sage. A brilliant analysis showing similar themes across national boundaries, some very challenging chapters, authoritative and erudite.

Pritchard C (1995) *Suicide the Ultimate Rejection? A Psycho-social Study*. Buckingham: Open University Press.

Brings together practice and social policy, showing the impact, at patient/family level, of socioeconomic changes and how the practitioner is in danger of being scapegoated, and at the end of the continuum, people can die.

United Nations (1948) *Declaration of Human Rights*. New York: UNO.

A brief 10 page document which is truly the universal basis for human rights, the pursuit of social justice and on reflection, the relative deterioration of the position of the citizen. An infallible challenge to any political party who further erode human rights, and by today's standards might be thought to be radical.

REFERENCES

Barclay GC (Ed) (1991) *A Digest of Information on the Criminal Justice System*. London: Home Office.

Bassett P (1994) Middle-Class job worries could cost the Tories dear. *Times* London, 17 August.

Brudney KL and Dobkin JH (1992) Resurgent tuberculosis in New York City. Human immune deficiency virus, homelessness and the decline of tuberculosis programmes. *American Review of Respiratory Disease* **144** (4): 745–748.

Creighton S (1993) Children's homicide: An exchange. *British Journal of Social Work* **23**(6): 643–644.

Department of Commerce (1993) *Statistical Abstract of the United States* 13th edition. National Data Series Washington DC. DOC.

Department of Employment (1974–1994) *Employment Gazette* January. London: DOE.

Department of Health (1992) *Health of the Nation: A strategy for England and Wales*. London: HMSO.

Dieskstra RFW (1991) Suicide and parasuicide: A global perspective. In SM Montgomery and NLM Goeting (Eds) *Suicide and Attempted Suicide Risk Factors: Management and Prevention*, pp. 16–37. Southampton: Duphar Medical Relations.

Dooley J (1990) Prison suicide in England and Wales. *British Journal of Psychiatry* **156**: 40–45.

Dooley D, Catalno R and Serxner S (1989) Economic stress and suicide: Multivariate analysis of economic stress and suicidal ideation. *Suicide Life Threatening Behaviour* **19**(4): 337–351.

HM Treasury (1979–1994) *Planned Government Expenditure 1993/4–1996/97* London, HMSO.

House of Commons (1992) *All Party Parliamentary Select Committee Report* Hansard, HMSO.

Howard M (1994) Annual Conference Speech, Brighton. *Conservative Party News Release* London: Conservative Party Central Office.

Hudson B, Roberts C and Roberts C (1993) *Training for Work with Mentally Disordered Offenders*. London: CCETSW.

Judd K and Benzeval E (1993) Health in Equalities: New concerns About The Children of Single Mothers. *British Medical Journal* **306**: 677–680.

Klein R (1995) *The New Politics of the NHS* 3rd edn. London: Longman.

Lawson R and Wilson JW (Eds) (1994) *Poverty, Inequality and the Future of Social Policy*. New York: Russell Sage.

Marshall EJ and Reed JL (1993) Psychiatric morbidity in homeless women. *British Journal of Psychiatry* **160**: 761–768.

Morrell DC, Green J and Savill R (1994) *Five Essays on Emergency Pathways: A Study of Acute Admissions to London Hospitals*. London, King's Fund Institute.

Pritchard B (1995) Personal communication. Manager Neurosurgical Theatres, Southampton University Trust Hospital.

Pritchard C (1990) Suicide, unemployment and gender variations in the Western World 1964–1986: Are Anglophone women protected from suicide? *Social Psychiatry Psychiatric Epidemiology* **25**: 1–8.

Pritchard C (1992a) Is there a link between suicide in young men and unemployment? A comparison of the UK with other European Community countries. *British Journal of Psychiatry* 160: 750–756.

Pritchard C (1992b) What can we afford for the NHS? An analysis of Government expenditure 1974–1992. *Social Administration Policy* **26**(1): 40–54.

Pritchard C (1993a) Re-analysing children's homicide and undetermined deaths as an indication of improved child protection: A reply to Creighton. *British Journal of Social Work* **23**(6): 645–652.

Pritchard C (1993b) Kindestotungen: Die estremeste Form der Kindesmisshandlung: Ein Internationaler Verleigh zwichen Bay/Klein-kindund Kindestotungen als ein fur den Schutzen dieser Gruppen. *Nachrichten Dienst* **72**(3): 65–72.

Pritchard C (1995) *Suicide the Ultimate Rejection: A psychosocial study*. Buckingham: Open University Press.

Pritchard C and Clooney D (1994) *Single Homeless in Dorset: Fractured Lives & Fragmented Policies*. Report to Dept of Environment, Bournemouth, Bournemouth Churches Housing Association.

Pritchard C and Taylor RKS (1978) *Social Work: Reform or Revolution?* London: Routledge and Kegan Paul.

Pritchard C, Cotton A and Cox M (1992) Mental illness, drug and alcohol abuse and risk of HIV infection in young adult clients of the probation service. *Social Work Social Science Review* **3**(2): 150–162.

Reed Committee (1994) *Report of the Committee of Mentally Abnormal Offenders*. London: Department of Health.

Scott J (1993) Homelessness and mental illness. *British Journal of Psychiatry* **162:** 314–324.

Seebohm Lord Frederick (1988) *The Seebohm Report. Twenty Years On*. Policy Studies Institute.

Stewart J and Stewart M (1993) *Social Backgrounds of Young Offenders*. Association of Chief Probation Officers: London.

Thatcher M (1987) Annual Conservative Association Conference, Buxton. *Conservative Party News Release* London. Conservative Party Central Office.

Titmuss R (1968) *Commitment to Welfare* London: Allen & Unwin.

United Nations (1948) *Universal Declaration of Human Rights*. New York; UNO.

Warnock Baroness Mary (1993) Children in Educational Need – 13th Annual Lecture Dept Social Work Studies, University of Southampton.

Whitehead M (1990) *The Health Divide: Inequalities in Health in the 1980's*. Harmondsworth: Penguin.

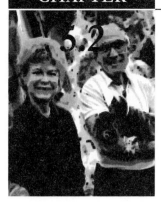

5.2

VALUE FOR MONEY

David Cohen

KEY ISSUES

- Principles of economics
- Resource scarcity
- Efficiency
- Objectives of community care policy
- Cost–benefit analysis
- Marginal analysis
- Cost-effectiveness analysis
- Cost utility analysis

INTRODUCTION

This chapter explains why considerations of value for money are important in determining how far community care policy should be pursued and how the resources devoted to community care could best be deployed. Its framework is that of economics and it provides an alternative way of looking at the sometimes unpleasant choices which resource scarcity makes necessary. A brief description of the techniques of economic appraisal is given together with examples, but the chapter's main aim is to show how application of the thinking behind economic appraisal can be of value even when the techniques are not rigorously applied. Community nurses should be able to apply this thinking to the problems and issues they face.

Value for Money: the Need to Ask the Right Questions

Government documents may give the impression that the recent shift toward more community care is motivated solely by concern for the well-being of patients, but many commentators (see, for example, Harrison *et al.*, 1990) have accused the government of having 'mixed motives', noting in particular the increasing need to control public expenditure. This begs the question 'is community care cheaper than institutional care?'

Unfortunately, the answer to this question is not straightforward and depends, *inter alia*, on whose perspective is taken and which costs are included (for a discussion of the difficulties of costing community care see Knapp, 1993). From the perspective of the National Health Service, community care is almost certainly cheaper because many costs are borne by local authority social services and by social security. From the perspective of the public sector as a whole, community care may be cheaper because many costs are borne by patients and their relatives and much care is provided by unpaid informal carers. From the perspective of society as a whole the answer is unclear. While determining whether or not community care is cheaper than institutional care may be informative, the question is largely irrelevant for purposes of evaluating community care policy because saving money is not its explicit objective.

A better question, and one which would recognize the health and welfare objectives of policy as well as government's natural concern to control public expenditure, would be 'does community care offer better value for money?' Or expressed slightly differently, is community care more cost-effective than institutional care? Yet, as will be explained more fully below, unless this question is asked about specific client or clinical groups then it too is largely irrelevant for policy evaluation since the NHS will never provide only residential with no community care nor only community with no residential care. Both clearly have a place and the question is not whether one is 'better' than the other, but whether the current *balance* between residential and community care is the right one. Since recent policy is seeking to shift the balance, an approach to assessing value for money which examines the effects of moving the boundaries of care is needed.

The remainder of this chapter will argue that economics provides just such an approach and at least ensures that the right questions are asked so that the right information is obtained and judgements are made about the right things. It will show how the principles of economics can be used both to examine the balance between community and other forms of care and to evaluate whether resources currently devoted to community care can be used more efficiently.

The Growing Acceptance of the Thinking of Health Economics

The basic tenet of health economics is that resources for health creation are *scarce* relative to the demands made on them. This means that resource allocation choices between competing claimants are inescapable. Put in a less attractive way, health care rationing is inevitable.

Until recently, this economist's view was largely shunned by health professionals who tended to argue that their duty is to provide the most effective health care possible. Considerations of cost are not only anathema to their whole way of thinking but using information on costs in decision-making would compromise their ethical principles (see, for example, Loewy, 1980). Such rigid opposition is becoming less commonplace.

In the UK the purchaser and provider functions of the NHS were separated in 1991. Purchasers were given budgets, instructed to assess the needs of the populations they served, and told to purchase health care services to meet those needs from the given budgets. It became immediately evident that the budgets could not purchase enough health care to meet all needs fully, immediately and in the most patient friendly way. Some form of prioritizing appeared to be necessary.

At a recent conference organized by the British Medical Association, the King's Fund and Patients' Association (Smith, 1993) Virginia Bottomley made a revolutionary claim for a British Secretary of State for Health that 'Setting priorities is an issue for every organization'. Although there was a good degree of vocal opposition, conference delegates later carried a motion 'This house believes that rationing in health care is inevitable'. It is most unlikely that such a motion would have even been debated, let alone passed, had it been considered at a similar conference ten years ago. Why the change in attitude?

Clearly, defining the populations which will receive health care paid from fixed budgets was instrumental in highlighting the economist's premise that resources are scarce, but why not just call for bigger budgets? Christine Hancock, secretary of the Royal College of Nursing, said at the above conference 'If doctors and nurses are seduced by the idea of rationing they give politicians the perfect excuse not to increase resources' (quoted in Smith, 1993).

Many who accept the need for rationing would probably also like to see additional resources devoted to the NHS, but there are a number of reasons why extra funding will not make the problem go away. Aside from the obvious higher costs of dealing with an ageing population, health care technology is advancing at a rapid and increasing pace. New pharmaceuticals, diagnostic procedures, equipment and surgical techniques among many other advances, mean that some patients who were previously untreatable can now benefit from treatment. Very low birthweight babies, for example, did not have a need for treatment until the technology of neonatal intensive care units was developed. Today they have a need.

New advances are also allowing patients who could previously be treated to now be treated better, but normally at higher cost. As the pace of technological advance is unlikely to decrease, the gap between met need (what we are achieving) and total need (what we could achieve in a world of infinite resources) will widen. Constantly increasing funding is therefore needed just to keep the gap from widening further and as long as society has other needs too (for education, defence, law and order, not to mention private consumption needs) closing the health needs gap completely is not possible.

For these reasons, there has been a recent shift in focus in the evaluation of health interventions from questions such as 'do they work?' to 'are they good value for money?' Consequently there is a growing interest in economics.

Basic Principles

For present purposes health economics may be regarded as a discipline whose way of thinking is more important than its range of techniques. As stated above, the main principle is that of resource scarcity; 'In the beginning, middle and end was, is and will be scarcity of resources' (Mooney, 1992).

Money versus Resources

In common usage the terms 'money' and 'resources' are often used interchangeably. In economics they have different meanings. Resources contribute to the production of healthier people either directly (e.g. nurses, doctors, drugs, dressings, equipment) or indirectly (e.g. administration). Money gives a command over resources, but will not make people healthier unless used to pay for resources. Some resources such as volunteer workers or informal carers do not incur money costs. Most health care resources do. Thus more resources normally means more money expenditure.

Opportunity Cost

Because of scarcity, devoting resources to X means sacrificing the benefits that could have been produced in Y. Economists regard the cost of X in terms of the benefits sacrificed from Y, and use the term opportunity cost to emphasize this notion of opportunity forgone.

Opportunity costs are not necessarily the same as money costs. Moving a nurse from A to B may mean no change in the nursing wages bill, but if the move to B means sacrificing the benefit she used to provide in A, an opportunity cost is incurred. By the economic way of thinking, cost always means opportunity cost and is one of the features which distinguish economic appraisal from financial appraisal.

Efficiency as a Criterion for Choice

Scarcity means that we cannot do everything we would like to do and resource allocation choices are inescapable. Economists have long argued that when choices are being made, the criteria used should be stated explicitly. The economist's preferred criterion is *efficiency* which is about maximizing the benefit to available resources but efficiency is never presented as the be all and end all of resource allocation. Inefficient allocations can be defended on political, public relations, ethical, equity or other grounds, but inefficiency carries a price since (by definition) inefficient allocations mean less total benefit than could have been achieved.

The Cost-Benefit Approach

All health care activities involve the use of resources which are expected to produce benefits but at the same time incur opportunity costs. The process of comparing gains (benefits) with sacrifices (costs) is called the cost-benefit approach. Its decision rule says to only do those things where the value of the gain exceeds the value of the sacrifice. Failing the cost-benefit test does not mean that the potential benefits of a programme are not worth some amount of cash, but that the cost of pursuing these benefits in terms of other benefits which will have to be forgone cannot be justified.

Applying the Cost-Benefit Approach: Cars for Community Nurses

The most difficult part of a formal cost–benefit analysis is determining what to included as 'benefits', deciding how they should be measured and valued, and comparing them with benefits forgone elsewhere. Nevertheless, as stated above, economics can be regarded first and foremost as a way of thinking which can be a valuable aid to decision-making even without formal application of the techniques. The usefulness of the cost-benefit *approach* even without a full-blown economic appraisal is illustrated in the following example.

In 1983, Lothian Health Board began to question why community nurses and health visitors who apparently once provided a satisfactory service by walking, cycling or using public transport to visit their patients, were increasingly regarding a car as a virtual necessity for the job. The question was generated by a concern that a large and growing proportion of the community nursing budget was being spent on transport rather than directly on patient care. Did the current expenditure on transport represent good value for money? For a variety of reasons an answer was needed quickly and a full and costly economic appraisal was not practical. It was decided nonetheless to examine the issue in a cost–benefit framework.

The first problem encountered was the reluctance of the community nurses and health visitors to participate. They shared the commonly held belief that economics is about economizing and therefore assumed that the objective of the study was to save money by taking their cars away. They argued that the study was inappropriate and unnecessary because they 'needed' their cars. The following passage illustrates how translating such commonly heard statements into economic language can help frame the issue in a way more consistent with economic thinking.

> Economic appraisal is based on the idea that there are always alternative uses for resources and that there are always choices to be made. When one hears it argued that in some particular circumstance there is no choice – Nurse Jones must have the use of a car – then it is implied that Nurse Jones currently provides a service which benefits patients in the community. If she did not have the use of a car and had to rely on other

forms of transport, she could not possibly do as much. The resulting loss of benefit to the community would be so great relative to the savings in transport costs as to be not worth considering. Put another way, there is unlikely to be any other use to which the freed resources could be put which could compensate for the loss of the benefit resulting from withdrawal of Nurse Jones' car. (Cohen and Yule, 1984).

Stated this way the questions that needed addressing were:

- How much money would be saved by providing nurses with alternative transport?
- How much additional travel time would this imply, i.e. how much less time would be available to care for patients?
- What would be the loss of benefit associated with less time with patients?
- What benefits could be produced by using the saved money to expand other services?

It was decided that crown car users with the lowest annual mileage and private car users with the lowest miles per visit ratios would be included in the study. Seven district nurses and eight health visitors were identified. On the basis of their knowledge of the local geography, etc., and in consultation with the nurses and health visitors concerned, nursing officers were asked to identify the most appropriate alternative form of transport and estimate the implications for extra travel time.

Benefit loss was estimated by converting the extra travel time into numbers of home visits forgone, but as explained below in 'Different objectives, different techniques of appraisal', loss of services can be a misleading proxy for loss of health benefits. Although crude, the results indicated that 1.38 district nurse home visits or 1.06 health visitor home visits would be lost for every £1 saved.

The issue of 'what is a visit worth?' was addressed by asking a wide range of other service providers to describe what they could achieve if they were given additional funding. Their answers, scaled to reflect extra benefit per pound, could then be compared with the perceived benefit attached to the home visits which would be forgone by removing car user status from the identified community nurses and health visitors.

It is not possible to state objectively whether the value of the benefits from the present level of expenditure on transport exceed the value of the benefits forgone elsewhere. This requires a value judgement. The advantage of applying the economic framework is that the trade-offs are clearly identified, thus ensuring that judgements are made about the right things.

In this case, the appraisal bore out the initial feelings expressed by the nurses. Now, though, instead of the uninformed statement that community nurses 'must have cars', we see an investigation using economic principles, albeit on a crude basis, which indicated that the benefits derived from current expenditure on transport exceeded the opportunity costs. This means that the present level of provision of cars for nurses was in fact good value for money.

Importance of the Margin

Most health care decisions involve changing the scale of an activity rather than doing it or not doing it. Accordingly, the appropriate cost–benefit question is normally not 'do the benefits justify the costs' but rather 'do the extra benefits justify the extra cost'.

The reason why this focus on the margin is so important is that relationship between *marginal* (extra) benefits and marginal costs can change dramatically as the scale of activity changes. For example, the first community nurse assigned to an area with no previous provision will allocate her time where need is greatest, i.e. on those patients who will benefit most from her care. Adding a second nurse will increase *total* benefit but as the most needy cases are already being seen, marginal benefit will be less. Adding more nurses will increase total benefit by progressively smaller amounts or to use the jargon, there will be decreasing marginal benefits. In an ideal world of infinite resources, nurses would continue to be added until all needs of patients in the community were met fully, immediately and in the most patient friendly way possible. In a world of finite resources nurses should continue to be added so long as the marginal benefit they produce exceeds the marginal cost of employing them, i.e. to the point where the ratio of marginal benefit to marginal cost equals one. In this example, constant marginal cost and falling marginal benefit mean this equality will be reached before all needs in this community are met.

Unfortunately, expanding every activity to the point where the marginal benefit/marginal cost ratio equals one is rarely possible because of budget constraints. In such cases expansion of A can only be achieved by transferring resources from B. Whether or not the transfer is justified on efficiency grounds depends on whether the extra benefits from expanding A are greater than the loss of benefits from contracting B? If so, then the transfer will increase total benefit with total cost unchanged. Overall efficiency is achieved when no further transfers which meet this condition are possible. This occurs when the ratio of marginal benefit to marginal cost is equalized across all activities.

Applying the Marginal Approach: Care of the Elderly

In the late 1970s Grampian Health Board's Care of the Elderly Programme Committee identified an imbalance in the services provided to elderly people in the community, in residential homes and in hospital which it wished to see redressed. The cost of caring for patients in alternative settings is clearly one factor in deciding on the best balance between these forms of care.

It initially appeared that the cost implications of moving patients from one form of care to another could be determined using routinely collected cost data. For example, if the cost per patient week is £1500 in hospital and £300 in the community, then it would appear that moving a patient from hospital to community care would save £1500 − £300 = £1200.

The problem with this reasoning is that these are *average* costs which were derived by dividing the total cost of caring for all patients in each setting by the total number of patients receiving care in that setting. The cost of caring for *individual* patients, however, can vary greatly depending on their respective needs. In the case of hospital care, for example, total costs include the cost of caring for very high dependency patients who would never even be considered for a move to community care. If a group of patients is to be moved from hospital to community care, the relevant questions are 'what is the current cost of caring for these patients in hospital and what would be the cost of caring for them in the community?' Average cost data is irrelevant to these questions. The problem in practice, though, is that average cost data is normally readily available while the relevant *marginal cost* data is normally not and has to be collected specifically for the purpose.

In the Grampian illustration (Mooney, 1978), health professionals were asked to identify 'marginal populations', i.e. those patients most suitable for shifts between the different forms of care. Hospital patients, for example, were classed as being suitable for residential home care, suitable for care in the community, or suitable for continued hospital care. Each marginal population was then described in terms of various need characteristics such as the proportion having frequent falls, night confusion, locomotor difficulties, mental impairment and so on, and their ability to perform day-to-day tasks with and without assistance. The cost of caring for each marginal population in the current setting and the relevant alternative setting could then be estimated.

As in the example of cars for community nurses, the results did not provide firm conclusions of what should be done, but rather identified the trade-offs upon which value judgements would have to be made. The study showed the true cost implications of altering the balance of care, which could then be considered against descriptions of the people who would actually be affected. This is another example of how application of the framework, even a crude manner, can be greatly informative.

Different Objectives, Different Techniques of Appraisal

A major problem in any evaluation is that 'effectiveness' cannot be measured without an explicit statement of objectives; effective at doing what? If the objective is to improve or sustain the health of patients, then the most effective form of care is that which produces the most health gain. But what about the preferences of patients? What about the effect on the patients' relatives or informal carers? What if delivery of the most effective form of care is judged to be inequitable, unethical, or goes against a political objective?

Cost–benefit analysis (CBA) examines whether, or to what extent, a given objective is worth pursuing. It does this by weighing gains (benefits) against sacrifices (costs), normally using a 'social welfare' view which includes all costs regardless of who bears them and all benefits regardless to whom they accrue. If, for example, community care confers benefits (positive or negative) on informal carers, then a cost-benefit analysis using a social welfare view would have to include them.

It is, however, often the case that the issue is not to determine whether or to what extent to pursue an objective, but more simply *how* to pursue it. In these cases cost-effectiveness analysis (CEA) can be used to find the least costly way of achieving some much more narrowly defined benefits. For example, an objective to reduce blood pressure (BP) in hypertensives, could be addressed by a CEA comparing alternative interventions and measuring benefits in terms of units of BP reductions. The programme with the lowest cost per unit reduction is the most cost-effective.

This much simpler analysis, however, only allows comparison of alternative ways of pursuing the specific objective to reduce BP. It does not indicate whether spending £x on reducing BP represents better or worse value for money than spending £x on something else. Normally, the narrower the objective, the simpler the appraisal but the less informative the results.

If raised BP is regarded as a risk factor in stroke and other life threatening conditions, then it is possible to view the objective of BP reduction programmes in broader life saving terms. In this case, a CEA would compare different blood pressure reduction programmes in terms of cost per life saved. This will involve a more complex appraisal because while BP can be accurately measured, translating today's reduced BP into tomorrow's lives saved involves greater use of assumptions and estimations.

The advantage of the more complex CEA, though, is that in addition to indicating the most cost-effective way of reducing BP, the results allow cost-effectiveness comparisons of BP reduction with all other life saving interventions thus indicating whether or not BP reduction programmes represent better or worse value for money than other life saving interventions.

This CEA would still be limited, though, because only life saving programmes can be included in the comparisons. It cannot show whether BP reduction represents better value for money than programmes which improve the quality of life without necessarily extending it.

This problem can be overcome by broadening the object to take in both life extension and quality of life improvements – or stated more generally to produce 'health'. The advantage would be that the cost-effectiveness of all interventions, whether preventive, curative or caring, can be compared in terms of cost per unit of 'health' produced. The problem, of course, is that while years of life saved can be counted (measured), 'health' cannot.

Because of this, health care *services* are often used as a proxy for health on the assumption that more service equals more health. This can be dangerous, however, as not only is the assumption not always true, but it is implied that the relationship between service provision and health gain is constant. In the cars for community nurses study, for example, it was evident that the more home visits were to be lost the greater would be the loss of benefit associated with each additional lost visit.

Thus while the published study (Cohen and Yule, 1984) measured benefit loss in terms of lost visits, Lothian Health Board could only make a decision about whether or not to reduce expenditure on transport by asking the nurses to describe in the best terms possible what these forgone visits meant in terms of the health of the patients concerned.

Although directly measuring health changes is clearly no easy task, it is not an impossible one and there are numerous alternative tools available for doing so (for a good review see Bowling, 1991, and Chapter 3.1 of this volume). Some of these yield multidimensional health *profiles*, others undimensional health *measures*. Since health itself has many dimensions (pain, distress, disability, etc.) the unidimensional measures are inevitably imperfect because combining dimensions involves attaching weights (values) to the different attributes of health. For example, does relieving one person's pain represent a greater or lesser health gain than reducing another person's distress?

The great advantage of using unidimensional health measures, however, is that they provide the effectiveness measure described above which allows all interventions on all groups of patients for all conditions to be compared in terms of cost per unit of effectiveness.

A unidimensional health measure favoured by many economists is the quality adjusted life year (QALY) which is based on the assertion that all health gains can be expressed in terms of extra life years (LY) or improved quality of life (QA) or some combination of the two. Thus all interventions produce QALYs. Since resources are finite, total QALY production is maximized when resources are allocated *on the margin* to those interventions producing the greatest number of QALYs per pound spent. Because QALYs and similar measures are based on the utilities (values) attached to different health states, studies which use them as the measure of the effectiveness are called 'Cost Utility' analyses (CUA).

Cost/QALY league tables are being drawn up which can help inform, but never dictate, resource allocation decision-making (see, for example, Maynard, 1991). Unfortunately we are unaware of any CUAs in the area of care in the community.

Applying the Cost-Effectiveness Technique: a Community Care Initiative for the Elderly Mentally Infirm

In 1983 the (then) Department of Health and Social Security made £6 million available to support a policy objective of maintaining elderly people with severe or moderate organic disorders at home rather than in long-term institutional care. One of the innovative projects it funded was a Family Support Unit (FSU) in South Tees which offered respite care, day care, evening care and special occasional residential care to support the carers of elderly mentally infirm people. Given the stated objective which made no explicit reference to the quality of life or other health effects of the policy, a study was undertaken to compare the cost-effectiveness of community care, including the FSU with conventional community care (Donaldson and Gregson, 1989).

Time spent in the community (the unit of effectiveness) was calculated as the number of days between assessment and either admission to long-term care or death while living at home. Patients in the FSU group spent a mean of 664 days in the community compared to 492 days for the controls. The cost of community care with the FSU was considerably higher at £6.60 per patient day compared to £2.30 for the controls. Combining this with information on time spent in the community meant that community care with the FSU cost £3200 per patient more than community care without. This £3200, however, allowed an extra 172 days in the community which would have cost £7912 if these patients had spent the time in a long-term hospital bed instead.

Is community care with an FSU more cost-effective than community care without? Given the above objective the answer is clearly yes. However, since effectiveness was only measured (quite correctly in these circumstances) in days spent in the community, the authors hedged their conclusion by stating that the FSU is cost-effective '. . . if it is assumed that clients and their carers find time spent at home in the community at least as desirable as long term hospital care' (p. 205).

If the health status of the two groups had been monitored and the results expressed in (say) cost/QALY terms, then the study would have shown whether community care with FSU is a more cost-effective way of pursuing a health objective than community care without. Comparing these results with cost/QALY information from other interventions would show whether a transfer of resources on the margin from these other interventions to more provision of FSU would be justified on efficiency grounds.

As a separate exercise this study also examined the costs and benefits to carers of the FSU and discussed the issue of health authority/local authority transfers to fund FSUs.

CONCLUSION

The messages from this chapter are simple. Scarcity means that decisions on the appropriate level of resources devoted to community care and the way in which those resources are deployed both require value for money information. Value for money, however, cannot be assessed without clear reference to the broad objectives of policy or the narrower objectives of specific interventions. Too often these objectives are either poorly defined or, possibly for political or other reasons, intentionally misleading.

Examining whether or not community care is cheaper than institutional care is not a straightforward task but on its own is only worth doing if the stated objective of policy is to save money. If objectives are more health orientated, then other questions need to be asked.

Economics provides a framework based on sound principles which allow issues of value for money to be addressed in a scientific way, while emphasizing that the values attached to the various benefits of care can never be determined objectively. Since value for money is by definition a value judgement, economic appraisal can never be a substitute for decision-making. Examining issues using the economic way of thinking, or more formally applying the techniques of economic appraisal, can, however, greatly aid such decision-making.

SUMMARY

- The key economic issue is *not* whether or not community care is cheaper than the alternatives, but whether or not it is a more efficient way of delivering health care.
- Similarly, the issue is not all community care versus no community care, but whether or not the *balance of care* should be shifted further toward community care.
- The above questions are addressed within economics by accepting that resources for health care are scarce and therefore resource allocation decisions (i.e. priorities) are inescapable.
- One key criterion for prioritizing is 'efficiency' which attempts to maximize the benefit to available resources.
- Four techniques of economic evaluation: cost minimization, cost-effectiveness, cost utility and cost–benefit analyses can help to assess the efficiency of changes in the balance of care toward community care.

DISCUSSION QUESTIONS

♦ How would you respond to someone who stated that the health of your patients must be 'beyond considerations of cost'?

♦ What arguments could you use in support of a request for funding for some new equipment which you know will greatly benefit your patients.

♦ Why should you be sceptical about the claim that a measure of the success of the NHS is the fact that it is treating more patients than ever before?

♦ From a nurse's perspective what are the key issues of community care requiring economic appraisal and why?

FURTHER READING

Cohen D and Henderson J (1988) *Health, Prevention and Economics*. Oxford: Oxford University Press.

Mooney GH (1992) *Economics, Medicine and Health Care*, 2nd ed. Brighton: Wheatsheaf.
These two publications explain the principles of health economics more fully.

Drummond MF, Stoddart GL and Torrance GW (1987)

Methods for the Economic Evaluation of Health Care Programmes. Oxford: Oxford University Press.
Describes the techniques of economic appraisal.

Drummond MF and Maynard A (eds) (1993) *Purchasing and Providing Cost-Effective Health Care*. Edinburgh: Churchill Livingstone.
Explains the relevance of economic principles to the reformed NHS.

Netten A and Beecham J (Eds) (1993) *Costing Community Care: Theory and Practice*. Aldershot: Ashgate Publishing.

Discusses problems and methods for costing community care programmes.

REFERENCES

Bowling A (1991) *Measuring Health: A Review of Quality of Life Measuring Scales*. Oxford: Oxford University Press.

Cohen D and Yule B (1984) The case for community cars. *Nursing Times: Community Outlook*. May 9: 173.

Donaldson C and Gregson B (1989) Prolonging life at home: what is the cost? *Community Medicine* **2**(3): 200–209.

Harrison S, Hunter DJ and Pollit C (1990) *The Dynamics of British Health Policy*. London: Unwin Hyman.

Knapp M (1993) The costing process: background theory. In A Netten and J Beechan (Eds) *Costing Community Care: Theory and Practice*. Aldershot: Ashgate Publishing.

Loewy EL (1980) Letter. *New England Journal of Medicine* **302:** 6970.

Maynard A (1991) Developing a health care market. *Economic Journal* **101:** 1277.

Mooney GH (1978) Planning for balance of care of the elderly. *Scottish Journal of Political Economy* **25**(2): 149.

Mooney GH (1992) *Economics, Medicine and Health Care*, 2nd Edn. Brighton: Wheatsheaf.

Smith R (1983) *British Medical Journal* **306:** 737.

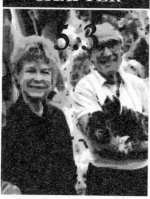

ACHIEVING HEALTH GAINS

Elizabeth Gould

KEY ISSUES

- Health gain
- Measuring health status
- Needs assessment
- Community perspectives
- Target setting
- Multi-agency collaboration
- Benchmarking

INTRODUCTION

The expression 'health gain' has only appeared in health service literature in recent years; what does it mean and how does the concept of achieving health gain affect the way health professionals practise? This chapter aims to clarify the prerequisites for achieving health gain.

Firstly, knowing where you are starting from and agreeing on a definition of health. What is the current health status of the population you serve; what resources are available to meet their health problems and how does the community itself perceive its health needs?

Secondly, what improvements in health are you trying to achieve? From a thorough understanding of the starting point should emerge goals or targets for improved health which are appropriate, measurable and achievable.

Thirdly, how are you going to get from the starting point to the destination? The route you take will depend upon the availability of strategies known to be effective together with their cost, their social and clinical acceptability, and their practical feasibility. Along the route there will be challenges to overcome: the lack of evaluation of many health care interventions; the difficulties of defining and measuring relevant outcomes; the need for multi-agency collaboration and for monitoring progress and highlighting good practice. Each of these elements is a complex area of study in its own right. As a practitioner the key to achieving health gain is to remain constantly critical of what you do, why and how you do it, and questioning whether there are more effective ways of maximizing health benefit. See Chapter 3.3, for further discussion.

This chapter offers three outline case studies which describe very different ways in which health gain can be achieved:

- Through the fluoridation of water supplies as a strategy against dental caries.
- Through the promotion of breastfeeding as a way of improving maternal and early child health.
- Through cardiac rehabilitation as a health service intervention aimed at improving the quality of life of those who have suffered from a myocardial infarction.

The Meaning of Health Gain

The expression 'health gain' appears to have originated in the Welsh Office's strategy for improving the health of the people of Wales (Welsh Office, 1989) and was cited in that strategy as being the key criterion for judging the effectiveness of a health service. Since then the expression has found increasing popularity and is to be found in other strategic health service documents (DOH, 1991). It must be recognized that it acquired currency in the UK at a time of extensive health service reforms. Driven largely by the need for cost control, a number of major organizational changes were made (DOH, 1989b) including the introduction of an internal market whereby, as the guiding principle, those who manage services (the providers) compete to contract services with those who commission them (the purchasers). See Chapters 5.5 and 5.6 for further discussion.

In 1948 with the introduction of the NHS, Aneurin Bevan said that his role as a politician was '. . . To give you all the facilities, apparatus and help I can and then leave you as professional men and women to use your own skill and judgment without hindrance . . .'. (Bevan, 1975). This early faith in subjective clinical judgement has given way to a pressing need for providers of health services to justify how they make use of resources in terms of both effectiveness and efficiency. That is to say doing the right things (clinically effective things) in the right way (cost-effectively using resources). The term 'health gain' has largely become synonymous with effectiveness. Is an intervention effective in advancing and maximizing the health potential of an individual? Is it effective in raising the overall health of a population? Health gain is fundamentally about productivity in relation to health care, resulting in a better outcome than would have been achieved without the intervention. This may be in terms of reducing the risk of mortality – the recipient of the service lives longer, and/or reducing the severity or duration of morbidity – the quality of life of the recipient is improved.

The slogan which exhorts health services to 'Add years to life and life to years' may seem straightforward enough but actually conceals many complex issues. Health gain is a vague term in which many other concepts overlap. As Hunter (1993) points out 'Health gain is something of a catchall notion insofar as it embraces a number of issues and initiatives that are derived, sometimes loosely, from the National Health Service (NHS) reform agenda. Developments in needs assessments, in health outcomes, in listening to local people, in health services research and development programmes, and in articulating a health strategy, all in one way or another flow from and impact upon health gain.'

The Starting Point: How Big is the Problem?

Agreeing on a Definition of Health

Measurement of health status itself implies an underlying agreement about the nature of health (Bowling, 1991) but as Seedhouse (1986) has pointed out health is not a word with a single uncontroversial meaning. Negative definitions of health relate to the absence of disease or illness, and health problems as medical problems. Traditional indicators of negative health status include measures of mortality, disease incidence, sickness data. This may still be the most appropriate way in which to measure the health status of severely compromised populations (Bowling, 1991) where many of the basic prerequisites for health, such as peace, shelter, food, education, income, are absent. But in less extreme situations, measurement of health status necessitates an underlying concept of health which is positive, as in the World Health Organization definition – 'A state of complete physical, mental and social wellbeing, and not merely the absence of disease or infirmity'. Whilst this may be challenged as an unachievable ideal, it sets health into a broad context, moving outside the narrow confines of a medical paradigm. The need to see health in a social, economic, cultural and environmental context can be considered as central to the concept of a health gain. Seedhouse (1986) has suggested that amidst all the various theories and conflicting approaches to defining health, a significant common factor can be found, viz: 'All theories of health and all approaches designed to increase health are intended to advise against or prevent the creation of, or to remove, obstacles to the achievement of human potential'. By this token, achieving health gain, is about *addition*, (the adding of years to life and life to years) but it, can also be seen as a *subtraction*, breaking down the barriers to improved health status.

Measuring Health Status   The need to undertake epidemiological assessments in order to inform both short-term and strategic health planning is not something new. Prior to the reorganization of the NHS in 1974, Local Authority Medical Officers of Health had a statutory obligation to produce annual Public Health reports describing the health profile of the local population, analysing contributory factors and making recommendations for disease prevention and health promotion. These were largely discontinued after 1974 although following the Black Report (Townsend, 1988) there was a revival of interest in local health problems which linked social and economic conditions with health status. The Annual Report of the Director of Public Health Medicine on the state of public health in a particular region or district was reinstated in 1988. The completion of a community health profile has been a requirement of post-basic community nursing courses, while every medical general practice is required to submit an annual profile of the practice population together with performance data.

There are a number of guidelines available on how to compile a health profile (Twinn, 1990) but there is no universal prescription of exactly what information needs to be included; that will depend on the precise aim of the profile. Pickin and St Leger (1993) provide a useful guide to the sources of demographic and health data one could include in a comprehensive assessment of health status whilst others such as Burton (1993) use a definition of community profiling which is a more general description of the social, environmental and economic aspects of a given area.

Broadly speaking, the measurement of health status identifies health problems in a community and requires information on:

- *Demography*
  Age/gender distribution
  Ethnic groupings
  Household/family type
- *Disease patterns*

Mortality measures – death rates; crude and age specific
Summary mortality statistics – standardized mortality ratios
– expectation of life
Morbidity – short-term self-limiting illnesses to chronic conditions
* *Determinants of health (modifiers)*

Socioeconomic factors – e.g. unemployment, housing
Environmental factors – e.g. atmospheric pollution
Ethnic factors – e.g. racial effects on disease prevalence of sickle cell anaemia in
those of Afro-Caribbean origin
Cultural factors – e.g. religious beliefs of a community

There are ways in which a profiled population has specific characteristics of interest to nurses; for example a population may be all women who have undergone breast surgery, or all individuals who have continence needs. The principles are the same in that you need hard data – quantified information about the structure and characteristics of the group, as well as soft data which may be concerned with clients' perceptions of their needs and priorities.

Measurement of health status can be part of the wider process of health needs assessment, a process which has been given prominence since the introduction of the NHS reforms (DOH, 1989b). Pickin and St Leger (1993) describe this process as one of 'exploring the relationship between health problems in a community and the resources available to address those problems in order to achieve a desired outcome'. There are a number of needs assessment methodologies representing both medical and socioeconomic models (Frankel, 1991; Stevens and Raferty, 1991). The life-cycle framework starts with a population and looks at the needs of that population as it passes through life stages (Pickin and St Leger, 1993); a locality approach divides a population into geographical areas. Another approach is to use a framework of predetermined health gain targets (Hamilton-Kirkwood and Parry-Langdon, 1993).

Although health needs assessment is currently considered as a purchaser function, the principles behind it – which require a matching of available resources to existing problems in the most effective way – can be usefully applied by providers and practitioners.

The Community Perspective

Communities and the individuals within them are not just the passive recipients of health care; the need to involve the users of health services in decisions about those services has been recognized as a fundamental principle of primary health care. The 'Health for All by the year 2000' philosophy (WHO, 1981) put the community at the centre of health systems, defining need, setting priorities, planning and evaluating services.

During the late 1960s and early 1970s community participation was promoted in the developing world (Conyers, 1982) as a way of expanding accessibility to health services without necessarily increasing the costs. It arose from a recognition of the failure of existing health services to provide adequate care at realistic cost, and from the realization that improved health status was often linked to environmental, social and cultural issues which could be better dealt with by communities themselves than by a narrowly defined health sector. Participation by individuals and communities was suggested as a process of consciousness-raising and empowerment, in the belief that power gravitates to those who solve problems (Freire, 1972).

Community participation is the logical conclusion to involving people in health service planning; in the context of the British NHS this involvement is less extensive. It has been argued (Ong, 1991) that despite the fact that responsiveness to local views is a theme of the reformed NHS (Welsh Office, 1989), clients/patients/communities are seen simply as *consumers* of health services. Their views are sought in terms of their satisfaction with the care provided rather than as contributors to service development. Efforts to assess local perspectives through traditional patient-satisfaction surveys have been questioned (Dixon, 1993) and increasingly a variety of qualitative sociological research methods are used to involve local people in purchasing decisions (Popay and Williams, 1993). Systematic research strategies such as Rapid Appraisal (Ong, 1991) bring together individual research techniques in attempts to understand how people perceive their health needs. Such perceptions are based on underlying value systems which may be at variance with the value systems of those who provide the services. Local communities have been shown to have different priorities from those of providers (Ruffing-Rahal, 1987) as far as their perceived health needs are concerned.

Whilst there are sound democratic and moral reasons for involving communities in the decision making process, the process itself is not straightforward. Hunter (1993) asks whose values should count – those of clinicians, politicians, managers or the public? An agreed value system and a correlation, or at least a compromise, between the perspectives of the community and the providers, is essential if a health gain strategy is to be acceptable and workable.

The Destination: Choosing Appropriate Goals

Determining the starting point of our 'journey' to achieve health gain requires the incorporation of health needs assessment into a current profile of health status – but this is not without its complexities. Agreeing on appropriate goals which are measurable, acceptable and achievable (both to the community and to those who provide services) is the next step. Increasingly the process for this is the setting and monitoring of targets.

In 1985 the World Health Organization produced its strategy based on the overall aim of *Health for All* by the year 2000 (WHO, 1985), a goal which it had adopted at the 34th World Health Assembly in 1979. This strategy took the form of 38 specific targets with an emphasis on health promotion and disease prevention. Since then a wealth of targets has arisen. In Wales, the Welsh Health Planning Forum has issued Protocols for Investment in Health Gain which identify health gain areas – some, disease related, e.g. cardiovascular diseases, while others are specific to, for example, maternal and early child health (Welsh Health Planning Forum, 1991a, 1991b). In England the Green Paper *The Health of the Nation* suggests specific targets for health improvement (DOH, 1991).

Harvey (1992) assesses the arguments for and against target setting which may be summarized as follows:

Arguments for targets

- Targets are quantified indicators of achievement or failure.
- Targets inspire action and a sense of purpose.
- Targets stimulate debate and highlight the nature of major health problems in a population.

- Targets encourage rational purchasing of health services.

Arguments against targets

- Targets over-emphasize the destination at the expense of how to get there.
- Targets encourage guesswork.
- Targets over-emphasize health issues which are readily measurable at the expense of equally significant issues which are measurable only with difficulty.
- Targets can be over-optimistic and lead to distortion.
- Targets based on secular trends (We'll get there even if we do nothing!) lead to complacency.

Ideally, individual practitioners can develop their own targets, setting goals which are appropriate to current local health status and needs, and which are acceptable to the community. In reality, targe⬚⬚⬚⬚⬚⬚⬚⬚⬚⬚⬚⬚⬚ut, by a central agency, or the purchasing authorit⬚⬚⬚⬚⬚⬚⬚⬚⬚⬚⬚⬚⬚⬚ss. Despite the concerns that this generates (Trom⬚⬚⬚⬚⬚⬚⬚⬚⬚⬚⬚⬚rve as 'another piece of the jigsaw to try and get th⬚⬚⬚⬚⬚⬚⬚⬚

The Route: Strategies for Achieving Health Gain

Strategies for achieving health gain can be categorized into two elements – those which are therapeutic or rehabilitative, providing services to meet existing health needs; and those which are health promoting by improving health through action on lifestyles and environments, or preventive such as the implementation of screening services or immunization programmes. Obviously the type of strategy which is employed will depend on the health gain identified for achievement but all strategies will present challenges relating to (1) the need to move from input to output measures, (2) attribution and the need for multi-agency collaboration, recognizing that improvements in health do not depend on health services alone, (3) benchmarking – the need to obtain baseline data and to monitor practice. The significance of giving consideration to financial resource implications and the cost-effectiveness of a particular intervention, must obviously play a part in the choice of strategy. This aspect of planning and achieving health gain is considered in Chapter 5.2.

Outcomes: Moving from Input to Output Measures

In the past the focus of health service evaluation has been largely based on service inputs – the use of resources – and throughputs – activities or processes of care (Beck *et al.*, 1992). Such measurements can generally be stated in concrete terms: how many people received a particular intervention, how much time was involved and what did it cost? In using health gain as the key criterion for judging the effectiveness of health services, there is a need to move to outcome measures. Was the *outcome* worthwhile: did the intervention achieve what it was intended to achieve: overall did the intervention do more good than harm? The evaluation of interventions in terms of their outcome is more difficult to perform for several reasons and the complexity of outcome measurement is well documented (Beck *et al.*, 1992; Holland, 1983; Long *et al.*, 1992, 1993). Box 5.3.1 lists a number of outcome measures with their relative advantages and disadvantages:

Long *et al.* (1992, 1993) describe the serious practical difficulties in measuring the outcomes of some types of service:

- Those with 'low level effects' – consultations without clinical interventions. This

Box 5.3.1. Advice of outcomes

Proposed measure of outcome	Advantages	Disadvantages
Performance indicators	Routinely collected Wide range of indications available National and standardized Comparable Identify problem areas	Inaccuracies in data Timelines (time lags) Difficulties with analysis and interpretation Lack quality measures Not an absolute measure of performance Tend to relate to structure and progress
Mortality data e.g. Standardized Mortality Ratio (SMR) Potential Years of Life Lost (PYLL) 'Avoidable deaths'	Easy to produce, use routinely collected (OPCS) data Death certificates provide information about disease directly or indirectly leading to death	Death certificate may be subject to error Issues of association and causal inference (social and economic factors may affect death and not just physiological) Time lag Death is an uncommon outcome for most episodes of ill health In some cases death may be seen as a positive outcome
Morbidity data Generally measured by biochemical test, observed symptom rates and role performance e.g. number of days off work	Various forms of data collected: – Inpatient data – Outpatient data – Cancer registration	Large proportion of morbidity will not require hospital administration, yet it is the inpatient data which is the most detailed and routinely collected
Quality of life measures	(i) *Plethora of scales and indices* Measures of functional status Measures of psychological state Measuring social aspects of health Multidimensional indices and profiles Disease specific measures (ii) Economic measures of quality of life	– Tend to be time consuming and expensive
	QALYS: Theoretically yields a theoretical index to measure and compare health effects could aid policy-makers and clinicians in decision-making process, especially with respect to allocation decisions	– Such theories offer substantial methodological and ethical problems
Patient satisfaction Work currently being undertaken by various centres e.g. CASPE (has been highly criticized by Carr-Hill, 1992), Cardiff Business School (this project concentrating on maternity services)	Gives consumers a voice on quality of health care they receive and acts as a feedback mechanism. Assesses whether quality statements within a particular contract have been satisfied or to identify any shortfalls in service	Patient satisfaction is a complex and elusive target with various problems, such as (i) opinions may not be reliable over time (ii) patients' answers often inconsistent (iii) cannot give views on technical aspects as they have insufficient knowledge

Box 5.3.1. (contd.)

Proposed measure of outcome	Advantages	Disadvantages
Medical audit used as a method of monitoring and controlling services especially clinical procedures. The development of clinical guidelines by way of audit is increasing	Is a useful tool for monitoring adverse events Can assess and improve the quality of patient care Enhances medical education (moves towards 'best practice' methods Can identify ways of improving the efficiency of clinical care	It is unlikely that clinicians will be willing to scrutinize their work for the purpose of evaluating contracts Clinicians will also be wary of any activity that they perceive as infringing on clinical freedom.

Source: Welsh Office: Contracting for Health Gain Project. Cardiff.
Reprinted by permission of The Welsh Office.

is a feature of many community nursing contacts where the use of interpersonal skills to support clients is often difficult to evaluate.

- Those where the start and end of a treatment or intervention are unclear, for example in rehabilitation programmes.
- Those where several interventions are being conducted simultaneously.
- Those where many variables are interacting over the long term. This is often the case in health promotion activity where it may be virtually impossible to demonstrate a causal link between a health promoting intervention and a specific outcome.

Clark and Henderson (1983) described the difficulty in attributing an outcome to a particular intervention in the field of preventive health where a positive intervention aims for a negative outcome. Immunization of a child against polio should prevent it contracting the disease – 'It is logically impossible to prove causation for an event which did not happen; the best one can do is to replace proof by an estimate of probability' (Clark and Henderson, 1983: 274).

Establishing evidence of causal associations between an intervention and an outcome is important if we are to decide which interventions are likely to achieve health gain and which are not. However, there is an acknowledged lack of research based evidence to support many health care interventions which have become part of accepted health service provision (Cochrane, 1972). For evaluation to have scientific rigour it requires the use of research methods which have the following approximate hierarchy for reducing bias:

- Clinical impressions
- Cases/case-series without formal controls
- Studies with historical controls
- Case-control studies
- Non-randomized concurrent controls
- Randomized controls

However, even these, applied to the evaluation of long-term outcomes and particularly preventive health programmes, may be unsatisfactory (Clark and Henderson, 1983), and there is a risk that interventions which are complex and long term in their outcomes may bear the brunt of disinvestment.

Attribution and Multi-Agency Collaboration

To what do we attribute improvements in the health status of a population? Was the health gain *really* due to health care intervention or could there be other factors involved? Put in another way, what *is* the relationship between the input, the process, and the outcome? We cannot assume that a process is responsible for all its outputs (Long *et al.*, 1992, 1993), or, conversely, that the outcome is the result of the process. The need to see health in a social, cultural, economic and environmental context is central to the concept of health gain, and therefore initiatives to improve health cannot be considered as the exclusive territory of health professionals.

Consider, for example, the following inputs which may possibly contribute to avoidable road traffic accidents and the benefits to health gain which could result from changes in habits or policies, with consequent reduction in accidents:

- *Individual*. Stress; alcohol and drug abuse; driving experience.
- *Socio-economic*. Resources for safety measure implementation; traffic engineering; vehicle requirements; transport policies.
- *Cultural*. Attitudes towards alcohol use/driving; legal system/penalties; seat belt legislation.
- *Ecosystem*. Terrain; climate, population densities.

McKeown and Lowe (1967b) suggested that changes in the health status of the British population during the second half of the nineteenth century and early part of the twentieth century were largely due to rising incomes and material advances, in which they implicitly included better food, housing, education, rather than changes in health input through medical discoveries. Although their views have been challenged, there remains the fundamental recognition (Hunter, 1993) that health status is not the result of health care alone but that other policy fields and services may be more important and instrumental in achieving certain aspects of health gain. This has implications at government level where commitment to health gain might involve the diversion of resources from 'health services' into other areas such as improvement of housing stock, food policies, the introduction of traffic calming measures.

'The integrating, synthesizing focus of health gain may constitute its chief appeal for those anxious to mobilize healthy alliances which deliberately seek to blur professional and organizational boundaries' (Hunter, 1993: 103). Multi-agency collaboration at an organizational policy level is outside the influence of most individual practitioners whose contribution to multi-agency working will be at a practical teamwork level. Even here, the collaborative approach is not without its difficulties. Issues such as the following can mean that the meeting of community needs is subordinated to the assertion of professionalism:

- Inter-professional rivalry
- Authority/power differentials
- Conflicting agendas
- Differing priorities
- Role ambiguity
- Differing resource inputs

McMurray (1993) asks 'What mechanisms exist in the community to promote collaboration between health care providers, the education, the environment, industry and housing sectors? Are community-wide concerns represented by the different sectors on committees and task forces? What are the gaps in efforts across the sectors?' The need to share information, agree on divisions of labour and ensure policies are compatible, with a common aim, are the basic requirements of multi-agency collaboration on an everyday level. In this way health gain targets may be seen as an appropriate way of identifying goals.

Benchmarking

Achieving health gain requires not only improvements in health status, but also improvements in the quality and performance of the interventions themselves. The process of finding and implementing best practice, or benchmarking, is not new but has only recently been introduced as a systematic approach to health service evaluation. Benchmarking is 'A continuous process of measuring products, services and practices against leaders, allowing the identification of best practices which will lead to sustained and superior performance' (Bullivant and Naylor, 1992), and is essentially about problem solving, using marketing principles of understanding your business, identifying your consumer needs, recognizing those who can influence demand and performance, and organizing your services to meet expectations. The key elements of benchmarking have been described as Planning, Analysis, Action, Review (NHS Wales, 1992). NHS reforms have meant competition between provider units, and now more than ever there is a need to seek out good practice and adapt and integrate it into specified strategies. The first step in being able to demonstrate improvement, lies in the ability of a service, or a practitioner, to describe clearly the current position or starting point.

Outline Case Study 1. Achieving Health Gain Through Public Health Measures: Fluoridation and Dental Caries

What is the Starting Point?
- Dental caries or tooth decay affects children and adults, and together with gum disease accounts for most of the British national expenditure on dental health (Smith and Jacobsen, 1989).
- Experience of tooth decay shows a clear correlation with social class – the lower socioeconomic groups experience higher levels of disease (Welsh Health Planning Forum 1992).

What is the Destination?
Oral health targets relate to reduction in the number of decayed, missing and filled teeth in a population.

What Strategies are Available to Reach the Destination?

Dietary Measures
- A diet high in refined sugars leads to the accumulation of dental plaque which harbours the microorganisms that act on the mineralized tissues of the teeth, resulting in cavity formation (Murray and Rugg-Gunn, 1982).
- A reduction in the volume and frequency of refined sugar intake will reduce the incidence of dental caries. This requires behavioural changes on the part of individuals, influenced by social and cultural attitudes (Welsh Health Planning Forum, 1992).
- Dietary supplements in the form of fluoride drops can be given with good effect on an individual basis. This requires a long-term commitment from parents and children.

Dental Hygiene
- Toothbrushing with fluoridated toothpaste is to be encouraged.

Fluoridation of Water Supplies
- The weight of scientific and epidemiological evidence supports the view that at levels of one part per million, fluoridation of water supplies is a completely safe

and effective measure in dental caries prevention (DHSS, 1969; Knox, 1981; Murray and Rugg-Gunn, 1982).

- The World Health Organization has declared that fluoridation should be the cornerstone of any national programme of dental caries prevention (WHO, 1975).
- Water fluoridation appears to remove inter-social class differences in dental caries experience (Carmichael and French, 1984).
- Water fluoridation has been shown to be cost-effective (Fidler, 1977; Jackson, 1987).

Discussion Points

1. Opposition to fluoridation has focused partly on unsubstantiated health concerns (Knox, 1981) and partly on the issue of individual autonomy in relation to the state (freedom of choice). Consider whether the state has a duty to minimize suffering by collective decisions to benefit the public health (achieve health gain) or whether population based health measures are an innocent-looking form of totalitarianism.

2. In Britain the Water (Fluoridation) Act 1985 gave power to health authorities to request fluoridation of water supplies by water authorities. At that time less than 10% of the UK population were receiving fluoridated water (Smith and Jacobsen, 1989). Consider the political changes and practical difficulties which have made the likelihood of agreements on fluoridation remote.

Outline Case Study 2. Achieving Health Gain Through Behavioural Change: the Promotion and Maintenance of Breastfeeding.

What is the Starting Point?
- The consensus of medical opinion is that breastfeeding has clear health benefits for both mother and infant (Cunningham, 1977; Howie *et al.*, 1990).
- In 1990 only 63% of British women with newborn babies initiated breastfeeding. (White *et al.*, 1992).
- Social attitudes in Britain are not always encouraging to breastfeeding women (NOP, 1993).
- Partners and family are important in influencing women's infant feeding decisions (Hally, 1981; Rosseau, 1982; Jones, 1983).
- Health professionals themselves can be ambivalent about promoting breastfeeding for fear of making women who choose to bottle feed feel guilty (Bruce *et al.*, 1991).

What is the Destination?

The World Health Organization has called on governments to set up appropriate national targets for breastfeeding in the 1990s (WHO, 1990). Wales, for example, has recommended that by 1997 80% of women should choose to breastfeed and that 75% of them should continue for at least six weeks (WHPF, 1991b). Local targets have to be adjusted so that they are achievable in relation to the current local breastfeeding rates.

What Strategies are Available to Reach the Destination?

Improving Health Professional Input
- Is the breastfeeding advice health professionals give consistent?
- Are women given the amount of health professional support they want?
- Do all health professionals support the breastfeeding ethos?
- Are all health professionals aware of current best practice guidelines?

Providing Information Education	• Does breastfeeding appear in the health education programmes in schools? • Are partners/family welcome at antenatal preparation sessions? • Is infant feeding information distorted by the commercial interests of breastmilk substitute manufacturers?
Encouraging Social Support for Breastfeeding	• Do the media portray breastfeeding in a positive light? • Are local shops and institutions welcoming to breastfeeding mothers? • Are there local peer group support networks? • Do employers make provision for employees to continue breastfeeding when they return to work?
Influencing National Policies	• Does the welfare food system discourage women from trying to breastfeed? • Are there any financial incentives for women to breastfeed? • Is maternity leave provision adequate to promote and maintain breastfeeding?
Discussion Points	1. What would you consider to be the extent of health professional influence on the promotion and maintenance of breastfeeding? 2. Are health professionals justified in their concerns over being thought judgemental in promoting breastfeeding? Consider this in relation to other health promotion issues, e.g. smoking, misuse of drugs.

Outline Case Study 3. Achieving Health Gain Through Rehabilitation: Cardiac Rehabilitation

What is the Starting Point?	Ischaemic heart disease, which involves the deposition of fatty plaques on the walls of the coronary artery system, is the most common single cause of premature death in men over 45 years of age in Western societies. Following myocardial infarction, self-assessed health status has been found to be dramatically reduced.
What is the Destination?	• Reduced levels of disability for postmyocardial infarction patients. • Improved quality of life for those patients.
What Strategies are Available to Reach the Destination?	Rehabilitation is a form of tertiary prevention, the aim of which is to limit damage, prevent recurrence and restore quality of life. It has been suggested (Chua and Lipkin, 1993) that cardiac rehabilitation programmes are cost-effective and should be made available to all who would benefit.
Psychological Aspects	• Allaying of fears, reducing anxiety. • Developing individual coping skills. • Rebuilding confidence of patients and carers.
Educational Aspects	• Promoting a healthy lifestyle. • Encouraging behaviour changes, e.g. smoking, diet.
Social Aspects	• Encouraging a gradual return to former activities.
Physical Aspects	• Improving exercise tolerance. • Encouraging a gradual return to former activity levels.

Discussion Points

1. What outcome measures might be appropriate for a cardiac rehabilitation programme?
2. How does achieving health gain through rehabilitation fit in with the view that prevention is better than cure?

CONCLUSION

It has been the aim of this chapter to identify some of the implications of using health gain as the underlying value base for health service provision.

The summary highlights the main issues, and the role of the practitioner is implicit throughout.

Many of the strategic decisions on service provision will be outside the control of practitioners and indeed of provider units, as purchasers and ultimately politicians determine the planning agenda, albeit in consultation with others. However, decisions on how to actually bring about the desired improvement in health status are within the practitioner's scope of practice. Confronted with a particular health deficit or a potential barrier to health in a specified population, deciding on the most effective intervention for implementation must take account of other quality issues such as social acceptability, equity, efficiency, appropriateness and accessibility. Approaching health issues from a health gain perspective requires practitioners to evaluate their work critically in terms of benefits to clients, patients and communities and as such is a useful framework for practice.

SUMMARY

- Health gain is fundamentally about improving health status.
- Seeing health in a social, economic, cultural and environmental context is central to the concept of health gain.
- An assessment of current health status, together with available resources, is a prerequisite to the identification of acceptable, appropriate, health gain targets.
- Community values and perspectives are important in planning and implementing a health gain strategy.
- Using health gain as a guiding principle requires a shift in focus from process to outcomes.
- Multi-agency collaboration is often essential to achieving health gain.
- Benchmarking can be used to identify best practice, to improve one's own performance and to demonstrate progress towards goals.

DISCUSSION QUESTIONS

♦ 'A strict adherence to a health gain approach may conflict with publicly held views which wish to see services offered or attempts made to save lives regardless of the expense involved or the likelihood of success. And who is to say they are wrong?' (Hunter, 1993a: 104). Consider this statement in the light of limited Health Service resources.

- ◆ What criteria would you use to decide between two alternative strategies to improve health? Use an example from your own experience.

- ◆ Consider the view that solving problems of disease is not the same as creating health. Are they both aspects of health gain?

- ◆ Consider one of the important components of your own professional role. What health gain may be achieved in carrying out that aspect of your work? What outcome measures would be appropriate?

- ◆ Consider a health problem pertinent to your client group in terms of the key questions identified below (Source: 'Strategy for Health', Trent Regional Health Authority).

  — How big is the problem?
  — What possible health promoting, preventive, therapeutic or rehabilitation strategies could be pursued?
  — How effective is each of these options?
  — How expensive are they?
  — How many local people might benefit?
  — What services will produce the greatest improvement in health?
  — Is everyone agreed that these are priorities?
  — What practical obstacles and opportunities are there for introducing these changes?

FURTHER READING

Bowling A (1991) *Measuring Health - A Review of Quality of Life Measurement Scales*. Milton Keynes: Oxford University Press.
Comprehensive analysis of qualitative outcomes.

McKeown T and Lowe CR (1966) *An Introduction to Social Medicine*. Oxford: Blackwell.
The shape of health services has changed a great deal since this was written; nevertheless it provides a historical perspective to the provision of health care.

Pickin C and St Leger S (1993) *Assessing Health Needs using the Life Cycle Framework*. Buckingham: Open University Press.
Presents the life cycle framework as a means of organizing the assessment of the health needs framework. Identifies routinely available sources of information.

Smith A and Jacobsen B (1989) *The Nation's Health: A Strategy for the 1990's*. London: King's Fund.
Reviews recent progress in public health, interprets trends in health and identifies measures likely to be effective in improving public health.

REFERENCES

Atkinson S (1991) Targets, targets everywhere. *HFA 2000 News*. 16: 3-5. Faculty of Public Health Medicine.

Beck E, Lonsdale S, Newman S *et al.* (Eds.) (1992) *In the Best of Health? The Status and Future of Health Care in the UK*. London: Chapman & Hall.

Bevan A (1975) Cited in Watkins B *Documents on Health and Social Services; 1834 to the present day*. Methuen.

Bowling A (1991) *Measuring Health - A Review of Quality of Life Measurement Scales*. Milton Keynes: Open University Press.

Bruce NG, Khan Z and Olsen NDL (1991) Hospital and other influences on the uptake and maintenance of breastfeeding: the development of infant feeding policy in a District. *Public Health* **105**(5): 357-368.

Bullivant J and Naylor M (1992) Best of the best. *Health Service Journal* 27 August.

Burton P (1993) *Community Profiling: A guide to identifying local needs*. School for Advanced Urban Studies, University of Bristol.

Carmichael CL and French AD (1984) Social class and caries experience. *Community Dental Health* **1**: 47–54.

Carr-Hill R (1992) Measuring patient satisfaction. *Journal of Public Health Medicine* **14**(3): 236–249.

Chua TP and Lipkin DP (1993) Cardiac rehabilitation. *British Medical Journal* **306**: 731–732.

Clark J and Henderson J (Eds) (1983) *Community Health*. Churchill Livingstone.

Cochrane AL (1972) *Effectiveness and Efficiency: Random Reflections on Health Services*. London: Nuffield Provincial Hospital Trust.

Conyers D (1982) *An Introduction to Social Planning in the Third World*. New York: John Wiley.

Cunningham AS (1977) Morbidity in breastfed and artificially fed infants. *Journal of Paediatrics* **90**: 726–729.

Department of Health (1989a) *The Health of the Nation*. London: HMSO.

Department of Health (1989b) *Working for Patients*. London: HMSO.

Department of Health (1991) *The Health of the Nation*. London: HMSO.

Department of Health and Social Security (1969) *The Fluoridation studies in the UK and the results achieved after eleven years*. Report on Public Health and Medical Subjects. 122.

Dixon P (1993) Some issues in measuring patient satisfaction. *The Bulletin of the Community Consultation and User Feedback Unit*. CCUF Link, WHCSA, Cardiff. Dec.

Fidler PE (1977) A comparison of treatment patterns and cost for a fluoridated and non-fluoridated community. *Community Health* **9**: 103–113.

Frankel S (1991) Health needs, health care requirements, and the myth of infinite demand. *Lancet* **237**: 1588–1590.

Freire P (1972) *Pedagogy of the Oppressed*. Harmondsworth: Penguin.

Hally MR (1981) *A Study of Infant Feeding Factors Influencing Choice of Method*. Health Care Research Unit, University of Newcastle-upon-Tyne.

Hamilton-Kirkwood L and Parry-Langdon N (1993) The Needs Agenda: Health Needs Assessment. *The Bulletin of the Community Consultation and User Feedback Unit*. CCUF Link, WHCSA, Cardiff. August.

Harvey I (1992) In: Targets, Targets Everywhere. In: Director of Public Health Medicine. *The Health of South Glamorgan*, The Annual Report of the Director of Public Health Medicine, South Glamorgan Health Authority.

Holland W (Ed.) (1983) *Evaluation of Health Care*. Oxford: Oxford University Press.

Howie P, Forsyth J, Ogston S *et al.* (1990) Protective effect of breastfeeding against infection. *British Medical Journal* **300**: 11–16.

Hunter D (1993) The mysteries of health gain. In: *Health Care 92/93*. London: King's Fund Institute.

Jackson D (1987) Has the decline in dental caries in English children made water fluoridation both unnecessary and uneconomic. *British Dental Journal* March, **7**: 170–173.

Jones DA (1983) The attitudes and practices of infant feeding and the effect of a Lactation Nurse on the success of breastfeeding. PhD Thesis. University of Wales College of Medicine.

Knox EG (1981) *Fluoridation of Water and Cancer*. London: DHSS.

Long AS, Bate L and Sheldon TA (1992) The establishment of UK clearing house for assessing health service outcomes. *Quality of Health Care* **1**: 131–133.

Long AS, Dixon P, Hall R *et al.* (1993) The Outcomes Agenda, Contribution of UK Clearing House on Health Outcomes. *Quality in Health Care* **2**: 249–252.

McKeown T and Lowe CR (1966) *An Introduction to Social Medicine*, 1st edn. Oxford: Blackwell Scientific Publications.

McMurray A (1993) *Community Health Nursing: Primary Health Care in Practice*. Melbourne: Churchill Livingstone.

Murray J and Rugg-Gunn,A (1982) *Fluorides in Caries Prevention*. Wright.

National Opinion Poll Survey (1993) *Men's Attitudes to Breastfeeding*. London: NOP.

NHS Wales (1992) *Benchmarking for continuous improvement and superior performance in the NHS*. Revised notes of guidance. NHS Wales.

Ong BN, Humphris G, Annett H and Rifkin S (1991) Rapid appraisal in an urban setting; an example from the developed world. *Social Science in Medicine* **32**: 909–915.

Pickin C and St Leger S (1993) *Assessing Health Need using the Life Cycle Framework*. Buckingham: Open University Press.

Popay J and Williams G (1993) In C Pickin and S St Leger (Eds) (1993) Chapter 4 in *Assessing Health Need Using the Life Cycle Framework*. Buckingham: Open University Press.

Rosseau L (1982) Influence of cultural and environmental factors on breastfeeding. *Canadian Medical Association Journal* **127**: 701.

Ruffing-Raffal MA (1987) Resident/provider contrasts in community health priorities. *Public Health Nursing* **4**(4): 242–246.

Seedhouse D (1986) *Health: The Foundations for Achievement*. Chichester: Wiley.

Smith A and Jacobsen B (1989) *The Nation's Health: A Strategy for the 1990's*. London: King's Fund.

Stevens A and Raferty J (1991) *Assessing health care needs*. A DHA project discussion paper. NHS Management Executive, Dept of Health, London.

Townsend P and Davidson N (Eds) (1980) The Black Report in *Inequalities in Health*. London. Penguin 1988. Edited version of the Report of the Working Group on Inequalities in Health by Black D, Morris JN, Smith C and Townsend P.

Trent Regional Health Authority (1992) *Strategy for Health: A Consultation Document*. Internal publication.

Tromans P (1992) Purchasing for Health Gain – Contracts based on Strategies. In: Director of Public Health Medicine. *The*

Health of South Glamorgan. The Annual Report of the Director of Public Health Medicine, South Glamorgan Health Authority.

Twinn S, Dauncey J and Carnell J (1990) *The Process of Health Profiling*. London: Health Visitors Association.

Welsh Health Planning Forum (1991a) *Protocol for Investment in Health Gain: Cardiovascular Diseases*. Cardiff: Welsh Office, NHS Directorate.

Welsh Health Planning Forum (1991b) *Protocol for Investment in Health Gain: Maternal and Early Child Health*. Cardiff: Welsh Office NHS Directorate.

Welsh Health Planning Forum (1992) *Protocol for Investment in Health Gain: Oral Health*. Cardiff. Welsh Office NHA Directorate.

Welsh Office NHS Directorate (1989) *Strategic Intent and Direction for the NHS in Wales*. Cardiff: Welsh Office.

White A, Freeth S and O'Brien M (1992) *Infant Feeding 1990*.

A Survey carried out by the Social Survey Division of OPCS on behalf of the Dept of Health, the Scottish Home and Health Dept, The Welsh Office and the Dept of Health and Social Services in Northern Ireland. London; HMSO.

World Health Organization (1946) *Preamble to the Constitution: Meeting, New York*. Geneva: WHO.

World Health Organization (1975) *Fluoridation and Dental Health*. WHO Chronicle 23 505–12. Geneva: WHO.

World Health Organization (1981) *Global Strategy for Health for all by the Year 2000*. Geneva: WHO.

World Health Organization (1985) *Targets for Health for All – Targets in support of the European Regional Strategy for Health for All*. WHO Regional Office for Europe: Copenhagen.

World Health Organization (1990) *Innocenti Declaration on the Protection, Promotion and Support of Breastfeeding*. Geneva: WHO.

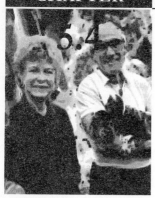

SCIENCE OR SOCIAL CONTROL?

Michael Hardey

KEY ISSUES

- Influences on practice
- Expert knowledge
- Surveillance and social control
- Holistic health

INTRODUCTION

This chapter considers how the development of scientific knowledge and the growth of the health professions have influenced the practice of community nursing. The work of any professional group is claimed to be non-judgemental and based on a defined set of expert knowledge that is grounded in scientific research. In recent years there has been much emphasis on the nature of the nursing knowledge base and an increasing debate about evidence based medicine. At the same time more attention has been paid to how care is delivered and to the reactions of patients, clients or customers. This new discourse of 'patients, clients and customers' is significant because it implies a shift in power from the health professions to those they provide care to. However, community nurses are also expected to monitor and assess clients for signs of deviant or potentially dangerous behaviour. The specialist knowledge of practitioners and the potential gap between the educational, cultural and material experiences of practitioners and many of their patients/clients makes it important to examine their role as agents of social control.

The Emergence of Community Health Work

It has been suggested that in the first decade of the twentieth century there was a moral panic over the health and fitness of the population (Weeks, 1981). This alarm about the state of the nation's health emerged at one level from the evidence of Booth and Rowntree who provided detailed reports of the conditions of the poor. Such surveys provided powerful evidence that countered the view that the poor were exclusively responsible for their impoverishment and often unhealthy lives. The evident physical defects revealed by attempts to recruit men for the Boer War (1889–1902) made it clear that the health of the working class was also a matter of national security. It should be remembered that in this period that led to the First World War there were fears that Britain's economic and military position could not be maintained in the face of competition from Germany and North America if it had a weak, inefficient workforce subject to illness and disease. The development of the biomedical sciences and the medical profession provided another significant dimension to the creation of the health panic. Biomedicine had mapped out the links between lack of cleanliness and disease and these ideas had been transmitted to a growing middle class audience through the work of doctors and the popular journals of the time. Furthermore science had shown that disease did not respect moral worth or social class and could all too easily escape from poor communities into the general population. The spread of biomedical knowledge such as the germ theory of disease beyond the domain of experts led some to suggest that a 'new concept of dirt' (Starr, 1982) emerged in this period. Earlier public health reforms had increased life expectancy but had failed to make similar inroads into infant mortality and chronic diseases such as tuberculosis (McKeown, (1979). In particular germ theory suggested that common conditions such as infant diarrhoea (a major cause of infant death) were preventable if proper hygienic measures were followed in the home. Cleanliness was not hard to achieve in those households that could afford to employ domestic workers but it was far more difficult achieve modern standards of hygiene in overcrowded and dilapidated homes that often had to share facilities, such as toilets, with neighbours.

The problem of persistent ill health led to the setting up of the Interdepartmental Committee on Physical Deterioration that reported in 1904. This committee heard a wide range of evidence and made a series of recommendations that are regarded as marking the inception of modern state social policy. The report concluded that poor child and consequent adult health was the result of 'ignorance and neglect on the part of the parents' rather than material disavantage. Responsibility for the provisioning and care of the household could be located in an individual – the wife and mother – while the emphasis on 'ignorance' identified the problem as one located amongst those households on the economic and social margins. Thus the Interdepartmental Committee called for 'some great scheme of social education'. This was based on the idea that the problem was one of 'maternal inefficiency' in that the working class mother did not know or failed to recognize what was now regarded as good health and domestic practices. The report noted that there were ad hoc arrangements in some parts of the country that provided women 'visitors' to give advice to poor families about health and hygiene. Through this report and consequent legislation, the range of charitable 'visiting' services was drawn into state control and the basis for contempary community nursing was established. State regulation and employment of community health occupations transformed the service from a voluntary activity with little or no training (the superior skills and abilities of the middle class wife and mother were regarded as more than sufficient) to one which training and a recognized clinically based qualification became necessary.

Community based health provision emerged into the post-war welfare state as a universal service with close links to acute sector nursing from which the majority of practitioners began their careers. Community based health care was no longer a philanthropic service provided by 'ladies' but a relatively low status and low paid female occupation (Dingwall *et al.*, 1988). Traditional concepts of gender and domestic relationships that stressed order, cleanliness and discipline provided the framework for the development of community nursing and its subordinate relationship with the medical hierarchy. Although now a universal service on paper, community health provision defined 'community' in a way that identified it largely with those who lived on the economic and social margins. In particular, much of the time of practitioners was to be spent dealing with problems amongst people who lived in the new towns and the large social housing experiments of the postwar years. The underlying philosophy of the practitioner–client relationship remained one of voluntarism, trust and collaboration despite the frequent gap in economic and social position.

Knowledge, Power and Practice

The development of biomedical and sanitary knowledge led to early schemes to provide poor families with health and hygiene information. The mission of the early community health workers was to spread the gospel of contemporary sanitary and medical knowledge. Scientific knowledge developed rapidly, especially in the areas of biology, nutrition and psychology. As noted above, by the end of the Second World War state intervention had become legitimate and was generally regarded as necessary if not desirable to ensure a stable and healthy society.

The natural sciences represent the triumph of modernism in their representation of the world as made up of 'facts' which operate according to discoverable laws. This may work for material objects but as 'scientists' have discovered, human beings are more complex. In the nineteenth century the science of phrenology believed that it could predict potential criminal behaviour from the shape of human heads. In the 1950s psychiatric research led to the use of lobotomies for patients with mental disorders. In 1974 The American Psychiatric Association decided to take a vote of its members to decide whether homosexuality should still be seen as a disease (Kennedy, 1983). What these examples suggest is that 'science' itself is a human product and as such may 'get it wrong' even after years of research.

A key reason why the scientific work noted above 'got it wrong' was that human beings attach meanings to their actions which they understand through a set of symbols we commonly call language. They do not behave like inanimate objects but are constantly interacting with their environment. Their beliefs may at times appear rather strange if not contradictory, for example when a researcher asked women about their health many: replied 'yes' to the question 'do you feel fit and well?' In answer to the next question, 'What ailments do you suffer from?', the same women listed a whole series of problems including anaemia, headaches, consumption, rheumatism, prolapse of the womb, bad teeth and varicose veins (Spring-Rice, 1939: 69). Thus 'meanings' are important if we are to understand human behaviour and to take an analytical approach to the science on which practice is based.

The work of Foucault (see Foucault, 1970, 1972; Smart, 1985) argues that knowledge is generated and utilized in modern societies to regulate the population. Knowledge is therefore essentially defined as power over others. The development of biomedical and psychological knowledge involved a process of interactions between 'experts' in which, for example, diseases were defined, classified and brought under control. These expert discourses took place in a framework of rules that defined who could take part and what form the debate took. This framework is commonly referred to as the scientific method which it is claimed is capable of revealing 'facts' which would remain hidden under different approaches. For example, two mothers without an 'expert' education will talk about child care in everyday language and use 'common sense' rather than academic 'theories' to support their arguments. From this it should be evident that those who are able to lay claim to legitimate areas of knowledge also have the power to shape the form of enquiries and who or what is included in the discourse. Foucault's work also highlights the role of language in defining meaning and shaping knowledge. Without entering into the complex area of metaphysics (an example of excluding the reader from this discourse!) it should be noted that biomedicine, psychology and all the other domains of knowledge not only use language differently but also invent new words with their own complex shades of meaning that demand an understanding of, for example, medicine to comprehend properly. Furthermore these terms may enter wider vocabularies. For example, medical discourse refers to 'diagnosis', 'illness', 'problem families', 'therapy' and 'cure' which are accepted as morally neutral terms that may involve the categorization of deviant behaviours and the social control of them.

From Foucault's standpoint modern society is characterized by a constant struggle over power and the ability to impose meanings on others. Foucault undertook a number of studies of the power/knowledge struggles in the disciplines of psychiatric medicine, sexuality and criminality. He drew attention to how the development of biomedical knowledge and psychiatric medicine generated a power/knowledge platform from which experts could decide what was appropriate for others. Powerful tools have been developed since the early surveys of Booth and Rowntree to study the population and monitor its health. Thus, information about the infant mortality rate gave rise to changes in health visiting. Power/knowledge produces and feeds off ever more discreet and detailed mechanisms of surveillance of both populations and individuals. 'Biopolitics', as Foucault called the process, draws attention to the links between apparently abstract and neutral science and the exercise of power and politics. Such knowledge is used in the education of practitioners and informs various attempts to define 'quality' and outcomes of practitioner interventions. Thus, community health workers may be viewed as engaged in the work of biopolitics. They are also engaged in a discourse with 'experts' which helps shape the generation of further knowledge through research and other activities.

The development of psychiatric knowledge had important implications for community health work and did much to create the space for the growth of social work. In particular by describing 'normal' development and behaviour this area of expert knowledge also defined the 'abnormal'. The theories of Freud maintained that the nuclear family and especially the gender divisions within were essential to the future mental health of children. Bowlby (1953) revised Freud's work to produce the 'maternal deprivation' model which highlighted the impact of a child's early years on future behaviours. Childhood came to be regarded as a time that demanded a high level of care and nurturing in which the child learned appropriate behaviours. Bowlby's thesis become highly influential and reinforced existing notions of 'maternal inefficiency' already used in practice. Bowlby claimed that continuous and proper 'mothering' was essential to the development of healthy adults. Spock and other popular writers disseminated similar mother centred ideas to a wide audience. For both community nursing and the expanding profession of social work Bowlby's theory provided an individualistic explanation of social problems based on inadequate mothering. It also challenged explanations that might focus on structural factors such as economic insecurity, inadequate housing etc., that shaped the lives of many clients. The incorporation of maternal deprivation theory into professional practice and increasingly into popular culture added a further dimension to the post-war changes in the economic and social role of women. As Michell suggests, 'from now onwards appeal to maternal guilt vied with the political exploitation of the economic situation to keep women at home . . . we learnt that a person sucked his emotional stability literally with his mother's milk' (Michell, 1975: 228).

The emphasis of psychoanalytic theories on mother–child bonding contributed to the classification of 'normal' cognitive and emotional development with associated mechanisms to allow experts to assess 'healthy' development. The growth of knowledge therefore identified and categorized new pathological conditions and behaviours which practitioners were expected to prevent, identify and 'cure'. In particular it provided the foundation for the classification of families as 'normal' or 'deviant'. The presence or absence of a conventional male head of the household was an evident indicator of 'deviant' and problematic status.

The development of community nursing can be seen as part of the strategies devised under biopolitics to impose regulation and control on the population and especially those located on the economic and social margins. In particular, this has involved surveillance of poor or unconventional families as well as treatment and care of the sick. The utilization of psychoanalytic theories, particularly in school nursing and health visiting, provided the means to assess and monitor child development and helped to define what constituted 'good mothering'. This enhanced surveillance role has led a number of writers to describe community health practitioners as involved in the 'policing of the family' (Abbott and Sapford, 1990; Dingwall and Robinson, 1993).

Continuity and Change: Practice and Clients

The relative 'ignorance' and the inability of those located on the economic and social margins to manage in a modern urban society has been seen as the major cause of social and health problems. Although the material conditions of the general population have been transformed since the opening of the century there remain significant social and economic divisions (see Townsend *et al.*, 1992).

> Social class inequalities for men, and probably also women, have widened since the 1950s, both relatively and absolutely; and they are now probably greater than at the start of the century. (Editorial, 1986)

Such social divisions have been reinforced by racial and geographical factors. There is now a considerable dislocation between the opportunities and choices open to those on the economic and social margins and the majority of the population which remains in relatively secure employment. Between 1979 and 1987 it is estimated that the number of people living in poverty more than doubled (Oppenheim, 1990). A disproportionate number of these households contained children or elderly people. In 1987 over a quarter of all children in Britain lived in households that were below the poverty line (DSS, 1990). This growth in the number of households living in poverty led to the suggestion that society was become increasingly polarized. While the majority of the population had experienced increased living standards and more opportunities for leisure and consumption, a significant minority were experiencing worse real incomes and less access to adequate housing and amenities such as shops and inexpensive leisure facilities.

During the past decade there have been various attempts by the government to link moral failure with dependence on welfare and thus further marginalized groups such as lone parents (see Hardey and Crow, 1991). The importation of the 'underclass' thesis from the United States provided the ground for revisiting the 'deserving/undeserving' categorization of the poor. In particular, recent debates about lone mothers and the claimed association with 'poor mothering' and consequent future criminality of children has created the basis for the further stigmatization of this group. Such debates have the effect of 'blaming the victim' and emphasizing individual self-help to overcome structural problems. Material marginality has been increasingly defined by locality so that parts of cities or particular regions may contain a concentration of deprived households and an associated lack of resources (see Walker and Walker, 1987). Such concentrations of disadvantage are reflected in health data such as the postneonatal mortality statistics which demonstrate that the inner city area of Birmingham experiences nearly three times the mortality of more affluent areas (Woodroffe *et al.*, 1993).

Government statements such as *Health of the Nation* (DOH, 1992) in England noted that the health education and health promotion role of community nursing is central to achieving various 'health gains'. This reflects the established emphasis of governments on individual health behaviours and choices and the failure to properly consider health inequalities or their causes. There are echoes here of the nineteenth century argument that poverty was the responsibility of the individual and not related to wider factors such as unemployment, pollution and so on. Smoking behaviour amongst the disadvantaged, and in particular mothers reliant on state benefits, provides a good example of an area that is regarded as a potential health gain target. Smoking was highlighted as a deviant behaviour for which targets for reduction were set by the *Health of the Nation* (DOH, 1992). At one level smoking by mothers with few economic resources appears 'irrational' and deleterious to both infant and adult. Health education has sought to address such behaviours for many years and practitioners have been expected to discourage the activity. However, a deeper analysis of smoking behaviour suggests that it is a coping strategy for disadvantaged mothers who have to cope with material deprivation and the stress of life on the economic and social margins (Graham, 1993). Graham argues that it is necessary to understand how poverty within families influences health behaviours. She notes that women are not only expected to undertake the role of 'housekeeper', but are also assigned the role of 'health-keeper', particularly in relation to the purchase and preparation of food and housework related to hygiene. In deprived households mothers and children may spend a lot of time in a home where the immediate social and physical environment is hostile and reflects physical and psychological problems. Women may cut down on food for themselves rather than go without cigarettes because:

> . . . smoking can be both necessity and luxury; a necessity that enables a women to maintain her role as family health-keeper and a luxury that symbolises her participation in the lifestyle of the wider society, cigarettes offer moments when, however temporarily, the experience of relative poverty is suspended (Graham, 1990: 216-217)

This suggests that not only will health advice fail to have an impact, it may also undermine the client–professional relationship by making overt the gap in experiences and expectations between them. The example of smoking illustrates how complex health behaviours are and the inadequacy of assuming that health choices are only a product of individual irresponsibility, ignorance or irrationality. Studies of food choices and income level show that families in receipt of low incomes are aware of what constitutes a healthy diet but that they are unable to afford such a diet (see Chapter 2.5).

From Foucault's thesis it is apparent that community nursing practice is defined, shaped and measured according to specific scientific discourses and structures. In particular the women centred nature of practice serves to reinforce the traditional family forms and gender divisions. Furthermore advice or education is not value free and notions of proper health behaviours or caring practices may implicitly include theories and values that fail to address the real needs of clients. In line with the heritage of the 'mother's friend' philosophy, community practitioners have retained an approach based on cooperation if not collaboration with the client. This also reflected the patient and care centred philosophy of the 'new nursing' (Salvage, 1985) that emphasized a holistic philosophy of care and the collaboration between nurse and client. A 'therapeutic alliance' (Olds and Kitzman, 1990) that is based on trust and facilitates effective interventions into the private domain of the domestic life home remains something of an ideal when communities are so divided by inequalities of opportunities and material circumstances.

CONCLUSION

In a way similar to that under which a new concept of dirt (Starr, 1982) has been said to have emerged in the late nineteenth century it can be argued that the late twentieth century is witnessing the emergence of a new concept of 'holistic health'. This formulation of health is broader than the traditional, medically defined one and embraces social, economic, psychological as well as bodily well-being. It is informed by the discourse of choice and individuality and underpinned by a broad philosophy of holism.

For the majority of the population this new holistic health model reinforces their role as consumers of health care who are able to make active health choices and have developed informed health behaviours. However, for those who live on the economic and social margins holistic health emphasizes their lack of opportunities while the new politics of health and welfare stress their own responsibility for their plight.

Holistic health also reflects contemporary nursing discourse with its emphasis on clients rather than patients, participation in care and health gains. The recent shift in the relative importance of primary and secondary care provides the opportunity to further extend the role of community nursing. This suggests that the boundaries around social work and community nursing may become increasingly blurred. Throughout the 1980s social work has been accused of being overtheoretical by the government and the profession may be going through a period of change and restructuring which redefines the work of those dealing with social problems outside the criminal justice system as 'health work'.

New holistic health problematizes the lives of those who are economically and socially marginal and may also bring together those professions that are involved in working with the disadvantaged. At present, community nursing remains a universal provision and it is with the relatively advantaged clients who have an income and security that the full potential of holistic health can be realized. However, the reorganization of health care may encourage this group of clients to seek care outside the NHS. Community nurses may therefore become increasingly focused on dealing with economic and social problems that arise out of increasing economic and social inequality. The degree to which the practitioners will be defined and see themselves in working with or for the disadvantaged, as opposed to being part of a system developed to control and contain this population, is open to question.

SUMMARY

The chapter discussed the following issues:
- The development of expert knowledge in community nursing.
- The surveillance of the more economically and socially marginal clients.
- The role of community nurses in the delivery of care.

DISCUSSION
QUESTIONS

♦ To what extent is community nursing engaged in regulating and controlling the poor?

♦ Will community nursing merge with other occupations engaged in working with the least advantaged to form a residual health and social service?

♦ Is 'client collaboration' and 'choice' a myth when coping with those living on the economic and social margins?

FURTHER READING

Morgan M *et al.* (1985) *Sociological approaches to health and illness* London: Routledge.

This text is interesting in the way it integrates social theory with concerns about health and the delivery of health care. It is particularly useful for those wanting a good theoretical introduction although it is beginning to be a little dated in places. It is less strong on social and nursing policy.

Stacey M (1988) *The Sociology of Health and Healing* London: Unwin Hyman.

Something of a classic text that remains very good on the development of nursing and other health professions. The text is quite dense but it rewards a careful read by providing a rigorous linking of gender related issues to the delivery of health care.

Nettleton S (1995) *The sociology of health and illness* Cambridge: Polity Press.

A general textbook that provides some up to date material and highlights some of the current debates about health. It is particularly good at examining issues to do with the rise of holistic health care and the implications this may have for the health professions.

Jones LJ (1994) *The social context of health and health work* London: Macmillan.

A recent textbook that offers a general introduction to social policy and sociology for health professionals. It covers a lot of ground in a way that is accessible to those without a strong background in the social sciences.

REFERENCES

Abbott P and Sapford R (1990) Health visiting: policing the family? In P Abbott and C Wallace (Eds) *The Sociology of the Caring Professions*. Bristol: Falmer Press.

Bowlby J (1953) *Child Care and the Growth of Love*. Harmondsworth: Penguin.

Department of Health (1989) *Caring for People: Community Care in the Next Decade and Beyond*. London: HMSO.

Department of Health (1992) *Health of the Nation: a consultative document*. London: HMSO.

Department of Social Security (1990) *Households below Average Income: a Statistical Analysis 1980-87*. London: HMSO.

Dingwall R and Robinson, KM (1993) Policing the family?

Health visiting and the public surveillance of private behaviour. In A Beattie *et al.* (Eds) *Health and Wellbeing: a reader*. London: Macmillan.

Dingwall R, Rafferty M and Webster C (1988) *An Introduction to the Social History of Nursing*. London: Routledge.

Editorial *Lancet*. (1986).

Foucault M (1970) *The Birth of the Clinic*. London: Tavistock.

Foucault M (1972) *The Archaeology of Knowledge*. London: Tavistock.

Graham H (1990) *Hardship and Health in Women's Lives*. Chichester: Wheatsheaf.

Hardey M and Crow G (1991) *Lone Parenthood*. London: Harvester Wheatsheaf.

Kennedy I (1983) *The Unmasking of Medicine*. Allen and Unwin: London.

McKeown T (1979) *The Role of Medicine*. Oxford: Oxford University Press.

Michell J (1975) *Psychoanalysis and Feminism*. Harmondsworth: Penguin.

Office of Population Censuses and Surveys (1992) *Mortality Statistics, Perinatal and Infant: Social and biological factors series* DH3 No23. London: HMSO.

Olds DC and Kitzman H (1990) Can home visiting improve the health of women and children at environmental risk? *Paediatrics* **86:** 108–116.

Oppenheim C (1990) *Poverty: the facts*. London: Child Poverty Action Group.

Salvage J (1985) *The Politics of Nursing*. Oxford: Heinemann.

Spring-Rice M (1939) *Working-class Wives: Their Health and Conditions*. Virago 1981 edition.

Smart B (1985) *Michael Foucault*. London: Tavistock.

Starr P (1982) *The Social Transformation of American Medicine*. New York: Basic Books.

Stedman-Jones G (1971) *Outcast London*. Oxford: Oxford University Press.

Townsend P, Davison N and Whitehead M (1992) *Inequalities in Health*. Harmondsworth: Penguin.

Walker A and Walker C (1987) *The growing divide: a social audit 1979–1987*. London: Child Poverty Action Group.

Weeks J (1981) *Sex, Politics and Society: the regulation of sexuality since 1800*. London: Longmans.

Woodroffe C et al. (1993) *Children, teenagers and health: the key data*. Buckingham: Open University Press.

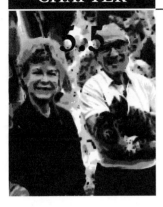

MARKETING AND THE NHS

Judy Edwards and Elizabeth Muir

KEY ISSUES

- Pressures for change in the NHS
- The creation of an internal market
- The philosophy and process of marketing
- The concepts of customers, users and beneficiaries

INTRODUCTION

This chapter describes the guiding principles of marketing, the context in which a marketing philosophy developed within the NHS and considers both the positive and the negative implications of adopting marketing strategies within a health care system.

Pressures for Change in the NHS

The shape of the National Health Service (NHS) has been continuously evolving since its inception but the early idealism has, in recent decades, given way to the stark realities of managing the dynamics of health care in an era of competition and innovation. In this new environment, choices and decisions have to be made in the face of changing public expectation and the problems associated with redistributing resources to give equality of access and equity in service development across the NHS. This is having to be achieved amidst significant demographic change where many users of health care resources are less able to identify and manage their own health care needs and less likely to be familiar with advances in medicine and associated technology. These essentially management issues have had to be addressed in a fluctuating economic climate with a continuous squeeze on public expenditure. At the same time there has been a major shift of emphasis from traditional acute secondary care settings, to local community based services and primary care, as technological and scientific developments have transformed treatment regimes.

The Creation of an Internal Market within the NHS

Nothing in the past has been as radical as the organizational changes resulting from the NHS Management Enquiry conducted by Roy Griffiths in the early 1980s and the White Papers *Working for Patients* (DOH, 1989a) and *Caring for People* (DOH,

1989b) which followed a few years later. Both aimed to improve the overall performance of health and social care: the first by delegating specific responsibilities to general managers for the planning and control of service performance – seeking public opinion in the process – and the second by motivating improvements through a quasi or internal market. This was considerably different from the buying and selling between district health authorities (DHAs), which had been going on for some years. For social care, the term used for the market was 'a mixed economy', since the intention was to change the balance of provision so that the role of non-statutory or independent providers of care was increased in comparison with that of statutory providers.

The assumption underlying the development of a government regulated internal marketplace in health care was that it would encourage people to look at what they were doing from different perspectives. In so doing, it was anticipated that there would be a contribution to resolving some of the problems besetting the NHS. These problems were not so much to do with increasing costs as to do with the inability to find an appropriate economic framework which would create 'the right incentives to encourage the efficient delivery of care' (Hudson, 1994: 6).

The commercial market is based on a number of suppositions, which if met, allow shoppers/customers/consumers not only a wide range of choice but the opportunity to promote their own values and obtain what is for them, the best product or service, at the best price, according to individual priorities. As choices are made to buy – or to refrain from buying – those who offer goods or services are stimulated to produce ever better quality and less expensive goods to attract more business; or to provide goods/services with unique or specialized characteristics which meet customer needs at prices they are prepared to pay. In such circumstances, not only are people able to buy what they consider to be the best that is available, at the most reasonable price, but they can also opt to forgo the purchase of one item, in order to retain sufficient resources to purchase another.

From a service provider, or product development point of view, it will not only be critical to find out about minimum statutory or legal requirements but also whether current needs are already being met, or have changed, so that resources are not wasted in developing the quality of something which is either no longer required, or is already satisfying demand. It will be of equal importance to identify which elements of a product or service give it 'added value' to an actual or potential customer.

In a free marketplace, special conditions are needed to be effective in relating needs to provision and to coordinate the various activities involved. One theory – which would support privatization – argues that markets work best when there is unregulated competition, with many purchasers and providers (Gabe *et al.*, 1991: 39). That is to say, when there are many buyers, providers are less likely to be exploited by a single purchaser (a monopoly purchasing situation). And if a competing provider does not offer what is wanted, it is likely to founder; and if modifications are not made to the products or services on offer, the particular provider would ultimately go out of business. Such modifications to a product or service – to ensure survival in the face of competition – may be as much to do with ensuring actual and potential customers are fully and properly informed of the anticipated benefits of what is on offer, as to do with making adjustments to meet current or new quality and price requirements. Another theory – which would be against privatization – suggests that market regulation is needed to ensure that an adequate number of customers and suppliers exist in the first place.

Considering whether or not marketing can or should be applied to the NHS means having to confront a number of objections which arise as a consequence of the special institutional peculiarities of the NHS and the inherent distaste for some of the business discipline's marketing language. However, while the potential advantages should not be oversold, neither should marketing be rejected simply because of its commercial connotations. The underlying purpose of marketing is to improve communication: finding out about what is wanted, identifying and promoting the key features and associated benefits of a product or service and increasing business effectiveness by highlighting minimal usage, concentrating on reducing wasted costs and focusing resources on preferred options.

It must, however, be acknowledged that it would seem strange to any health care professional, to be exploring a process which aims to promote or *increase* 'the business' of health care when budgetary control and cost-effectiveness through targeting (rationing) are expected to *reduce* the level or direction of that business. It must also be acknowledged that in identifying preferred options within a health care system, the health needs of some individuals or groups may not be adequately addressed.

The Philosophy of Marketing

According to the Institute of Marketing, there is a basic philosophy which underpins all marketing activity. This philosophy contends that all the resources of an organization and all its activity should be focused on the process of anticipating, identifying and satisfying customer needs for the benefit of that organization. In simple commercial markets, people (customers) give something – usually money – in exchange for goods or services they believe they need. One aspect of 'the benefit' to the organization can be easily measured in terms of profit. In public service markets, third parties become involved in the exchange of money on behalf of people deemed to be in need of a service. Taxes, for example, are paid to the government which are then allocated as budgets to commissioning health authorities and fundholding GP practices (customers), for the purchase of services. Within the province of health care, in addition to the financial aspects of service provision, the expected benefits to the organization can be identified from objectives such as those identified in the report of the Royal Commission on the NHS (1979: 9–12), some of which are reiterated in more recent white papers. These objectives include:

- encouraging and assisting individuals to remain healthy;
- ensuring equal entitlement to services;
- providing a broad range of services to a high standard;
- ensuring equal access to these services;
- providing health care free at the time of use;
- satisfying reasonable public expectations for health care;
- providing a national service responsive to local needs.

Other objectives of the NHS are related to the provision of community care for the mentally ill, the elderly infirm and the mentally and physically handicapped. In addition could be added the European targets evident in the WHO policy of *Health for All 2000* (1985, targets 27,31) as well as those highlighted in *The Health of the Nation* (DOH, 1991) and the Health Gain Protocols of the Welsh Health Planning Forum (1991–1994). As mentioned above, there is also considerable concern to minimize public costs as part of a strategy to reduce the role of the state in the UK economy. While this is publicly recognized, it is not 'proclaimed as loudly as the claim that government now spends more on the NHS than ever before' (Sheaff, 1991: 2–3). In practice, the importance of cost control is revealed in managerial responsibilities and in the significance given to Resource Management Initiatives.

The issues which surround the philosophy of marketing are those concerned with creating a model of an organization and the debate centres on such questions as:

- What sort of organization is needed?
- What range of services should be offered to whom?
- How should the services be presented to prospective customers?
- What sort of relationships should be formed with those who use and receive services?
- In what ways should comparisons be made with other service providers?

These are all questions which have relevance for community nursing services and need to be considered in the light of local conditions and government policies. See Chapter 4 in this section for a more detailed discussion of policy issues and their implications for the development or modification of community nursing services.

Some Quality Issues

In the context of marketplace dynamics, there will be a number of strategic options available to change or improve the position of a service. The ones chosen will depend upon the underlying philosophy of the organization and on the resources available. It is at this point that managers critically assess not just the financial and material resources available but most importantly of all, the skills, attitudes, experience and expertise of the workforce. Human resources are fundamental to the successful provision of a service through the day-to-day contact with customers and users. It is because marketing objectives focus on the relationships between people, where the action of one group influences the knowledge or actions of another, that it is critical for all employees to play their individual parts in promoting the benefits of what is on offer – and be both skilled and motivated to do so.

The competitive atmosphere created by the purchaser/provider divide means there is a constant need to balance quality standards with the prices needed to generate the necessary income to provide a range of desired services at the required standard. Again it will be important to differentiate between quality markers which are significant for those who use and receive a service from quality markers which are important to purchasers. The overall philosophy of an organization will also be significant since it will influence the nature and structure of its internal relationships, as well as how people outside the organization perceive it. It is in just this sense that every individual working for an organization plays an important part in developing relationships which enable others to identify with it in a positive way.

The Process of Marketing

According to Piercy (1992: 21) 'The marketing process is common to virtually all forms of economic or social organisation'. The whole process is so interlinked that if any part of it starts to fail or is not carried out to the same standard and expectation as the rest, then the whole is in jeopardy. It is thus vital that everyone in an organization understands the purpose and process of marketing as well as their roles within it. Community nursing services are no different from many other organizations, in that within the marketplace for services there is a constant tension between the demands of 'the user' and those of 'the customer'. (Remember that in marketing terms the customer is always the one who pays the bill.) Contrary to some assumptions about marketing, the purchaser/provider divide in the NHS does not exclude the user or the recipient of the service from being influential but rather puts them at the heart of the marketplace (Box 5.5.1).

Customer Satisfaction

It is the role of commissioning authorities to assess the health needs of the population and to develop appropriate purchasing plans and related service objectives. GP practices, whether fundholding or not, will need to be familiar with such plans so that, where relevant, they are incorporated into priorities for the practice business plan. In turn, those involved in the design and provision of community nursing services need to be familiar with the plans and objectives of individual practices so that negotiated service specifications are responsive to requirements. Once service objectives have been negotiated and agreed, the individual community nurse providing a service is in a position to identify activities and responsibilities which will be sensitive to the particular characteristics of the population served and represent cost-effectiveness with reference to the available nursing resources. In order to ensure that all activity is focused on the marketing objectives and that there are no dilemmas in terms of resource allocation, these activities and responsibilities should link with job descriptions and annual performance appraisal.

Since the marketing process is continuous, it may be entered at any one of the various levels shown in Box 5.5.2. In essence the marketing process is all about creating change: getting from where an organization (or a fundholding practice) is now, to where it wants to be, in say two years time. From a community nursing perspective, that means being able to describe the current position of the service in

Box 5.5.1. The marketing exchange process

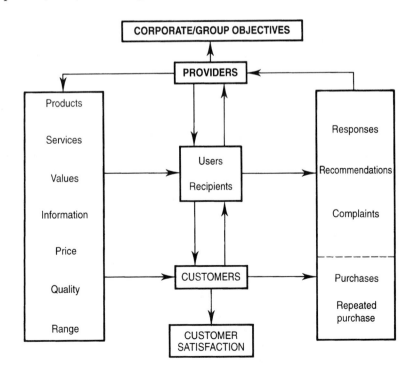

a way which is helpful to those who want to know more about what is on offer and in particular, how it is (and could be more) beneficial to those who use it. It means having a very clear understanding of the essential 'business' of the service, its key features and the associated benefits. The next chapter will be dealing with the practical application of these aspects of marketing.

The combination of devolved management responsibility to local commissioning authorities for assessing local health needs and for purchasing appropriate health care – together with competition between service providers – is expected to result in greater efficiency by the elimination of waste, by promoting innovation and by increasing value for money. However, once a scenario is in place which involves different agencies negotiating for health service contracts, the amount and speed of change becomes rather difficult to control and the consequences difficult to predict. It is against this backcloth of uncertainty and change that an understanding of the philosophy and process of marketing can be of particular value to those involved in community and primary health care nursing. Developing an awareness of factors influencing purchasing decisions at a local level is one way to begin to understand the marketing process. Keeping in touch with the views of community health councils, for example, and being familiar with GP practice based health and social profiles and the Annual Public Health Report, will also promote understanding of the likely focus and direction of health care developments at a local level. See Murray and Graham (1995) for a comparison of methods to assess health needs in one small neighbourhood.

The Nature of the Marketplace

The dynamics of the marketplace are, in part created by the tensions which exist between the changing roles within it. The separation of 'providers' from 'commissioners' for instance, meant that the former had to predict future demands

Box 5.5.2. The marketing process

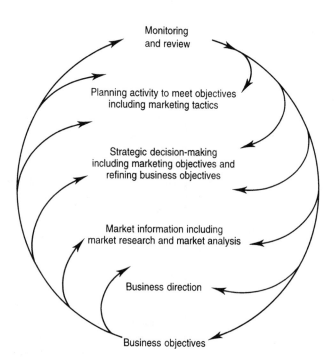

Monitoring and review

Planning activity to meet objectives including marketing tactics

Strategic decision-making including marketing objectives and refining business objectives

Market information including market research and market analysis

Business direction

Business objectives

for services, identify the strengths and weaknesses of current services in relation to competitors, and find out what must be done to secure a successfully negotiated contract. The acquisition of trust status for community units became part of this business planning process. It meant that community nurses became employees of the trust rather than the health authority and that the fundamental role of the manager is to meet the trust's (NHS) objectives and ensure the presence of an efficient delivery system. This usually means obtaining more health care benefits, while maintaining high quality services. The problem for doctors and nurses is that they are often taught to offer the best of care to 'each' patient/client, with little reference to the overall needs of the wider population. Again, in a local primary care setting, skills are used for the benefit of 'each' individual or family, in keeping with the particular primary care team's priority goals.

Adopting a marketing perspective is not to suggest that meeting the health needs of an individual and a population are mutually exclusive but it does suggest that doctors and nurses, in directing their attention to the needs of individuals, should do so in the context of how best to manage their time, skills and resources for the benefit of whole groups of individuals who may need different kinds/levels of health care. This would also include some concern for the amount of time available, so that the workload of health professionals is seen in the context of patterns of need, minimizing the impact of predictable peaks and troughs.

Tensions can also arise when long-term plans are made by people who are many levels removed from the day-to-day shorter-term requirements of community nurses and the users of their services. This means that a shift in communication is needed so that overall long-term budgets are broken down into short-term budget allocations. It is important that such communication is two way so that errors in budgetary breakdown can be amended and that there is sufficient flexibility to divert funds when justified. That means that where one section receives a specific budget in one year, it does not automatically mean receiving the same the following year plus or minus a percentage. A new budget should be negotiated based on previous experience and the best calculation of what is likely to happen in the future.

Value for Money

In an ever changing marketplace where the organization and delivery of community nursing services will vary from place to place, what is happening in 1996 will not necessarily be happening two or five years later. The changes will not just be concerned with what is being provided by whom, but how that provision is being managed and where the different responsibilities lie. The internal market in health care offers a new mechanism for shaping the rationing process, with commissioning managers being in a position to exert leverage by the possibility of purchasing from providers offering better value for money.

'Value for money' is a familiar concept to anyone with cash to spend and in that sense points to the variation between potential purchasers regarding the most likely appeal of specified products or services, in particular circumstances. That is to say, there is an assumed common awareness of when it is important to pay more, in order to gain, for example, reliability and quality or to gain something unique, which meets a special need. From a marketing perspective the critical issues are how best to convey the special features of a service which denote uniqueness, or reliability and quality; how best to assess the 'cost' of reduced quality and how best to describe the resulting benefits of that service so that they reflect customer requirements.

Competition

Writers on the American experience of competitive health care suggest that one way to compete more effectively is to increase specialization so that the distinguishing features of a service are more clearly differentiated. Other alternatives include forming cartels to fix prices; changing/modifying a service to reduce the costs, thus making it more attractive to potential purchasers; and shifting the cost of part of a service on to others. Chapter 2 in this section explores the concept of 'value for money' in health care in greater detail and deals with some of the practical issues as they affect community nursing services.

Competitive tendering, decisions about priorities and the development of service/contract specifications have become part of a system which makes rationing decisions more overt and open to public scrutiny. It is perhaps worth remembering that the NHS has never been able to meet all patient needs on demand. This dilemma has been made worse by the effects of an ageing population, by medical advances resulting in an increasing range of conditions which can be treated and by a more sophisticated public with unrealistic expectation of medical treatment rather than self-care and with perhaps unrealistic expectations of what is reasonable to provide from available resources. The more recently acknowledged health needs of carers also need to be seen against a more mobile population, more women in the workforce, changing family structures, fewer opportunities for the development of parenting skills and political decisions about whether or not to increase tax contributions to health care.

Customers, Users and Beneficiaries

As indicated above, every organization, every part of the NHS, all those health care services in the community have 'customers', those who contract and purchase services. It may be difficult sometimes to decide exactly who they are but it is essential that they and their requirements are identified. Purchasing plans, health authority priorities and health and social profiles are now in the public domain and should be familiar to all those interested in planning for the future development of community nursing services. Those elements of fundholders' business plans which have relevance for nurses in primary care settings, are also more readily available. The provision of health care for example, requires long-term planning: professionals have to qualify, technology needs to be developed and buildings have to be modified, designed and completed. The successful continuation of an organization – in this case a community trust – is dependent upon its ability to satisfy current customer needs and to anticipate needs for the future so that satisfaction with provision is maintained. A community trust will have to consider the thrust of government policies, the priorities of the Region or Office (Scottish, Welsh, Northern Ireland Offices) the views of fundholding practices, as well as the health and social profile of the local population.

Customers – those who pay for health care services – need to be separated from the host of service 'beneficiaries' such as patients, clients, carers and relatives and service 'users' such as social services, schools, voluntary agencies, commercial organizations and other health care providers. 'Customers' make purchasing decisions based on health policy, experience, perceived need, and an evaluation of what is currently provided and what can reasonably be provided in the future. Box 5.5.3 shows the steps in that decision-making process.

Box 5.5.3. The
purchasing decision
process

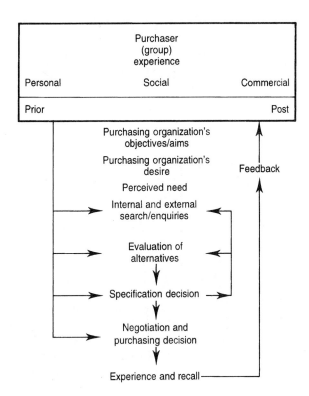

The marketplace, which is where the 'buying and selling' happens, is a constantly changing and dynamic arena. Every purchasing decision made, every contracted service provided, every visit to a neighbouring health authority or health care unit, every public health report, every discussion with a community health council (those who represent the 'customer's customers') will perhaps influence the way a purchaser perceives needs and how they may be met. Because the whole contracting process is relatively new territory for many people, it is possible that those likely to be negotiating for community nursing services, such as fundholding practices, may not be very clear about what is already being provided and what extensions or modifications are possible within available resources. It is worth remembering that while health authorities have had a longstanding planning function, it is only recently that they have been required to assess the health needs of the population served and to base commissioning for services on that assessment. The level of sophistication required to accomplish such a task, may take some while for all to achieve (Charlwood, 1990: 10). The most critical thing to establish is the degree of mismatch between what is required and what is already on offer. In this situation, the importance of communicating effectively about the key features and associated benefits of a service will be particularly significant, if the true value of that service is to be recognized.

Marketing and Communication

Marketing is a business discipline which has evolved in an attempt to create some order out of the seeming chaos of the marketplace (Greenley, 1989: 110–163). Those concerned with marketing must be both in the midst of the activity and be able to stand well back from it, in order to gain an overall view of the position and performance of the organization. Not only is the marketing process dynamic, it focuses particularly on relationships and communications. It is both a philosophy and a managed process; this does not mean that marketing is the specific job of managers, only that the processes involved need to be managed. Whether individuals participate in the thinktank philosophy of marketing, the creation of an internal organizational marketing culture, or a particular aspect of the marketing process (such as dealing with potential customers or providing services based on customer and user needs), there are specific marketing techniques which may be adopted, to understand, to maintain, or to improve the position of a service. (These are dealt with in more detail in the next chapter.)

No health professional is a stranger to the concept of marketing nor to some of the processes involved. Community nurses, for example, are familiar with individualizing care, with quality assurance and performance review and with the significance of effective communication to ensure that services respond to need. It is particularly in this area of communication that an understanding of marketing processes can contribute best to analysing some of the key influences on the future development of community nursing. It is not unusual, for example, for fundholding GPs not to know what they want from community nursing services, and the traditional way nurses and health visitors describe and explain their contribution is not usually undertaken with fundholding practice objectives in mind. Community nurses themselves tend to focus on elements of the nursing process, on the value of holistic care and the importance of developing research based practice, using language which is unlikely to demonstrate the full value of the service to those who have 'business objectives' in mind.

One of the advantages of the marketing process is that it draws attention to the different perspectives of those who receive or use a service and those who purchase or review the performance of a service. If the value of a service is to be recognized, the benefits resulting from its distinctive features have to be described with these different perspectives in mind. Hopton and Dlugolecks (1995), for example, draw attention to the way patients' perception of need for primary care services can be useful in setting priorities and thus influencing community and primary health care nursing. Adopting a marketing perspective helps in the improvement of communication skills and in ensuring that the unique features of a service are emphasized and that the benefits of those features are explained according to the perceived priorities of different audiences.

General business direction and business objectives are determined by government policies. However, local service provision and development is determined in the context of overall requirements translated into demographic variation, differences in health priorities of local populations and the facilities and resources available. The marketing process helps managers design and deliver services which are responsive to customers and to local user needs. However, strategic decisions made in that process are based on experience and knowledge of the marketplace. That means that information is needed from a variety of sources in order to build up a picture or model of customer requirements, user needs and experiences and competitor activity. Analysis of such information can help to identify trends, to focus on opportunities for service development, to recognize potential threats to existing services or to plans for expansion.

Health intelligence, from the NHS provider perspective, is largely derived from the published business plans and purchasing intentions of commissioning authorities. The exercise of business planning has been defined as the process by which 'organisations put their mission and aims into quantified plans to be achieved over several years' (Elphick and Dillarstone, 1990: 200). These authors point out that the business plan begins with a 'market assessment' and that this assessment is different from and in contrast to 'needs assessment'. The former requires information about what and where existing services are being provided to whom, and at what cost and volume. In this sense the market model of health care makes prioritization more explicit, where in the past it would have been largely obscured by waiting lists and by the clinical freedom of doctors (Hunter, 1993). The latter requires an agreed format to assess health status and the need for available health services. Buchan *et al.* (1990: 240) suggest that a simplified version of a DOH definition of a population's need for health services would include 'those for whom an intervention produces benefit at reasonable risk and acceptable cost'.

Without access to those aspects of the business plan and purchasing intentions which have implications for service development, community nurses will be in no position to identify or explore options for modification or expansion. Without a proper consideration of what constitutes quality or value for money from a purchasing perspective, as well as from a user or patient perspective, community nurses may fail to highlight those features and associated benefits of the service likely to have most appeal. Potential sources of competition may also be missed or ignored. The elements of 'professional quality' highlighted by Ovretveit (1992: 63) should be added to those which Maxwell (1984: 1470) assigns to important features of a service: acceptability, equity, appropriateness, efficiency, effectiveness and accessibility. In the context of communication about the potential benefits of a service, it is perhaps worth noting that Koch (1990) sees 'acceptability' as the driving force which will 'be a major quality predictor of success', including in turn the care, the information given, the manner in which information is communicated and the physical environment in which all this is achieved. This is reinforced by the NHS Management Executive paper entitled 'Local Voices' (1992) which states that making health services more responsive to the needs and views and preferences of local people is central to the new role of health service commissioners.

From a marketing perspective, communication is the central issue if the needs/wants of consumers are to be matched to the services on offer. When the results of health intelligence gathering are being collated for planning purposes, it will be critical to establish how the benefits of a particular service are perceived by those participating in the contracting process, as well as by those who receive services. This will have particular relevance where there are potential sources of competition and the position of a service has to be defined in relation to others in the marketplace.

The contracting process and the clinical audit were intended to be the mechanisms to push up the quality of health care and the means to review all aspects of service delivery. They were to achieve this on the one hand by encouraging everyone to become much more critical about established practices and the effectiveness of clinical and other caring activities, and on the other hand by requiring community nurses, for example, to be more imaginative about developing outcome measures that go beyond the quantity of things being done, to include a range of quality outcomes which represent a high standard of nursing care whether or not the recipient of the service is expected to recover or improve their health, regain independence, improve their quality of life or die in dignity. For example, at six monthly intervals, a community nursing service could take responsibility for asking a small random sample of service beneficiaries what they thought were the best and worst aspects of the service which had been provided/offered. In this way, aspects of service satisfaction could be monitored and modifications made where deemed most appropriate.

Whether or not a market oriented health care system is likely to reduce overall expenditure in the long term – and there are those who do not believe that it will – there are now significant opportunities for community nurses to review the focus and direction of their activities and to look again at the style and thrust of what is said and written about their services, so that customer and user dimensions are incorporated into that process.

SUMMARY

- The internal market for health care arose from policies devolving and separating responsibilities for assessing health needs, planning and prioritizing, negotiating contracts and providing health care services. The discipline of marketing has been considered in terms of its underlying philosophy and the processes involved, some of which already form part of any community nursing service.
- Marketing offers new and more overt mechanisms for shaping service developments, for justifying the rationing of health care and for assessing value for money. It is argued that the communication issues which comprise core components of marketing, are useful to those concerned with developing community nursing services, since they specifically draw attention to the differing perspectives of those who commission services, provide services, use or receive services.

DISCUSSION QUESTIONS

- ◆ Identify some of the ethical issues which could arise where health care services are offered on a commercial basis.

- ◆ Consider some of the potential difficulties likely to arise in the application of marketing to health care, particularly in relation to patient/client choice.

- ◆ Identify priority health service goals for your area and review how these are being addressed by a specified community nursing service. Identify one measurable and achievable health improvement goal associated with your service.

- ◆ Consider the way in which the following people might view the quality of a community nursing service:
  (a) a patient/client who is 'receiving' the service;
  (b) a social services department who is 'using' the service;
  (c) a commissioning authority who is 'purchasing' the service.

- ◆ Locate a community nursing service contract and consider ways in which it might be linked to a practice business plan. How might the contract need to be adapted to meet the needs of a specific practice population with which you are familiar?

♦ Locate a community Health Council Annual Report and consider its content in relation to an associated Annual Report from the local commissioning authority.

♦ Given current budgetary constraints, what is the nature of the tension between meeting the health needs of a local population and achieving equity in health service provision? How could such tensions be resolved?

♦ What information should be used to describe the current 'position' of a community nursing service?

♦ Consider ways in which the position of the service might be improved.

FURTHER READING

Chisholm J (Ed) (1990) *Making Sense of the New Contract*. Oxford: Radcliffe Medical Press.
Provides an interpretation of the contractual requirements within the GP terms of service contract with the NHS. Although directed at a GP audience this is essential reading for any organization or individuals attempting to 'sell' their community care services to GPs.

Clark H, Chandler J and Barry J (1994) *Organization and Identities: Text and Readings in Organizational Behaviour*. London: Chapman & Hall.
Provides an accessible introduction to organizational behaviour with discussion points suitable for group development. Aspects within the book of culture and quality, individuals and identities, flexibility and stress, and the professions are particularly relevant.

Greenley GE (1989) *Strategic Management*. Hemel Hempstead: Prentice Hall International.
Part two of this book 'Analysing the Environment' is particularly interesting and even though examples are taken mainly from the experience of large product marketing corporations, the relevance of the analytical processes to community health care service is apparent. The small section on 'Marketing Strategy' provides a useful model which classifies the broad managerial issues of marketing.

Maxwell RGI (1989) *Marketing*. London: MacMillan Professional Masters.
An accessible overview of marketing which does not need to be read from cover to cover. This book clearly explains the component parts of the marketing process; many of which are relevant in community nursing services.

Piercy N (1992) *Market-Led Strategic Change: Making Marketing Happen in Your Organization*. London: Butterworth-Heinemann.
Although written in the context of commercial organizations, this book has much relevance to those within community nursing services who are involved in developing marketing strategies *and in making them happen*.

Sheaff R (1991) *Marketing for Health Services*. Milton Keynes: Open University Press.
This is a solid book which covers the managerial aspects of marketing within the NHS. Chapters 3 and 4 on objective setting and market research, in particular, are relevant and useful for those involved in community health care.

REFERENCES

Buchan H, Gray M *et al.* (1990) Needs assessment made simple. *Health Service Journal* Feb 15, 240–241.
Charlwood P (1990) Figuring out the finances of the N.H.S. reforms. *Public Finance and Accountancy*, Nov 2, 11–13.
DOH (1989a) *Working for Patients*, Cm 555. London: HMSO.
DOH (1989b) *Caring for People*. London: HMSO.

DOH (1991) *The Health of the Nation*. London: HMSO.

Elphick C and Dillarstone P (1990) Order out of chaos. *Health Service Journal* Feb 8, 200.

Gabe J, Calnan M and Bury M (1991) *The Sociology of the Health Service*. London: Routledge.

Greenley GE (1989) *Strategic Management*. London: Prentice Hall.

Hopton JL and Dlugolecks M (1995) Patients' perception of need for primary care services: useful for priority setting. *British Medical Journal* **310:** 1237-1240.

Hudson B (1994) *Making Sense of Markets in Health and Social Care*. Sunderland: Business Education Publishers.

Hunter D (1993) *Rationing Dilemmas in Health Care*. London: NAHAT.

Koch H (1990) Obstacles to total quality in health care. *International Journal of Health Care Quality Assurance* **3**.

Maxwell R (1984) Quality assessment in health. *British Medical Journal* **288:** 1470-1472.

Murray SA and Graham LJC (1995) Practice based health needs assessment: use of four methods in a small neighbourhood. *British Medical Journal* **310:** 1443-1448.

NHS Management Executive (1992) Local Voices - the views of local people. *Purchasing for Health* January.

Ovretveit J (1992) *Health Service Quality. An Introduction to Quality Methods for Health Services*. Oxford: Blackwell Scientific Publications.

Piercy N (1992) *Market Led Strategic Change*. Oxford: Butterworth-Heinemann/Chartered Institute of Marketing.

Report of the Royal Commission on the NHS (1979) London: HMSO.

Sheaff R (1991) *Marketing for Health Services*. Milton Keynes, Philadelphia: Open University Press.

Welsh Health Planning Forum (1991-1994) *Protocols for Investment in Health Gain*. Welsh Office NHS Directorate.

WHO (1985) *Health for All by the Year 2000, targets*. Geneva: WHO.

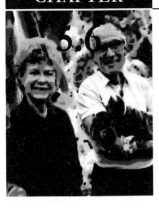

MARKETING AND SERVICE DEVELOPMENT

Judy Edwards and Elizabeth Muir

KEY ISSUES

- Creating and achieving change
- Characterizing a service
- Reviewing communication
- Identifying strengths, weaknesses, opportunities and threats
- Strategic marketing options

INTRODUCTION

The establishment of an internal market within the NHS, together with the subsequent influence of GP fundholders, means that there are a number of different ways in which a local population's health needs may be met. The potential for competition, created by the purchaser/provider split, also means that elements of cost, service quality, geographical spread, together with the range and level of service provision, can all be far more flexible than previously allowed. One service provider, for example, may organize and develop its services in the face of its actual and potential competitors, by having the workforce more highly qualified and experienced so that they can take total responsibility for complex programmes of nursing care. Another provider might decide to offer a much wider range of skills and expertise in more locations. Both would be aiming to demonstrate increased service attractiveness, in comparison with competitors.

In essence, the marketing process is all about creating change; getting from where an organization is now (in this case the NHS; and fundholding practices in particular) to where it wants or needs to be in, say, two years' time. Of course, in a dynamic marketplace, competitor activity, changing health needs of a population, medical and technological developments and government health policy priorities constantly influence the opportunities for service development. This means that the 'where we want to be' aspect of the equation changes over time. It is also prudent to ensure that there is a real understanding of 'where we are now' in a way which includes the advantages and the deficiencies of current service provision. A review of this kind should also include decisions to make relevant changes within the overall structure of the trust, as well as the framework for contracting and delivering community nursing services. Changing the culture within a trust or within fundholding practices may be a critical part of this process.

Characterizing a Service

The range of nursing care available outside hospitals, and within the NHS, to support public health and primary care objectives, means that there should be different ways of describing the services on offer. How this is done will in part depend on the source of funding and in part on those unique features of a service which reflect the expected benefits to those seeking to negotiate a contract (Edwards, 1993). For example, a trust may offer a home based 24 hour district nursing service with specialist support and aids, depending on local needs. For a GP fundholder that could mean continuing palliative care is available for the terminally ill. It could also mean a reduction in avoidable house calls and hospital admissions. In a similar vein, a community psychiatric nursing service offering short-term respite care and an emergency admission service could represent added value by reducing the risk of breakdown in packages of community care.

Where fundholding is concerned, coordinating primary health care nursing re-sources will become critical for efficient budgetary control (Audit Commission, 1992). That means each nurse/health visitor should be able to interpret available health and social profiles to predict the priority nursing or health visiting needs of the practice population. The next stage involves identifying effective research based strategies to meet those needs within available resources and communicating appro-priately about the potential implications of directing resources to one group rather than another. The unique features of a service can then be described in terms of: (i) how they will effectively meet the priority health needs of defined groups within a practice population, and (ii) how they will make a substantial contribution to the business objectives of the practice and enhance the overall quality of primary health care. It is not possible, however, to promote the actual and potential value of a service unless the business objectives of the practice (or at least those which have im-plications for primary health care nurses) are known and understood.

In the light of government involvement with the provision of health care services, the general business direction and objectives are already determined (See, for exam-ple, *The Health of the Nation* DOH, 1992) and every nurse in the community should be familiar with them and with relevant public health reports from the Department of Health (e.g. *Making it Happen*: 1995 and *The Health of the Nation: Targeting Practice*: 1993). Local health service provision is determined in the context of such national requirements translated into local policies, the health implications of popu-lation differences and the resources available within the local community.

Products or Service?

From a marketing point of view, key discussions have centred on such questions as: Does community nursing provision comprise a range of products (labelled for example 'wound dressing', 'male and female catheterization', 'developmental surveillance', 'drug monitoring', 'child protection') which require a high level of servicing support to enable the user to access them beneficially? Alternatively is what is being provided a service or range of services which sometimes include the supply of tangible products?

To understand marketing it is crucial to understand the differences in behaviour which surround the selling/buying transaction of 'a product' and those of 'a service'. In general terms when purchasing a product, the prospective customer goes to an agreed location (shop, warehouse) or follows a specific process (magazine, mail order catalogue, telephone), where a choice of products might be available which can achieve similar results (e.g. typewriter, wordprocessor, computer) and each product might have variations (colour, size). Products are tangible and can be inspected and compared. Prices are usually predetermined and set by the producer with limited scope for negotiation. In contrast, services comprise a range of intellectual and pragmatic activities which may be available but which are only provided on the basis of discussion and negotiation between the provider and their potential customer. It is not uncommon for the customer not to be the user and so there may also be negotiations and discussion between customer and user and market information based on the user's requirements. Decisions are frequently based on previous experiences and reputation; the price is related to what is used, but is an amalgam of rates set on what is possible to provide in the particular circumstances. Think about a hairdressing service, for example, and consider the basis for choosing a particular person or salon, rather than another, on a specified occasion. When is reputation, convenience, past experience or perceived value for money the most critical factor?

Significant differences between a product and a service, from the user's point of view, are that services cannot be reliably compared until after they have been experienced, and while a product can be returned, replaced or repaired, a service once received, cannot be returned and can only be modified.

It is generally accepted that community nursing comprises a range of services which are available at prescribed times and venues and which are provided as a unique package for each individual user. However, the 'customer' is actually purchasing the full range of services which are possible and which will be drawn on according to 'users' needs. The customer may well set limits regarding what is possible by setting geographical or financial limits; this may have repercussions as to the flexibility and quality of the service provided. For the rest of this chapter, the provision of community health nursing will be described as a *service*.

Reviewing Communication

It is not new for community nurses to modify their language when describing their services to different patient/client groups. People with different backgrounds and different needs will require a variety of information presented in an assortment of ways, depending on circumstances and the importance of understanding the full implications of the range and kind of services on offer.

How services are described and the language used will be dependent upon the audience and their existing or potential relationship with individual nurses or to a trust. So, for example, the way a health visitor might describe the maternal and child health services on offer, will depend on whether the 'audience' is a group of first time parents, other primary health care nurses, the practice manager, representatives of the local community health council, a social worker new to the area, or the media. The priority given to different features and associated benefits of the service will depend on the health visitor's assessment and perception of the different needs or requirements of each audience.

Effective communication means understanding the audience, their objectives and agendas (hidden or otherwise). In marketing terms it can be useful to think about audiences as customers of the information to be provided, and to group them into 'existing customers', 'potential customers', 'competitors', 'co-providers', 'users', 'influencers' and other groups which may be relevant to a specific service. A useful exercise for any community nursing service would be to list the relevant audience/customer groups and assign to them predicted aims, objectives and value judgements (see Box 5.6.1). A list of words or phrases might then appear to do with: quality, competence, price, image, reliability, reputation, comprehensiveness, flexibility, being on-tap or only available when required, a 24 hour service, mix of skills available, the level of training provided, ability to take responsibility for planning and evaluation, complexity of decision-making, saving time, providing a one-stop-shop, clinical effectiveness, availability at various locations, keeping people informed.

The particular marketing communication skill for this exercise primarily hinges on the ability to select the list of words related to the needs of a specific group; not by making assumptions but by asking questions and listening to and validating responses. Describing the actual and potential benefits of a service, in terms of meeting those specified requirements, is the next important step. If, for example, you have identified a GP practice as an existing customer and that the practice has some particular short- and longer-term objectives, you are in a good position to predict which features of your service are likely to be particularly valued (Box 5.6.2).

All services will have a unique range of features and the benefits of each feature will be many and varied. A community nursing service, for example, might be accessible by telephone across 24 hours and be able to undertake a wide range of complex nursing procedures. The benefits for newly discharged patients with complex treatment programmes (and for their carers) is the availability of competent help in symptom control and the reduction of anxiety/distress. For the fundholding practice it can mean a more efficient and cost-effective use of available expertise, as well as having the potential to reduce inappropriate use of expensive medical resources (Thomas, 1994).

Identifying Strengths and Weaknesses

Undertaking a SWOT analysis (strengths – weaknesses – opportunities – threats) can help to identify and clarify priority issues for the future development or modification

Box 5.6.1. Exercise 1

Community nursing service:			
Customer for information	Overall aim	Key objectives	Likely values

Box 5.6.2. Exercise 2

Community nursing service:	
Existing customer:	
Distinctive features of service	Predicted benefits to customer
1.	
2.	
3.	
4.	
etc.	

of a service. This will be an important activity if a service is to survive successfully in a rapidly changing environment. A SWOT analysis is simply a marketing technique which helps develop a model of a particular service in the context of the marketplace. Whilst the result is a 'snapshot' within an ever changing and dynamic health care system, it is a valuable tool for developing strategic options for service development and marketing communications. The process of carrying out a SWOT analysis, particularly in a team setting, can be extremely useful for promoting a better understanding of the marketplace in which the service is operating: members of a team can contribute to the model from their differing perspectives and positions.

Within community nursing services, a SWOT analysis may be carried out on all services which make up the whole, or on an individual service. Obviously a useful contribution may be made by analysing each service in turn and then collating those results into the overall model.

There are five elements to a SWOT analysis:

Strengths

The strengths of a service may be gauged by their uniqueness, the inclusion of quality standards and quality achievements (such as accessibility, availability, equity), evidence of value for money and clinical effectiveness, the degree of match to customer objectives, management structures which facilitate flexibility and change, positive comparison with competition etc. In total the strength of a service may be gauged by its scope, range and flexibility.

Weaknesses

The weaknesses of a service are not only the opposites of the strengths but specific areas of concern which prohibit development or immediate remedial action, e.g. inertia and fear of change; traditional information systems which fail to meet present need; past decisions concerning human resource planning and recruitment; education and training which is not keeping pace with health service development; geographical spread when what is required is dedicated primary health care nursing teams.

The strengths or weaknesses of a service are those internal aspects of the organization/trust/fundholding practice, such as financial and human resources, the structures, culture, communications networks, systems, equipment etc., which affect its capability to perform at an optimum level.

Threats

These are mainly from external sources such as changing user needs, increased competitor activity, government policy changes, purchaser decision-making (processes), media intervention.

Opportunities

Opportunities in the marketplace may be highlighted by competitor activity, purchaser decision-making and changing customer needs, modifications in the demography of a population, advances in medical knowledge, information technology or government policy development.

Opportunities or threats derive from influences outside an organization. Because there may be links between certain strengths and weaknesses within the community nursing service organization and between the threats and opportunities which exist in the marketplace, it is useful to highlight these in a way which provides a summation of the developmental priorities. (See Box 5.6.3.) This summary comprises the fifth element of the SWOT analysis: a statement which describes the present situation.

The exercise of a SWOT analysis is the basis of all marketing decisions and can be performed at individual, group, departmental, professional speciality or organization level. One of the crucial factors of such analysis is the honesty with which it is carried out, for the end result is a model of 'where we are now' within the context of the marketplace. From such a model can be seen areas for concern which need attention to protect the organization and key opportunities for growth and development.

The analysis, in its simplest form, comprises a list of the organization's (or individual community nursing service's) strengths and weaknesses in each of the outer boxes, together with the threats and opportunities within the community health service and primary care marketplace. These are then linked where relevant in the boxes A,B,C,D.

The information gathered in Box A, for example, will indicate those areas where an organization or service can clearly consider development. Box B indicates positive

Box 5.6.3. SWOT analysis

	Threats	Opportunities
Strengths	B	A
Weaknesses	C	D
Position statement:		

aspects of the organization or service, whereby threats in the marketplace may be counterbalanced or overcome.

Given that it is rare for an organization or service to be able to alter the outside influences of the marketplace, the real danger area is that of Box C which indicates a real need for internal change to combat threats. Of course the level of investment in such change will be dependent upon the potential impact of the threat. For example, the developing role of the practice nurse or community paediatric nurse may be perceived as a threat to the role of the district nurse or health visitor. The nature and size of the threat will in part be determined by the current image and reputation of the district nursing and health visiting services, by the degree to which they are adapting to the changing requirements of fundholding practices and whether or not there is evidence that they are responding effectively and efficiently to the priority health needs of the practice population.

Box D highlights an area where opportunities exist in the marketplace but they are of a kind which can only be capitalized upon if certain weakness within the organization or service can be overcome. Examples of changes needed here might include the development and availability of training programmes in response to advancing medical knowledge and technology; in staffing level adjustments to achieve greater efficiency in one part of the service so that expansion can be achieved in another; in reducing overlap between nursing services within primary care and in restructuring community nursing services in response to more reliable health and social needs assessment (Duggan, 1995).

Strategic Marketing Options

If one takes a 'snapshot in time' a community trust or a community nursing service, together with the individuals within it, should be providing a unique range of services based on population characteristics, health policy priorities and specific service objectives. The 'turnover' of a trust or a service, or an individual within it, might be considered as the number of times each of the range of services is provided. Of course in business financial terms this is then equated to the selling price of that provision. Financial profit is then the difference between this amount and the cost of providing the services.

In marketing terms, there is always a pressure to ensure that what is provided is done as cost effectively as possible, so that financial resources are focused on improving the quality, range and depth of service provision – and are not used up in inefficient and wasteful practices. This is not about choosing the cheapest, it is about achieving optimal impact in the light of identified health needs and policy priorities. Improving the quality, range and penetration of services, in line with user requirements, ensures service attractiveness to purchasers and thus competitiveness in the marketplace. (See Chapter 5.2 for a more detailed discussion of health economics.)

However, given that a community nursing service is operating efficiently, there is always a need to develop. An organization or trust may grow in one of two ways: either by introducing new or improved services (service development); or by providing the same services to new and different groups of people (market development).

Such 'strategic options' may well be summarized in the grid shown in Box 5.6.4 which can build up to demonstrate complete diversification, which is the provision of new services into new markets.

Box 5.6.4. Strategic options for development

		Services	
		Existing	New
Market groups	Existing	A	B
	New	C	D

Box A: Market Penetration

This is a strategy which requires selling most of the existing services to existing types of customer. In the reality of community nursing service provision, this can only be achieved by expanding one's geographical base and/or by offering service packages which expand the range of services purchased by individual customers.

Box B: Service Development

Given the 'ring fencing' of the NHS internal market, only a limited number of potential purchasers are perceived to be available. That means that one strategy for growth may well come from service development. As service providers recognize their particular strengths, they may refrain from offering certain services which are in competition with others, in order to invest resources in a particular 'niche' for which they have special and recognized expertise.

On the other hand, the development of new services in response to policies and commissioner priorities, should not only strengthen existing purchaser relations, but may also attract potential and new customers, although they will be of the same type.

Thus as a strategy, service development may result in reducing some elements of a service. Overall most services will be contracted to existing customers and development may attract new customers of the same kind.

Box C: Market Development

Market development is a strategic option involving contracting existing services to completely new types of customer. Community nursing and other health care services have traditionally – and within the concept of an internal market – provided services which are now purchased by health commissioning authorities and GP fundholding practices. They may decide, for example, to offer selected services to sections of the Armed Forces, both home and abroad; to private residential and nursing homes; to prisons and to large businesses and other organizations, in ways which have not been possible before.

Market development of this kind may require some changes to services or to the way they are provided but this should be at the level of service 'modification' rather than service 'development'.

Box D: Diversification

When a provider unit or trust embarks upon a strategy of developing new services for contracting with new types of customers, this is called diversification. Choosing an option of this kind may well arise as a result of successful service or market development. The managerial experiences of change, for example, may have led to the establishment of training and other consultancies which promote marketing skills and reduce the impact of competition. It may also have helped to pinpoint potential purchasing organizations, together with information about community health nursing requirements.

In the context of a dynamic health care system, there will be a number of different strategic options available. The options chosen will depend upon the underlying philosophy of the trust or service and the resources available. It is at this juncture that the manager or team leader not only critically assesses the budget and other material resources available but also the most vital resources which are the skills, experience and attitudes of the people employed. Such a resource is critical for the successful provision of services by virtue of the day-to-day contact with recipients, users or customers.

Previous discussion has sought to draw attention to some of the difficulties which can arise in an internal market where the primacy of financial objectives may be in conflict with identified health objectives. Nevertheless, the elements of the marketing process are likely to give community nurses a number of practical ideas to improve their communication about the special features and value of their services and to develop strategies which will enhance their position with actual and potential purchasers. In order to achieve the marketing objectives of a trust all employees have to be able to play their individual roles and be skilled and motivated to do so. In line with a marketing philosophy, all marketing objectives should focus on customer needs. Thus an understanding of the individual and collective purchasing decision processes is essential.

Marketing objectives must go beyond the decision to buy. Marketing is a continuous process: customers need to be satisfied with the current service and confident of service development in line with their own objectives, thus ensuring that they will continue to be customers. This is an area where there cannot be complacency and thus marketing objectives focus on endorsing the validity of the purchasing decision, enriching the practice experience of the service provided and involving them in service development.

Competition

Competition comes from other organizations who can also meet the needs of purchasers. The comparison between one service provider and another is based on a number of aspects of the service. For example, a typewriter, wordprocessor, computer or even a pen can all produce the written word on a page but how closely they are perceived as being in competition depends upon what the user actually needs, where, how often, at what quality and for what cost. Apparently disparate products such as a pen, watch, silver ornament or book may not seem to be in competition at all, unless one is looking for a gift when a colleague retires.

From a marketing perspective, competition means striving for service development and improvement to increase service attractiveness to potential customers and commissioning authorities. Again this focuses on the needs of the user and thus puts the patient/client at the centre of service development. The community nursing service which best enables a potential purchaser to meet the needs of its users is the most likely to be purchased.

There often exists the notion that the creation of a competitive marketplace results in a 'cut-throat' business environment where standards and quality are compromised for the sake of being able to provide a cheaper service. Whilst it cannot be denied that this might be the strategy of some provider units and those short-sighted purchasing authorities who have been tempted to purchase on the basis of price alone; it has been found in the commercial world that such a strategy is a very dangerous path to follow.

Competition, on the whole, helps organizations develop and refine their services to better fit what their existing and potential customers need. In the case of community nursing services this means a focus on the needs of patients, clients and carers and providing information about levels of health care that can be provided such that they match the needs of GP fundholding practices and commissioning health authorities. Taking time to make comparisons with other similar services provides the opportunity to review quality standards, the range and flexibility of services and the equity of provision.

Because the marketplace or the context in which community nursing services are provided is always changing, the organization or trust likely to be most successful is the one which plans and initiates service development. Effective marketing means building a series of 'unique selling points' for the services offered. Such uniqueness may come from being able to provide, as part of a range of services, one specialist highly skilled service which no other organization offers; being able to offer a service in a completely different way, which is more attractive to potential customers by being more effective/convenient/accessible for patients/carers/clients.

Opportunities

Unless there is a major outbreak of disease, the health care needs of a population do not fluctuate but tend to change over time. However, at a local GP practice level, fluctuations may be seen as a result of the material environment such as a new housing estate or the closure of a local factory or mine. Otherwise change in the need for community nursing services may alter as a result of medical knowledge or technology, e.g. keyhole surgery, advances in anaesthetics which result in shorter stays in hospitals. Further change is brought about by local health authorities' interpretations of government policy which might result in long-distance travel to obtain certain types of treatment, particular strategies for 'care in the community', priority given to certain categories of the population and funding being directed into specific areas.

Within the framework of such changes, community nursing service development can arise as a consequence of research which leads to innovation and modification to existing services. But these should be considered in the light of knowledge about the anticipated needs of local health service commissioners, GP fundholding practices and local population characteristics - often reflected in caseload profiles. Remember that whilst the planning and development of services can be exciting and creative, it can also be very costly - not just in terms of reallocation of new and existing resources, but in terms of the potential disruption which occurs when information about change is mismanaged.

When there are periods of radical change, people in any organization can begin to feel uncertain about their roles and responsibilities. An effective communications system is critical to achieve desirable changes and that means different types of communication need to flow in more than one direction; upwards and downwards as well as horizontally. All too frequently hierarchical organizations (e.g. trusts or large GP fundholding practices) have systems which enable information to flow upwards and instructions to flow downwards but fail to provide avenues for ideas and responses to flow back and forth or for cross-referencing between units or services.

Planning for the Future

It is a managerial responsibility to develop future plans and it is important for everyone in the NHS to understand and have commitment to the overall objectives and to the nature and direction of change. But, it is not essential for everyone to have access to all parts of the plan. The presentation of the plan needs to be modified according to the roles individuals are expected to play in it. Thus a plan – whether the business plan of a GP fundholding practice or a community trust – can be broken down and 'cascaded' through an organization so that each person has a clear understanding of personal and professional achievements to be attained. The planned activity associated with these achievements can then be aligned to other aspects of monitoring and development such as annual performance appraisals, job descriptions and responding to education and training needs.

Plans can then be seen as the summary of activities which are expected to have an effect on the market position of a service. As such, it will be important to incorporate certain milestones, or points of progress, which can be regarded as the time by which certain agreed activities have taken place and intermediate objectives have been achieved.

The dynamics of the marketplace is in part created by the tensions which exist between the changing roles within it. The concept of budgetary control is now, for example, a more visible management requirement. Problems exist when people who become responsible for budgets have the training to enable them to manage the financial aspects of budgetary control, but not the personal development which enables them to cope with the new responsibilities of budget management. Management which is limited to the application of accountancy criteria for the delivery of health care services would ultimately be self-destructive (Coombs and Cooper, 1992). Even though information systems have been greatly improved, there is still little evidence to demonstrate significant cost differences between the average district general hospital in the UK (Loveridge, 1992) and, there is still a long way to go to unravel the 'imponderables' of the various elements of diagnostic and treatment procedures (Ellwood, 1990).

Tensions can arise when plans are made on a long-term basis by people who are many levels removed from the day-to-day shorter-term requirements of community nurses and the users of their services. This means that a shift in communication is needed so that overall long-term budgets are broken down into shorter-term allocations. Such communication must be 'two way' so that errors in budgetary allocation can be identified and amended with sufficient flexibility to enable funds to be diverted as needed. Where this occurs, it is vital to highlight the transaction so that errors are not repeated and new budgets are based not only on what has gone before, but on the best knowledge of what is likely to happen in the future.

Further tensions can be predicted in relation to the perspectives adopted for planning and community nursing service developments. The nature of medical and nursing knowledge is likely, for example, to encourage specialization. However, within general practice there is considerable support for the generalist by virtue of the wide range of conditions presenting to these front line services.

There is no doubt that the significance of primary care, and the influence of GP fundholding practices in particular, will help to create new opportunities for innovation in both community nursing management and service development. However, there are inevitable tensions in the values held by those in management and those who are part of the health care delivery system itself – not least in the performance standards derived from such relatively alien disciplines as health and social welfare, and managerial economics. It may be worth noting in this final chapter that in a review of primary care in eleven Western nations, Starfield (1992) found total health expenditure to be generally higher in countries where health care systems are left to the vagaries of market forces.

For community nursing services looking to the future, the culture of the work setting is likely to provide a powerful determinant of the way services are likely to develop. The tensions generated by such different perspectives as public health population based planning and individual needs based service development may result in enhanced quality health care derived from new and different patterns of community nursing. The biggest problem may be finding the best way to ensure that those with the most clinical experience and the highest levels of clinical expertise do not become increasingly involved in resource allocation and the coordination of those with lower level skills and thus, more isolated from the patient or client and the actual delivery of care. At the end of the day, however, community nursing services are ultimately judged by those in receipt of nursing care or by other citizens in the political arena.

SUMMARY

■ This chapter has focused on the practicalities of the marketing processes with special reference to creating and achieving change which is necessary as community nursing services adapt to political agendas, new policy doctrines, the impact of new technologies and health care challenges.

■ The manner in which using marketing techniques can improve various aspects of communication is described, particularly with regard to conveying the actual and potential value of a service.

■ The elements of a SWOT analysis are considered in relation to options for further developments.

DISCUSSION QUESTIONS

♦ How would you describe the current position of your service with reference to:

(a) the practice profile or,
(b) the practice business objectives?

♦ What might be predictable sources of tension between the business objectives of a GP fundholding practice and the key objectives of a community nursing service?

♦ How would you describe the elements of your service which are utilized on a daily basis and those which are available but utilized only rarely?

♦ What might be regarded as the profit or predictable benefits arising from the range of services you provide? What kind of value would a fundholding practice place on those benefits and why?

♦ In the context of a GP fundholding practice, identify one element of a community nursing service which could be undertaken by another agency. What opportunities would then exist for improving or expanding other parts of the service?

FURTHER READING

Chisholm J (Ed) (1990) *Making Sense of the New Contract*. Oxford: Radcliffe Medical Press.

Greenley GE (1989) *Strategic Management*. Hemel Hempstead: Prentice Hall International.

Lawton A and Rose A (1991) *Organization and Management in the Public Sector*. London: Pitman.

Maxwell RGI (1989) *Marketing*. London: MacMillan Professional Masters.

Piercy N (1992) *Market-Led Strategic Change: Making Marketing Happen in Your Organization*. London: Butterworth-Heinemann.

Sheaff R (1991) *Marketing for Health Services*. Milton Keynes: Open University Press.

Smith I (1994) *Meeting Customer Needs*. Oxford: Butterworth-Heinemann.

Other Books of General Interest

Adler S, Laney J and Packer M (1993) *Managing Women*, Buckingham: Open University Press.

Deal T and Kennedy A (1988) *Corporate Cultures*. Harmondsworth: Penguin.

Decker B (1989) *How to Communicate Effectively*. London: Kogan Page.

Ehrenreich B and English D (1973) *Witches, Midwives and Nurses: A History of Women Healers*. Old Westbury, New York: Feminist Press.

Gabe J, Calnan M and Burry M (Eds) (1991) *The Sociology of the Health Service*. London: Routledge.

Haralambos M (Ed) (1985) *Sociology: New Directions*. Ormskirk: Causeway Press.

Haynes ME (1988) *Effective Meeting Skills*. London: Kogan Page.

Jones H (1994) *Health and Society in Twentieth Century Britain*. London: Longman.

Kennedy C (1991) *Guide to the Management Gurus*. London: Century.

Klein R (1989) *The Politics of the National Health Services*, 2nd Edn. London: Longman.

Mandel S (1987) *Effective Presentation Skills*. London: Kogan Page.

Martin DM (1994) *Manipulating Meetings: How to Get What You Want, When You Want It*. London: Institute of Management Pitman Publishing.

Pugh DS (Ed) (1990 New Edition) *Organization Theory: Selected Readings*. Harmondsworth: Penguin Business.

Roberts H (Ed) (1990) *Women's Health Counts*. London: Routledge.

Smyre P (1991) *Women and Health*. London: Zed Books.

Strage HM (Ed) (1992) *Milestones in Management*. Oxford: Blackwell Business.

REFERENCES

Audit Commission (1992) *Homeward Bound: A New Course for Community Health*. London: HMSO.

Coombs R and Cooper D (1992) Accounting for Patients: Information Technology and the Implementation of the NHS White Paper. In R Loveridge and K Starkey (Eds) *Continuity and Crisis in the NHS*. Buckingham: Open University Press.

DOH (1992) *The Health of the Nation – A Strategy for Health in England*. London: HMSO.

DOH (1993) *The Health of the Nation – Targeting Practice: The Contribution of Nurses, Midwives and Health Visitors*. London: DOH.

DOH (1995) *Making it Happen – Public Health: the Contribution, Role and Development of Nurses, Midwives and Health Visitors*. Report of the Standing Nursing and Midwifery Advisory Committee (SNMAC). London: DOH.

Duggan M (1995) *Primary Health Care A Prognosis*. London: Institute for Public Policy Research.

Edwards J (1993) *Marketing: A Way Forward for Community Nursing Services - A Resource Pack*. Cardiff: School of Nursing Studies.

Ellwood S (1990) Competition in health care. *Management Accounting*. April, 24-28.

Loveridge R (1992) The Future of Health Care Delivery - Markets or Hierarchies? In R Loveridge and K Starkey (Eds) *Continuity and Crisis in the NHS*. Buckingham: Open University Press.

Starfield B (1992) *Primary Care, Concept, Evaluation and Policy*. Oxford: Oxford University Press.

Thomas E (1994) Prime time: ensuring the most effective use of nursing time in primary care. *Primary Care Management* **4**(10): 6-9.

INDEX